A Neonatal Vade-Mecum

Edited by

Peter J. Fleming
MB ChB, FRCP, FRCP(C)
Consultant Paediatrician, Bristol Maternity Hospital, Bristol
Royal Hospital for Sick Children and Southmead Hospital

Brian D. Speidel
BA, MD, FRCP, DCH
Consultant Paediatrician, Southmead Hospital and Bristol
Maternity Hospital

Neil Marlow
MA, MB BS, MRCP, DM
Consultant Senior Lecturer, University of Bristol, Bristol
Maternity Hospital and Southmead Hospital

Peter M. Dunn
MA, MD, FRCP, FRCOG, DCH
Professor of Perinatal Medicine and Child Health,
University of Bristol, Southmead Hospital and Bristol
Maternity Hospital

Second Edition

Edward Arnold
A division of Hodder & Stoughton
LONDON   MELBOURNE   AUCKLAND

© 1991
Peter J. Fleming, Brian D. Speidel, Neil Marlow and Peter M. Dunn

First published in Great Britain 1986

British Library Cataloguing in Publication Data

British Library Cataloguing in Publication Data
A neonatal vade-mecum. – New. ed.
  1. Newborn babies
  I. Fleming, Peter J. (Peter John)
  618.9201

  ISBN 0–340–53869–4

Whilst the advice and information in this book is believed to be true and accurate at the date of going to press, neither the author nor the publisher can accept any legal responsibility or liability for any errors or omissions that may be made. In particular (but without limiting the generality of the preceding disclaimer) every effort has been made to check drug dosages; however, it is still possible that errors have been missed. Furthermore, dosage schedules are constantly being revised and new side effects recognized. For these reasons the reader is strongly urged to consult the drug companies' printed instructions before administering any of the drugs recommended in this book.

Typeset in Linotron Times by Rowland Phototypesetting Limited, Bury St Edmunds, Suffolk. Printed and bound in Great Britain for Edward Arnold, a division of Hodder and Stoughton Limited, Mill Road, Dunton Green, Sevenoaks, Kent TN13 2YA by Clays Limited, St Ives plc.

Contributors to the first edition

Zulfiqar Bhutta, MB BS, MRCP, Formerly Fellow in Neonatal Medicine, Bristol Maternity Hospital

David Carolane, MB BS, FRACP, Formerly Fellow in Neonatal Medicine, Bristol Maternity Hospital

Mary Colbeck, RGN, RSCN, JBCNS Course 400, Nursing Officer, Special Care Baby Unit, Bristol Maternity Hospital

Malcolm Donaldson, MB ChB, MRCP, Formerly Senior Registrar in Paediatrics, Bristol Royal Hospital for Sick Children

Mark Drayton, BA, MB BChir, MRCP, Formerly Senior Registrar in Neonatal Medicine, Bristol Maternity Hospital and Southmead Hospital

Timothy French MSc, MB BS, MRCP, Consultant Paediatrician, Musgrove Park Hospital, Taunton, Somerset

Andrew Long, MB BS, MRCP, MRCP(I), DCH, Formerly Research Fellow in Perinatal Medicine, Bristol Maternity Hospital

Helen Noblett, MB BS, FRACS, Consultant Paediatric Surgeon, Bristol Royal Hospital for Sick Children

Charles Pennock, BSc, MD, FRCPath, Senior Lecturer in Child Health, University of Bristol

Richard Primavesi, MB BS, DCH, MRCP, Formerly Senior Registrar in Paediatrics, Southmead Hospital

Barry Wilkins, MA, MB BChir, MRCP, DCH, Formerly Research Fellow in Perinatal Medicine, Southmead Hospital

Contributors to the second edition

P. Jeremy Berry, MRCPath, Consultant Perinatal and Paediatric Pathologist, Bristol Maternity Hospital (Chapter 25)

Mark Drayton, MA, MD, MRCP, Consultant Neonatologist, University Hospital of Wales (Chapter 10)

Timothy French, MB BS, MSc, MRCP, Consultant Paediatrician, Musgrove Park Hospital, Taunton, Somerset (Chapter 11)

Cameron Kennedy, MD, FRCP, Consultant Dermatologist, Bristol Royal Hospital for Sick Children (Chapter 22)

Peter Lunt, MA, MSc, MRCP, Consultant Clinical Geneticist, Bristol Royal Hospital for Sick Children (Chapter 24)

Richard Markham, MD, FRCS, Consultant Ophthalmologist, Bristol Eye Hospital and Bristol Royal Hospital for Sick Children (Chapter 23)

Robin Martin, MB, MRCP, Consultant Paediatric Cardiologist, Bristol Royal Hospital for Sick Children (Chapter 9)

Mary McGraw, MB ChB, MRCP, DCH, Consultant Paediatrician, Southmead Hospital (Chapter 16)

Helen Noblett, MB BS, FRACS, FRCS, Consultant Paediatric Surgeon, Bristol Royal Hospital for Sick Children (Chapter 12)

Charles Pennock, BSc, MD, FRCPath, Consultant Senior Lecturer in Child Health, University of Bristol (Chapter 31)

Bhupinda Sandhu, MD, MRCP, Consultant Paediatrician, Bristol Royal Hospital for Sick Children (Chapter 11)

John Walter, MSc, MD, MRCP, Lecturer in Child Health, University of Bristol (Chapter 13)

Barry Wilkins, MA, MB BChir, MRCP, DCH, Formerly Research Fellow in Paediatric Intensive Care, Bristol Royal Hospital for Sick Children (Chapter 17)

Michael Woolridge, BSc, DPhil, Lactation Physiologist, University of Bristol (Chapter 11)

Preface to the second edition

This second edition remains a **practical** guide to the care of the newborn baby, and has been expanded to include a number of areas of great importance which were not covered in the first edition, such as dermatology, ophthalmology, clinical genetics and pathology. Most chapters have been completely rewritten and we are especially pleased to have a detailed section on breast feeding now included in the chapter on Nutrition and Gastroenterology.

We hope the second edition will remain a useful pocket-sized companion for medical and nursing staff dealing with newborn infants.

We would like to acknowledge the many paediatricians who took the trouble to write to us with comments and suggestions after publication of the first edition. Many of these have been acted upon in producing this second edition.

We would particularly like to acknowledge the tireless efforts of our secretary, Mrs Angela Burge, without whose considerable efforts the second edition would not have come to fruition.

PJF
BDS
NM
PMD
1991

Contents

Preface v

List of abbreviations viii

1 Maternal conditions affecting the infant: High-risk pregnancy 1

2 In the delivery room 20

3 Birth trauma 39

4 Routine care of the newborn infant 46

5 Care of the high-risk infant 51

6 Congenital abnormalities 63

7 Transport of the sick newborn infant 80

8 Neonatal respiratory problems 86

9 Cardiac problems 108

10 Neurological disorders 131

11 Nutrition and gastroenterology 152

12 Neonatal surgical problems 178

13 Metabolic and endocrine problems 192

14 Perinatal infections 211

15 Haematological problems 224

16 Renal disease in the newborn 235

Appendix 250

17 Fluid and electrolyte therapy 253

18 Neonatal jaundice 260

19 Growth charts and gestational assessment 272

20 Care of the family 280

Appendix 285

21 Nursing care of newborn infants 292

22 Neonatal skin disorders 299

23 Ophthalmic disorders 309

24 Clinical genetics in the neonatal period 320

25 Perinatal pathology 329

26 Practical procedures 340

27 Follow-up after discharge 361

28 Drugs and prescribing 368

29 Medical audit 387

30 Medical ethics and the severely malformed or handicapped infant 400

31 Normal laboratory and physiological data 405

Index 419

List of abbreviations used

AFP	Alpha-Fetoprotein
AGA	Appropriate for gestational age
AIDS	Acquired immune deficiency syndrome
APH	Antepartum haemorrhage
ASD	Atrial septal defect
AV	Arterio-venous
BP	Blood pressure
BPD	Bronchopulmonary dysplasia
CAH	Congenital adrenal hyperplasia
CDH	Congenital dislocation of the hip
CHD	Congenital heart disease
CMV	Cytomegalvirus
CPAP	Continuous positive airway pressure
CSF	Cerebrospinal fluid
CT	Computer tomography
CTG	Cardiotocograph
CVP	Central venous pressure
CVS	Cardiovascular system
CXR	Chest X-ray
DIC	Disseminated intravascular coagulation
EDD	Estimated date of delivery
ETT	Endotracheal tube
FBC	Full blood count
FDP	Fibrin degradation products
FHR	Fetal heart rate
FiO_2	Fractional inspired oxygen concentration
GFR	Glomerular filtration rate
HIV	Human immunodeficiency viruses
ICP	Intracranial pressure
IDM	Infant of a diabetic mother
IMV	Intermittent mandatory ventilation
IPPV	Intermittent positive-pressure ventilation
ITP	Idiopathic thrombocytopenic purpura
IUGR	Intrauterine growth retardation
IVH	Intraventricular haemmorhage
IVU	Intravenous urogram
kPa	Kilopascals
LBW	Low birthweight (<2500 g)
LMP	Last menstrual period
LP	Lumbar puncture
MAP	Mean airway pressure
MCUG	Micturating cystourethrogram

NEC	Necrotizing enterocolitis
NEFA	Non-esterified fatty acids
NICU	Neonatal intensive care unit
$PaCO_2$	Arterial partial pressure of CO_2
PaO_2	Arterial partial pressure of O_2
PCV	Packed cell volume (= haematocrit)
PDA	Patent ductus arteriosus
PEEP	Positive end-expiratory pressure
PET	Pre-eclamptic toxaemia
PIE	Pulmonary interstial emphysema
PIP	Peak inspiratory pressure
PKU	Phenylketonuria
PTT	Prothrombin time
PVH	Periventricular haemorrhage
PVL	Periventricular leucomalacia
RDS	Respiratory distress syndrome
REM	Rapid eye movement (sleep)
ROP	Retinopathy of prematurity
RVT	Renal venous thrombosis
SaO_2	Saturation oxygen level
SCBU	Special care baby unit
SFD	Small for dates
SGA	Small for gestational age
SG	Specific gravity
SPA	Suprapubic aspirate (of urine)
SVT	Supraventricular tachycardia
T_i	Inspiratory time
T_e	Expiratory time
TB	Tuberculosis
$TcPO_2$	Transcutanenous oxygen tension
TOF	Tracheo-oesophageal fistula
TPN	Total parental nutrition
TORCH	Agents causing congenital infection: toxoplasma, rubella, cytomegalvirus and herpes
TTN	Transient tachypnoea of newborn
UTI	Urinary tract infection
VLBW	Very low birthweight (<1500 g)
VSD	Ventricular septal defect
WBC	White blood cell (count)
TP	Transpyloric
T_4	Thyroxine
TSH	Thyroid-stimulating hormone

1

Maternal conditions affecting the infant: High-risk pregnancy

---

High-risk pregnancy
Assessment of fetal growth and well-being during pregnancy
Detection of fetal abnormalities
Assessment of fetal well-being during labour
Management of preterm labour

Definition: 'A high-risk pregnancy is one complicated by maternal or fetal illness, obstetric disorder or drug therapy, and from which one may anticipate an ill or immature infant' (Halliday).

High-risk pregnancy

Hypertension in pregnancy

Hypertension (usually defined as a blood pressure greater than 140/90 on two separate occasions) is found in about 6% of all pregnancies and is a common cause of admission to the antenatal ward. It is also a major cause of maternal and fetal/neonatal morbidity and mortality. The main risks to the baby are from placental abruption, impaired growth and preterm delivery. In early pregnancy hypertension is associated with increased fetal loss, whilst the outcome if hypertension first appears later on in the pregnancy depends on whether or not the mother has pre-eclampsia (PET). The outcome for the baby is no worse than in normal pregnancies when the maternal hypertension occurs without PET. The best treatment for a mother with severe PET is to deliver the baby and the main risk to the baby is preterm birth. Maternal drug therapy may help prolong the pregnancy but exposes the baby to the side-effects of the drugs used. The more important adverse effects on the fetus and newborn of some commonly used hypotensive agents are given below.

Hydralazine	Thrombocytopenia
Diazoxide	Hypotension and fetal distress, thrombocytopenia and hyperbilirubinaemia, hyperglycaemia, hypertrichosis, alopecia, decreased bone age
Methyldopa	Reduction in sympathetic tone, transient neonatal ileus, small reduction in systolic blood pressure for 24–48 hours, smaller head size when used at 16–20 weeks, no long-term adverse effects
Labetalol (alpha- and beta-blocker)	Bradycardia, hypotension, hypoglycaemia
Beta-blockers	In general they may impair the capacity of the fetus to cope with intrauterine stress
Oxprenolol Atenolol Metoprolol	They may cause bradycardia, but cardiac reactivity is preserved
Propranolol	It may cause growth retardation, bradycardia, decreased cardiac reactivity, hypoglycaemia, respiratory distress syndrome and impaired autonomic responses
Diuretics	They are probably contraindicated. They reduce plasma volume and utero–placental blood flow

All these agents cross the placenta and are also excreted in breast milk in small amounts. Diazoxide should be regarded as a contraindication to breast feeding and diuretics should be avoided as they may decrease milk production. Breast feeding should be permitted where the mother is taking any of the other drugs on this list, unless in large doses, which carry a risk of hypoglycaemia and bradycardia for the infant.

Thyrotoxicosis

Mothers with thyrotoxicosis now or in the past, even if treated and now asymptomatic, may have circulating thyroid-stimulating IgG which crosses the placenta and may cause transient neonatal thyrotoxicosis. Maternal drugs (e.g. carbimazole) may cause transient neonatal hypothyroidism (Chapter 13, page 202).

Diabetes mellitus

(See Chapter 13, page 192.)

Idiopathic thrombocytopenic pupura (ITP)

(See Chapter 15, page 230.)

Tuberculosis

BCG immunization of the newborn is normally recommended where the infant:

(a) Is known to be a contact of a case of active respiratory TB.
(b) Belongs to an immigrant community characterized by a high incidence of TB.
(c) Will reside in or travel to any area where the risk of TB is judged to be high.

For these infants BCG should be given soon after birth and the infant need not be tested for sensitivity. The dose of BCG is 0.05 ml for infants under three months, given strictly intradermally and not subcutaneously, usually in the area over the insertion of the deltoid muscle. The tip of the shoulder should be avoided. At least three weeks should be allowed between the administration of BCG and any other live vaccine. No further immunization should be given in the arm used for the BCG for at least three months.

(a) Mothers with active or open tuberculosis

Immunize the infant with isoniazid-resistant BCG within a few days of birth and start isoniazid on day one. Continue isoniazid until the mother is sputum-negative for TB and infant has positive skin tuberculin test. Mother and baby should be kept separated until the mother has been on antituberculous treatment for two weeks (i.e. start treatment *before* delivery if possible).

(b) Mothers with healed or inactive tuberculosis

Perform chest X-ray and sputum cultures during pregnancy, as reactivation may occur. If there is no evidence of reactivation, give the infant BCG within the first week after birth (and arrange follow-up after 4–6 weeks to ensure successful immunization).

NB   Masks are of *no* value in preventing infection of the baby if the mother has active TB, and are unnecessary if she has not. Breast feeding is contraindicated only with active or open tuberculosis.

Epilepsy

Epilepsy may become worse or better during pregnancy.

Fits do not usually have significant adverse effects on the fetus unless there is severe maternal hypoxia.

The risk of fetal abnormality is increased to approximately 1 in 10 in women with epilepsy, whatever treatment they are receiving (including no treatment). The risk of abnormality may be higher in women receiving multiple-drug therapy.

Fetal abnormalities have been reported with all commonly used anticonvulsants.

The most common malformations reported are cleft lip and palate, congenital heart disease, and more recently in association with sodium vaporate, neural tube defects. Give folic acid 5 mg/day to all pregnant women on anticonvulsants. Prophylactic vitamin K_1 should be given, 10 mg daily, from 32 weeks' gestation, and the baby should be given 1 mg i.m. at birth to reduce the risk of haemorrhagic disease.

NB   Breast feeding is *not* usually contraindicated (see Chapter 11).

Systemic lupus erythematosus

There is an increased incidence of spontaneous abortion and peri-natal death, probably related to placentally transferred maternal IgG antibody. The fetus may present with cardiac involvement (fibroelastosis or heart block), haematological involvement (anaemia, leucopenia or thrombocytopenia) or rash. Thrombocy-topenia may respond to steroids (see Chapter 15, page 228).

Myasthenia gravis

Control may improve or worsen during pregnancy. Labour is usually normal. Twenty per cent of babies will experience a transient my-asthenic illness which may have a delayed onset and last for up to five weeks. The babies are hypotonic and have breathing and feeding difficulties. There is no contraindication to breast feeding. Symptoms are relieved by a test dose of edrophonium (Tensilon) 0.5 mg/kg i.m. Maintenance is with neostigmine 1 mg/kg six-hourly orally with feeds.

Anticoagulants

Anticoagulants may be used during pregnancy to prevent or treat deep venous thrombosis or pulmonary embolism and in women with artificial heart valves.

Warfarin is associated with a high abortion rate and is teratogenic (less than 5%). It is not secreted in significant amounts in the breast milk. Heparin is not teratogenic, but its use may be associated with increased fetal loss. It is not secreted in the breast milk. Its use is preferable to warfarin during pregnancy, especially within two weeks of delivery.

AIDS

Human immunodeficiency virus (HIV) is transmitted by sexual intercourse, infusion of infected blood products or needles shared by drug abusers. Heterosexual transmission of HIV is now rising rapidly.

Certain groups of women are at greater risk of HIV infection:

(a) Intravenous drug abusers
(b) Natives, residents or visitors of Central Africa or Haiti
(c) Sexual partners of HIV-positive or high-risk individuals
(d) Prostitutes

Testing for HIV in pregnancy should be offered to all women in these groups after counselling. High-risk women who refuse screening for HIV should be managed as if proven positive.

The risk of infection to staff or other patients is very low, provided appropriate precautions are taken in handling blood, lochia and other body fluids, from sero-positive women (e.g. use of gloves and impermeable protective gowns, disposable bedding etc.).

During pregnancy HIV infection may become symptomatic. In women who are clinically well before pregnancy, HIV sero-positivity does not necessarily affect pregnancy outcome for mother or baby. The risk to the infant is much higher if the mother is symptomatic during pregnancy. Overall, the risk of transmission of HIV to the infant has been estimated at 20–50%. Routine serological criteria are unhelpful in young children because of passively acquired maternal antibodies and more complex tests are available only on a research basis. Vaginal delivery and infectivity of breast milk have been implicated in HIV transmission to the baby, but there is inadequate evidence to advocate either elective Caesarean section or bottle feeding for all HIV sero-positive women. Such advice should take into account the medical, obstetric and social practice for each individual woman.

HIV-positive or high-risk mothers should not donate milk to human milk banks or to other infants.

The baby of an HIV-positive mother is only an infection risk as long as vernix or mother's blood is on his or her skin. It is therefore advisable to bath such a baby as soon as possible after birth, taking great care to ensure the baby is not cold-stressed.

Hepatitis B

Cross-infection precautions for hepatitis B must be taken in the delivery room for the following groups of patients whose infants should be given immunization after birth:

(a) Intravenous drug abusers
(b) Patients who have been resident in a mental institution
(c) Patients with chronic active hepatitis, cirrhosis or polyarteritis nodosa
(d) Patients who have had acute hepatitis within the past six weeks
(e) Sexual partner of a man who has been in prison in the past year
(f) All natives of the Far East (Chinese, Phillipino, Vietnamese etc.), Africans and Caribbean people born and raised in the country of origin
(g) Sexual partner of any of the above
(h) Mothers known to be hepatitis B surface antigen positive. If these mothers are e-antigen positive and e-antibody negative, the children are at especially high risk. If the e-antibody is positive and e-antigen is negative, the risk is low. The risk to infants of mothers with neither e-antigen nor e-antibody is intermediate.

Hepatitis B immunization

Infants of mothers in all the above eight groups should be given hepatitis B vaccine 0.5 ml i.m. shortly after birth and again at one and six months. Infants of mothers who are e-antigen positive and e-antibody negative should also be given human antihepatitis B immunoglobulin 200 international units by deep i.m. injection (NB *not i.v.*) as soon as possible after birth, not later than 48 hours. The first dose of hepatitis B vaccine should be given at a different site at the same time or within a few days.

Follow-up arrangements should be made to assess the serological evidence of immunity in all of these infants at the age of one year and at yearly intervals until the age of five years.

Haemoglobinopathies

Management of pregnancy

Screen all 'at-risk' women (from the Mediterranean, Asians, Africans and West Indians) for sickle-cell disease (Hb electrophoresis).

Screen all 'at-risk' women with apparent iron deficiency anaemia for thalassaemia.

Sickle-cell disease

Avoid iron. Give folic acid 15 mg/day, and prompt treatment of crises. Regular blood transfusions (3–4 units every 6–8 weeks) may help prevent crises. Very severe anaemia in late pregnancy may require exchange transfusions before labour.

Sickle-cell trait and heterozygote thalassaemia

Special management during pregnancy is unlikely to be required.

Antenatal diagnosis

Thalassaemia can be diagnosed by chorion villous biopsy (from 8 weeks) or endoscopic fetal blood sampling (at 18–20 weeks).

Postnatal diagnosis

Cord blood screening for at-risk groups is now in operation in some areas.

Thalassaemia can be diagnosed at birth by measuring globin-chain synthesis but, usually, diagnosis waits until 6–9 months when the level of HbF normally present at birth has fallen to levels at which it can be distinguished from the increased level found in thalassaemia.

Alpha-thalassaemia presents as hydrops fetalis and is incompatible with survival.

Alcohol

Fetal alcohol syndrome includes small-for-dates, mental retardation and a characteristic facial appearance (broad base to the nose, long upper lip and small lower jaw, epicanthic folds). It usually indicates alcohol consumption of 4–6 drinks/day (i.e. 40–60 mg alcohol), but can occur with less. (Some effects, e.g. withdrawal, possible with >100 mg alcohol/week). Alcohol is best avoided in early pregnancy. Withdrawal effects may include hyperactive infants and they may have fits (see Chapter 10, page 132).

Drug abuse

Addiction to any drug during pregnancy may lead to neglect of diet and self-care. The fetus will be at increased risk and may be growth retarded. In addition there are a number of specific problems associated with particular drugs.

Cocaine

Cocaine or amphetamine use in pregnancy may lead to a high rate of placental haemorrhage and stillbirth, prematurity and intrauterine growth retardation. The infants are at high risk of fetal distress and birth asphyxia. Cocaine acts as a sympathomimetic agent and has direct cardiovascular actions causing hypertension and vasoconstriction with toxic effects on the fetus, possibly mediated by placental vasoconstriction. Withdrawal effects may be tremors, irritability, abnormal sleep patterns and poor feeding initially. The babies may then become extremely drowsy and require tube feeding for a few days. Microcephaly and cardiac malformations have been described in infants of cocaine-abusing mothers.

Opiates

(For example, heroin, morphine, methadone.)

Antenatal attendance is usually haphazard, and there may be repeated maternal infections from the use of 'dirty' needles. Overdose may occur. Preterm delivery occurs in up to 50% of cases. The infant of an opiate abuser may have **severe** withdrawal symptoms, which usually appear at 24–48 hours but may come on later (particularly if methadone has been used, when withdrawal may appear up to 14 days after birth). **Early signs** are irritability, high-pitched cry, sneezing, sweating and tachycardia with loose stools. **Later signs** are diarrhoea and vomiting, dehydration and seizures.

Management during pregnancy   The pregnancy should be managed in conjunction with a psychiatrist specializing in the care of drug abuse. The advantages of switching to methadone (i.e. decreased infection risk) must be weighed against its more prolonged and severe withdrawal effects in the baby. If the mother and fetus can be adequately monitored, gradual withdrawal of the opiates during the pregnancy may be successful.

Management of the infant   Nurse in a quiet environment. Keep under close observation for **at least** 14 days. If necessary obtain a 'place of safety' order to prevent parents taking the child home against medical advice. Irritability and hyperactivity are decreased by wrapping the baby fairly firmly in blankets. A single dose of morphine (25–50 microg orally) may settle the infant but repeat doses should only be given with caution. Give chlorpromazine (1–3 mg/kg/day) if irritability is severe or it interferes with feeding. Treat convulsions as described in Chapter 10, page 136. Infants of mothers on methadone may have severe neonatal jaundice. Careful social assessment is necessary to decide if the child should be allowed to go home, including case conference, appointment of a Key Worker and provision for long-term follow-up in the community. In spite of these safeguards the outlook for the infant is not good. One in 10 will have died and more than 50% will have been taken into care by the age of two years. Breast feeding is contraindicated, as variable drug levels in breast milk may lead to unpredictable and possibly fatal late withdrawal effects on the baby.

Marijuana

Little evidence of harmful effects in pregnancy.

LSD

Reports of fetal abnormalities associated with its use in pregnancy may be related to contamination in illegally prepared LSD.

Cigarette smoking

The risks of preterm delivery, growth retardation and perinatal mortality are increased by 30%. No increase in congenital abnormalities occurs, but closure of the ductus arteriosus may be delayed. There is some evidence that children of mothers who smoked during pregnancy are at greater risk from respiratory disease in the first years of life, even if mothers gave up smoking after pregnancy. Smoking 20 cigarettes per day during pregnancy increases the risk of cot death fourfold.

Every effort should be made to dissuade mothers from smoking, especially in those at high risk.

Oligohydramnios

This may result from chronic leakage of amniotic fluid.

The fetus normally produces 300–800 ml/day of urine; thus, any cause of decreased urine production may lead to oligohydramnios (e.g. severe growth retardation, renal agenesis or dysplasia, urethral valves).

Oligohydramnios from any cause may result in *pulmonary hypoplasia and postural deformities* of the fetus (see Chapter 6, page 70, and Chapter 16, page 235).

Antenatal ultrasound scanning may enable the diagnosis to be made.

After birth examine the infant's urinary tract clinically and with ultrasound.

Polyhydramnios

Polyhydramnios is defined as an amniotic liquor volume greater than two litres. This may be associated with maternal factors (e.g. maternal diabetes) or fetal factors (e.g. oesophageal atresia, high intestinal obstruction, diaphragmatic hernia, choanal atresia, anencephaly, Down's syndrome, neuromuscular disorders, congenital nephrosis, osteochondrodystrophy, hydrops fetalis, Beckwith's syndrome or multiple pregnancy). Any condition causing decreased swallowing in the fetus may lead to polyhydramnios.

Forty per cent of infants born to women with polyhydramnios have major malformations.

All women with polyhydramnios should have a glucose tolerance test carried out and there should be a detailed ultrasound examination of the fetus.

Antenatal tapping of the excess fluid in severe polyhydramnios gives only a brief respite and may lead to placental abruption or preterm labour.

See Chapter 2, page 24, for management of the baby born to a mother with polyhydramnios.

Assessment of fetal growth and well-being during pregnancy

Assessment of fetal growth and well-being requires **accurate knowledge of gestation** including:

Date of LMP (plus length and regularity of periods)
Early bimanual examination
Date when fetal movements were first felt (very variable)
Early (<20 weeks) ultrasound scan (preferably 12–16 weeks)
Measurement of fundal height (Fig. 1.1, page 12)

Fetal well-being

This may be assessed by:

'Kick charts'
Cardiotocograms (CTG) (see the section on assessment during labour, page 14)
Placental hormone assays, e.g. Oestriol, human placental lactogen are unreliable and are now seldom used

Biophysical assessment

Biophysical assessment of liquor volume, fetal activity, fetal heart rate pattern and fetal breathing movements is a more sensitive indicator of fetal well-being or compromise which is increasingly used.

Detection of fetal abnormalities

Techniques

Ultrasound

Ultrasound is considered safe regardless of gestational age.

It is used increasingly to diagnose a number of structural fetal abnormalities (e.g. hydrocephalus, neural tube defects, congenital heart disease, exomphalos, obstructive uropathies, hydrops fetalis).

Chorion villous biopsy

This may be performed trans-vaginally or trans-abdominally at 9–11 weeks of pregnancy. It provides material for rapid chromosome analysis and DNA/biochemical studies. The risk of miscarriage after chorion villous biopsy is approximately 5%.

Amniocentesis

NB   Amniocentesis for diagnosis of fetal abnormality should **only** be carried out after careful parental counselling, usually on the understanding that termination will follow the detection of abnormality.

Risk of fetal loss after amniocentesis is 1–2%.

Fetal cells may be grown in tissue culture for chromosome or biochemical studies.

Amniotic fluid may be examined chemically (e.g. alpha-fetoprotein, AFP) or physically (e.g. spectrophotometry in severe rhesus disease) (see Chapter 18, page 260).

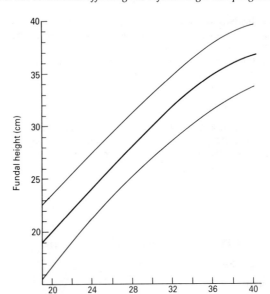

Fig. 1.1   Fundal height (±2s.d.) and gestation. (Adapted from Robinson *et al.*, 1990, *Brit. J. Obstet Gynaec.* **88** 115)

Chromosome abnormalities

The risk of trisomies rises with the mother's age (see page 325). The presence of a low serum AFP level in the mother suggests a high age-related risk of Down's syndrome; high or normal levels of AFP suggest a lower risk. Thus AFP is a useful adjunct in counselling prior to amniocentesis.

Neural tube defects (NTD)

Screening

Screening is used in some centres.

Maternal blood is taken for serum AFP level at 16–18 weeks gestation. If the AFP level is elevated the test is repeated, and if it is still elevated an ultrasound scan (to check gestation and fetal morphology) and amniocentesis are performed. If the amniotic fluid AFP is elevated and an abnormal acetylcholinesterase band is present, the parents are offered termination of the pregnancy.

Potential limitations of AFP screening The screening must be fully discussed with mother **before** serum AFP measured.

The pregnancy must be **accurately** dated at 16 weeks.

Normal screening **does not** rule out NTD (or any other abnormality).

Other conditions may cause raised AFP levels (e.g. twins, exomphalos, Turner's syndrome) and must be carefully sought with ultrasound examination.

Amniocentesis carries a 1–2% risk of fetal loss (80–90% of these will be **normal** fetuses).

If diagnosis of NTD is confirmed, a later termination (at about 20 weeks) will be necessary.

Most infants with severe NTD die in early infancy (see Chapter 10, page 148).

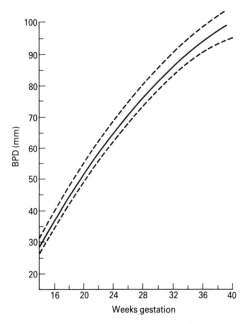

Fig. 1.2 Mean fetal biparietal diameter (BPD) plus 5th and 95th percentiles from 14 to 40 weeks gestation.

Assessment of fetal well-being during labour

Fetal heart rate

Fetal heart rate (FHR) is assessed by fetal stethoscope (adequate in low-risk patients).

Indications for continuous intrapartum monitoring of FHR
High-risk pregnancy (see Table 1.1)
Fetal bradycardia (<120) or tachycardia (>160)
Prolonged labour
Meconium in liquor
Induced labour
Abnormal presentation (e.g. breech)
Preterm labour
Hypotension
Epidural anaesthesia
Augmented labour

Table 1.1   Causes of high-risk delivery

1 Pre-existing medical conditions
Haematological – anaemia, haemoglobinopathies, idiopathic thrombocytopenic purpura (ITP), sickle-cell disease
Endocrine – thyrotoxicosis, diabetes mellitus, Cushing's disease
Cardiovascular – hypertension or heart disease
Respiratory – asthma, tuberculosis
CNS – epilepsy
Psychiatric illness
Others – e.g. SLE, myasthenia, ulcerative colitis, Crohn's disease
Malignant disease
Drug abuse
Renal – chronic or recurrent pyelonephritis, renal failure

2 Past obstetric history
Anatomic abnormality of uterus or cervix
Fetal or perinatal loss – abortion, stillbirth or neonatal death
Previous infant with major structural or metabolic abnormality
Previous preterm or complicated delivery
Previous infant with intrauterine growth retardation

3 Complications during this pregnancy
Age (< 17 or > 35 years)
Smoking
Drug abuse or therapy (including alcohol)
Hypertension/PET
Gestational diabetes mellitus
Infection (e.g. toxoplasma/rubella/cytomegalovirus/herpes (TORCH),
   urinary tract infection (UTI), viral infections with fever)
Prolonged or premature rupture of membranes
Preterm labour
Oligohydramnios
Polyhydramnios
Social problems

4 Fetal conditions
Multiple gestation (twins, triplets)
Growth retardation
Fetal abnormality detected on ultrasound scan or X-ray
Abnormal CTG ('non-stress test')

5 Complications of labour or delivery
Antepartum haemorrhage
Preterm delivery
Abnormal presentation (breech, face, transverse lie)
Maternal fever
Maternal hypotension
Cephalopelvic disproportion
Prolapsed cord
Deep transverse arrest
Fetal distress
   Persistent bradycardia or tachycardia
   Abnormal CTG
   Meconium in liquor
   Scalp pH <7.25
Forceps or ventouse delivery
Caesarean section

Monitoring may be by an ECG electrode on the presenting part (after rupture of the membranes) or ultrasound transducer on the mother's abdomen. Uterine contractions are recorded by a strain-gauge transducer strapped to the abdomen or (less commonly) by an intrauterine pressure catheter.

The print-out of FHR and uterine activity is called a cardiotocograph (CTG) (see Tables 1.2 and 1.3).

Cardiotocographs are more difficult to interpret in the second stage of labour. Brief large decelerations (>40 bpm) are not uncommon, but type 2 dips with loss of variability are potentially serious and prolonged bradycardia may warrant immediate delivery.

Table 1.2 Interpretation of cardiotocographs in the first stage of labour

Pattern	Description	Action
Normal	FHR 120–160 bpm; no significant change in FHR during contractions Baseline variability ('beat-to-beat variability') >5 bpm	None
Acceleration pattern	FHR increases at start of contraction, returning to baseline during or at end of the contraction; **normal pattern**	None
Loss of baseline variability	Baseline variability <5 bpm ('flat trace'); commonly indicates fetal hypoxia	Check fetal pH
Baseline bradycardia	FHR <120 bpm; abnormal only if accompanied by loss of baseline variability ± decelerations	Turn patient on her side; check fetal pH
Baseline tachycardia	FHR >160 bpm; abnormal only if persistent or accompanied by loss of baseline variability ± decelerations	
Early deceleration (type 1 dip)	Deceleration begins with onset of contraction; returns to baseline by the end of the contraction Deceleration is usually <40 bpm; it may be due to head compression or may be an early sign of hypoxia	None
Later deceleration (type 2 dip)	Deceleration with the lowest point beyond the peak of the contraction; the later the deceleration, the more serious its significance, especially if accompanied by loss of baseline variability ± tachycardia.	Check fetal pH immediately
Variable deceleration	Deceleration of irregular shape and large amplitude (>50 bpm) appearing at a variable time during the contraction; if this occurs with each contraction it suggests developing fetal hypoxia	Check fetal pH
Normal uterine contractions	3–4 contractions every 10 min; duration <75 sec (uterine catheter: baseline 5–12 mm Hg, peak 30–60 mm Hg)	None

Table 1.3 Interpretation of fetal blood pH

pH	Interpretation	Action
>7.3	Normal	None needed
7.25–7.29	Borderline	Repeat in one hour or if CTG is abnormal
7.20–7.24	Abnormal	Expedite delivery (consider Caesarean section or forceps delivery)
<7.2	Very abnormal	Immediate delivery

Recent evidence suggests that some infants, particularly those who are small-for-dates, may be severely compromised by hypoxaemia during labour in the absence of any significant fetal acidosis. **Thus a normal pH in the presence of other evidence of fetal stress (e.g. abnormal CTG, meconium staining) should be treated with caution.**

Management of preterm labour

Definition

Onset of regular painful contractions accompanied by effacement and dilation of the cervix after 20 and before 37 completed weeks of pregnancy.

Preterm labour accounts for 5–10% of births, but leads to 85% of neonatal deaths.

Contributory factors in preterm labour
Ante partum haemorrhage (APH)
Hypertension
Intrauterine growth retardation
Multiple pregnancy
Infection (e.g. amnionitis, pyelonephritis)
Premature rupture of the membranes
Uterine anomaly
Diabetes mellitus
Polyhydramnios
Maternal smoking
Heavy physical activity
Psychological stress

Management of preterm labour

Treat underlying cause (e.g. pyelonephritis).

If fetal welfare is compromised (e.g. amnionitis) then deliver the baby rather than inhibit the labour.

Monitor closely and consider Caesarean section for fetal distress if >26 weeks' gestation.

If <34 weeks gestation, consider inhibiting labour with infusion of β-sympathomimetic (e.g. ritodrine, salbutamol) unless contra-indicated (e.g. amnionitis, APH, pre-eclampic toxaemia (PET), maternal cardiac disease).

NB   There is a risk of early hypoglycaemia in infants born to mothers given sympathomimetic agents, therefore check the baby's blood glucose.

If labour can be inhibited, then transfer the mother with baby *in utero* to a unit with a special care baby unit (SCBU) or neonatal intensive care unit (NICU) (see Chapter 5).

The use of *steroids* to accelerate lung maturation is controversial.

Antepartum steroids: Although many clinicians remain cautious in their use, betamethasone or dexamethasone 12 mg i.m. repeated once after 12 hours has been shown to reduce the risk of respiratory distress syndrome (RDS) if delivery is delayed for 1–6 days. Con-traindications to steroid use include maternal fever, hypertension or PET, cervical dilation, rupture of membranes.

Premature rupture of the membranes in the absence of contractions

If gestation is less than 34 weeks, this is best managed conservatively (i.e. hospital admission and bed rest; weekly sterile speculum vaginal examination and high vaginal swab for culture).

If fever occurs, take blood culture from mother, start antibiotics and expedite delivery.

If labour starts more than 48 hours after membrane rupture, then do not attempt to inhibit if gestation is >30 weeks.

Prolonged (>2 weeks) drainage of amniotic fluid at <30 weeks' gestation, if it leads to oligohydramnios, may cause pulmonary hypoplasia; therefore, consider elective delivery after 10–14 days if there is oligohydramnios.

For management of the infant after prolonged rupture of membranes see Chapter 14, page 213.

Bibliography

Berkowitz, R. L. (Ed.) (1980). High risk pregnancy. In: *Clinics in Perinatology*, Volume 7, Number 2 (September). London: W. B. Saunders.

Brettle, R. P., Bisset, K., Burns, S. *et al.* (1987). Human immunodeficiency virus and drug misuse – The Edinburgh Experience. *Br. Med. J.*, **295**, 421–4.

Brock, D. J. H. (1982). *Early Diagnosis of Fetal Defects*.
    Edinburgh: Churchill Livingstone.
Crowley, P., Chalmers, I. and Keirse, M. J. N. C. (1990) The
    effects of corticosteroid administration before preterm delivery:
    an overview of the evidence from controlled trials. *Br. J. Obstet.
    Gynaecol.*, **97**, 11–25.
DHSS (1987). *Immunization Against Infectious Disease*. Amended
    Section Tuberculosis and BCG Vaccinations, September.
    London: HMSO.
DHSS (1988). *Immunization Against Infectious Disease*. London:
    HMSO.
Editorial (1988). HIV infection. Obstetric and perinatal issues.
    Lancet, **1**, 806–7.
Petrie, R. H. (Ed.) (1982). Fetal monitoring. In: *Clinics in
    Perinatology*, Volume 9, Number 2 (June). London: W. B.
    Saunders.
Polakoff, S. and Van Der Velde, E. M. (1988). Immunisation of
    neonates at high risk of hepatitis B in England and Wales national
    surveillance. *Br. Med. J.*, **297**, 249–53.
Report of the Royal College of Obstetricians and Gynaecologists
    Sub-Committees (1987). Sub-committee on problems associated
    with AIDS in relation to obstetrics and gynaecology. London:
    Royal College of Obstetricians and Gynaecologists.
Stirrat, G. M. (1986). *An Obstetric Pocket Consultant*. Oxford:
    Blackwell Scientific.

2

In the delivery room

Organization
Preparation before delivery
Management at birth
Special resuscitation problems
Aftercare in the delivery room

'At all times, in all maternity units, there must be someone available in the labour ward (or able to reach there within two minutes) capable of starting expert resuscitation by intubation or by bag and mask' (Extract from *British Paediatric Association Minimum Standards of Neonatal Care*, 1983).

Organization

Delivery room resuscitation is the most important responsibility of the paediatric staff. Much neonatal morbidity and mortality may be prevented by prompt and efficient action.

Responsibility of the neonatal medical team

(1) Ensure that *all* medical and nursing staff are familiar with and experienced in *neonatal resuscitation*. This includes preparation of appropriate protocols.
(2) Ensure that a *roster of trained staff* immediately available for resuscitation is posted in the delivery suite, the telephonists' office and the paediatric department.
(3) Ensure that delivery room staff *summon assistance in good time* whenever a resuscitation problem may be anticipated (Table 2.1).
(4) Ensure that *resuscitation equipment is available and working* (Table 2.2).

Table 2.1   Deliveries at which paediatric staff should routinely be present

Caesarean section
Breech delivery
Forceps (except simple 'lift outs')
Twins
Preterm delivery (<37 weeks)
Delivery after significant antepartum haemorrhage (APH)
Prolonged (>24 hours) rupture of membranes, or suspected amnionitis
   (e.g. foul liquor or maternal fever)
Polyhydramnios
Fetal distress (see Chapter 1)
Mother with severe pregnancy-induced hypertension
Mother a drug addict or alcoholic
Fetal disease or abnormality known or suspected
Rhesus disease
Delivery under heavy sedation or general anaesthesia
Mother with history of diabetes mellitus, myasthenia gravis
   thrombocytopenia, thyrotoxicosis, or other disease known to affect the
   fetus (see Chapter 1)

Two or more paediatric medical staff should attend
Multiple births
Delivery before 32 weeks' gestation (or if the baby is thought to be <1.5 kg)
Preterm (<37 weeks) Caesarean section

Preparation before delivery

The parents

Paediatric staff should ensure they are called to the delivery suite sufficiently early to introduce themselves to parents, explain what is happening or likely to happen and to answer parents' questions.

Always introduce yourself to the parents as soon as possible after your arrival in the delivery room.

The obstetric history

Obtain as full a history as possible from the mother, midwife or obstetrician and examine the mother's notes (see Chapter 1).

NB   Any drugs given to mother?
     Gestation? (? certain)
     Evidence of fetal distress?
     Prolonged rupture of membranes?
     Any relevant past obstetric or medical history?

Table 2.2 Delivery room resuscitation equipment

(A) Immediately available in every delivery room

Resuscitation trolley with overhead heater, lighting, stop-clock

Oxygen and air supply (with reducing valve, flow-meter, pressure blow-off device (set at 30 cm H_2O), pressure measuring device, e.g. manometer)

Connecting tubes to supply air/oxygen to bag and mask and (with side hole) to endotracheal tube (ETT)

Face masks (e.g. Bennett, sizes 2 and 3)

Resuscitation bag with fitting for face mask and ETT adaptor and blow-off valve (e.g. Ambu, Laerdal)

Two laryngoscopes, with preterm- and term-sized straight blades (e.g. Wisconsin or Magill) and spare bulbs and batteries

Endotracheal tubes (2.5, 3.0 and 3.5 mm) and connectors and fixation devices

Endotracheal tube introducer (nylon or metal)

Suction device and suction catheters (FG 4, 6, 8)

Sterile towel, scissors, cord clamps

Antiseptic cleaning solution (e.g. povidone-iodine, chlorhexidine)

Silver swaddler and warmed sterile towel

Intravenous cannulae, 3-way taps, connecting tubing

Sterile syringes (2, 5 and 10 ml) and needles

Oral mucus extractors

Adhesive tapes and safety pins

Sterile containers; specimen bottles for blood tests (e.g. full blood count, packed cell volume, electrolytes, sugar, bilirubin, blood group and Coomb's test)

Drugs
    Naloxone (20 microg/ml: *dose* 0.5–1 ml/kg i.m.)
    Vitamin K_1 (*dose* 0.5–1 mg i.m.)

Capillary blood sugar test strips (e.g. 'Dextrostix', 'BM Glycemie')

Stethoscope with infant endpiece

Alcohol swabs

(B) Available at all times within the delivery suite

Equipment for umbilical catheterization

Pneumothorax drains + Heimlich valves

10% glucose solution for infusion (500 ml)

Intravenous giving sets (paediatric)

Intravenous infusion pumps

Fresh frozen plasma

Fresh blood (group O, Rh-negative)

Drugs
    Glucose 25% (25 ml ampoules)
    Adrenaline 1 in 10 000
    Calcium gluconate 10%
    Sodium chloride for injection 0.9%
    Water for injection

Common neonatal conditions which may often be anticipated

(NB   See Chapter 1)

Preterm infant
   Menstrual history
   Obstetric observations

Small-for-dates (SFD)
   Past history of SFD
   Maternal pregnancy hypertension/vascular disease
   Placental insufficiency
   Evidence of intrauterine growth retardation

Congenital infection
   History of maternal infection during pregnancy
   Prolonged rupture of membranes (>24 hours)
   Signs of amnionitis (fever or offensive liquor)

Respiratory distress
   Preterm delivery
   Meconium in amniotic fluid
   Oligohydramnios
   Prolonged rupture of membranes
   Amnionitis
   Breech delivery
   Caesarean section without a preceding labour

Fetal sedation
   Maternal drug addiction
   Medical drugs given to mother during pregnancy, e.g. for
      pregnancy hypertension
   Analgesic drugs during labour
   General anaesthesia for delivery

Fetal 'concussion'
   Cephalopelvic disproportion
   Breech delivery
   Forceps or other extraction
   Difficult delivery
   Larger second twin
   Precipitate delivery

Fetal asphyxia
   History of chronic fetal distress and growth retardation
   Abruptio placentae
   Second twin
   Passage of meconium
   Other signs of fetal distress during labour (see Tables 1.2 and 1.3)

Hypovolaemia (fetal blood loss) (see Chapter 15)
   APH associated with placenta praevia/vasa praevia
   Post-amniocentesis
   Caesarean placental loss
   Twin-to-twin loss
   Early cord clamping

Congenital malformation
   Family history
   Prenatal diagnosis (see Chapter 1)
   Oligohydramnios
   Polyhydramnios

NB   *if the infant is below average weight for gestational age with a history of polyhydramnios, malformation is most likely. If the baby appears to be externally normal but there is a resuscitation problem, consider diaphragmatic hernia, oesophageal atresia or choanal atresia.*

Specific maternal-related conditions
   Rhesus and other haemolytic disease (see Chapter 17)
   Idiopathic thrombocytopenia (see Chapter 15)
   Transient myasthenia gravis (see Chapter 1)
   Neonatal thyrotoxicosis (see Chapter 13)
   Infant of diabetic mother (see Chapter 5)
   Maternal hypertension (see Chapter 1)

Check and prepare the resuscitation equipment

(a) Check that equipment is available and in working order
(b) Turn on overhead heater
     Ensure that warmed towels are available
     Ensure that the transport incubator is switched from 'stand-by' to 'ON'
(c) Ensure the delivery room is warm ($>24°$ C) and free of draughts
(d) Make other preparations: e.g. draw up naloxone into a syringe if the mother has recently received a narcotic such as pethidine

Management at birth

Time at birth

Start the clock.

Thermal care

(See Chapter 5, page 52).

Even healthy infants have difficulty in maintaining body temperature soon after delivery. Small, sick and sedated infants are particularly likely to become chilled. Their problems are greatly exacerbated by cold stress. Even mild chilling may double oxygen requirements and significantly impair prospects for intact survival.

Heat loss is minimized by immediately drying and wrapping the infant in a warm towel. In breech presentations this may be done even before the baby is fully delivered.

Other measures to keep the infant warm include the overhead heater, the incubator and silver swaddler. The latter should not be used under an overhead heater as they reflect radiant heat and reduce the effectiveness of the heater.

NB   A clothed infant may lose up to 85% of its total heat loss through the head, therefore use a bonnet to reduce heat loss during all prolonged resuscitations.

Assessment of clinical status

Apgar score

The status of the infant at birth is usually assessed by the Apgar score.

The Apgar score is recorded at 1 and 5 min after birth. The score is also recorded at 5-min intervals as long as the infant requires resuscitation. With experience, the score may be assessed in a few seconds. Once this skill has been acquired, it is useful also to record the score in the first few seconds after delivery, the heart rate being estimated by gently palpating the cord near the umbilicus. The status of the newborn infant at birth broadly falls into one of three groups:

Normal (Apgar score: 7–10)   A pink infant, often with blue extremities, who breathes or cries, has a strong heart beat of more than 100/min, a good tone, and has an active response to stimuli.

Mild/moderate birth asphyxia (Apgar score: 3–6) The infant is usually blue and apnoeic, with a fairly strong heart beat at a rate of 90–160/min; muscle tone is present but diminished, as is also the response to stimuli. Often referred to as *blue asphyxia*.

Severe birth asphyxia (Apgar score: 0–2) The infant is usually pale (or cyanosed) due to peripheral vasoconstriction. The heart rate is slow and often weak or even absent. Tone is flaccid, there is no response to stimuli, and the infant is apnoeic. Often referred to as *white asphyxia*.

The Apgar score

Sign	Score 0	Score 1	Score 2
Heart rate	Absent	Below 100/min	Above 100/min
Respiratory effort	Absent	Weak	Good, crying
Muscle tone	Flaccid	Some flexion of extremities	Well flexed
Reflex irritability	No response	Grimace	Cough or sneeze
Colour	Pale or blue	Body pink extremities blue	Completely pink

Cord blood pH

For babies born after evidence of fetal distress (Chapter 1) or those needing resuscitation, the cord blood pH may be an indicator of the severity of intrapartum asphyxia.

A normal cord blood pH in the presence of a low Apgar score may indicate that the infant was unable to respond to intrapartum asphyxia by anaerobic metabolism (e.g. because of poor glycogen reserves in light-for-dates baby). Some such infants may have suffered significant intrapartum asphyxia despite the normal pH.

Dividing the umbilical cord

Clamping the umbilical cord not only determines the distribution of blood between the infant and placenta but may also, while pulsation persists, cause major haemodynamic changes in the circulation.

In the past the umbilical cord was not clamped and divided until after the placenta had delivered, had lain alongside the baby for 10 or more minutes, and until after all umbilical cord pulsation had ceased. There is some evidence that such practice has advantages for normal adaption to extrauterine life.

However, modern obstetric practice usually involves division of the cord while the placenta is still *in utero*. In these circumstances, the optimum distribution of blood volume and the least haemodynamic disturbance are likely to be achieved by clamping the cord 30 sec after delivery of the baby. By this time the infant will usually have taken his first breath and will have received a partial placental transfusion.

Preterm infants, and especially those delivered by Caesarean section, are at special risk of maladaptation and require special management (see page 35).

After division the cord should be firmly occluded about 2 cm from the umbilicus using either a rubber band or a plastic disposable umbilical cord clamp.

Care of the airway

The upper airway

Obstruction of the upper airway is uncommon (but may occur after birth because of thick meconium, by a congenital abnormality or infected secretions). It is not a *primary* cause of apnoea. The clinical signs of airway obstruction are inspiratory retraction of the chest wall with poor or absent air entry.

The majority of babies do *not* require aspiration of the upper airway with a mucus suction catheter. It is usually sufficient to wipe the lips and nose with a piece of gauze. The use of a mucus catheter should normally be confined to aspiration of the nose or mouth. The tip of the catheter should *not* be inserted into the pharynx unless there is clear evidence of obstruction, in which case it should be done under direct vision with the aid of a laryngoscope. *More resuscitation problems are caused than are resolved by blind probing of the sensitive area around the entry to the larynx with a mucus catheter; the practice can lead to activation of reflex bradycardia, apnoea and hypotension.*

There is also no indication for passing a catheter into the stomach except to rule out suspected oesophageal atresia or in order to aspirate gastric contents for examination for infection.

When the upper airway is obstructed, the blockage is usually located in the nose and is due either to debris or to choanal atresia/stenosis. The patency of the nasal passages may be quickly tested by listening to each nostril in turn with the bell of a stethoscope, the opposite nostril being temporarily occluded.

The lower airway: meconium aspiration

(See page 32.)

Management of the normal infant at birth

Provided a quick inspection reveals no major resuscitation difficulty or any other problem, the baby should be handed at once to the mother. This may be done even before dividing the umbilical cord. The baby may be wrapped in a warmed towel or nursed skin-to-skin on the mother's body and then covered with a towel. If the mother intends to breast feed, the baby should be put to the breast. Such a practice not only improves the success of lactation but also helps to speed delivery of the placenta through the reflex release of oxytocin (see Chapters 4 and 11).

Management of an infant requiring resuscitation

Move to resuscitation platform

If the infant is of very low birthweight, or is clearly asphyxiated, or has not breathed within one minute of birth, then move the child to the resuscitation area, at the same time taking measures to avoid hypothermia (see page 25).

Positioning the baby

DO NOT place the baby in a head-down position. This common practice is itself responsible for much resuscitation difficulty by impairing diaphragmatic action because of the weight of the abdominal contents, by reducing pulmonary lymphatic drainage because of the raised central venous pressure, and by delaying the recovery of normal cerebral activity by causing raised cerebral venous blood pressure. Venous return to the heart, and hence cardiac output, may also be reduced in the head-down position, further contributing to cerebral venous congestion.

Therefore, place the infant in a gentle head-up position with support under the shoulders so that the neck is neither flexed nor extended.

Reassess the infant's status

If the infant is still apnoeic then decide whether the problem is 'blue asphyxia' (Apgar score 3–6) or 'white asphyxia' (Apgar score 0–2).

With blue asphyxia, attempt to stimulate respiration by flicking the feet or ears, by gently clearing the nose with a mucus catheter, or by skin stimulation with a warm, dry towel.

Use of an opiate antagonist

If the mother has received pethidine, morphine, heroin or other related opiates within the previous eight hours, give naloxone 10 microgs/kg promptly by i.m. injection into the thigh (0.5 ml/kg of Narcan Neonatal). Do not waste valuable time trying to inject naloxone intravenously. This specific antagonist given i.m. usually produces a response within 2 min. The dose may need to be repeated after 30–60 min. Naloxone may also be rapidly effective if given down the endotracheal tube.

Positive-pressure ventilation

Air/oxygen at pressures of up to a maximum of 30–35 cm H_2O should be administered to the airway at a rate of 30 puffs per minute using either a bag and mask such as the Laerdal or Ambu bag, or through an endotracheal tube. The purpose of the former technique is more to provoke the onset of respiration by reflex stimulation of pressure receptors in the lower airway than to inflate the lungs mechanically.

(i) *Using bag and mask* *All* medical and midwifery staff in the delivery suite should know how to use the bag and mask. The method is simple and non-invasive. It is the technique of choice for infants with 'blue asphyxia', partly because most of them respond well and also because infants with some tone are less easy to intubate. In addition, the intubation of lightly depressed infants may cause further reflex apnoea.

(ii) *Using endotracheal intubation* (see Chapter 26, page 350   Intubation is the preferred method for infants not responding within 1 min to bag-and-mask ventilation (rise in heart rate, improved colour, onset of respiration) and for those with more severe birth asphyxia ('white asphyxia').

Intubation should be carried out as a calm elective procedure. If the first attempt is unsuccessful recommence bag-and-mask resuscitation for 30–60 sec before a further attempt at intubation. **DO NOT ALLOW THE BABY TO BECOME COLD OR MORE HYPOXIC AS A RESULT OF REPEATED UNSUCCESSFUL ATTEMPTS AT INTUBATION.**

If the baby does not respond to intermittent positive-pressure ventilation (IPPV) within 30 sec, check that the tube is correctly placed and is not blocked or dislodged.

Always use a resuscitation bag or air/oxygen supply, with a blow-off set at 30–35 cm H_2O. **Do not** exceed flow rates recommended by the manufacturer (usually 2–3 l/min).

Once spontaneous respiration is established and the baby is pink, remove the endotracheal tube. **Do not** leave an open endotracheal tube (ETT) in place as this will impair oxygenation and may lead to apnoea by reducing functional residual capacity, increasing airway resistance and preventing grunting.

Cardiac massage

(See Chapter 26, page 358.)

If the heart beat is undetectable or the heart rate remains below 50–60 per minute despite positive-pressure ventilation, then cardiac massage should be commenced. This is done by placing the fingers around the chest, with one or both thumbs on the lower sternum which is then depressed by about 2 cm 100 times a minute. Compression of the sternum must not be violent, especially in preterm infants to avoid damage to the chest wall, heart or liver.

Persisting bradycardia or asystole with adequate ventilation

Give:

(1) Adrenaline 0.1 ml/kg of 1 in 10 000 dilution intravenously or via the endotracheal tube.
(2) Calcium gluconate 10% solution 1 ml/kg intravenously (use the umbilical vein for access).
(3) If no response to the above, give intracardiac adrenaline and calcium gluconate in the same dose.

Use of plasma

If the infant remains poorly perfused despite adequate ventilation give 10 ml/kg of fresh frozen plasma or plasma protein fraction over 20 min. Repeat once if necessary.

Use of sodium bicarbonate

Intravenous alkali ($NaHCO_3$ or THAM) is widely recommended for the asphyxiated infant. We firmly believe that its use is unnecessary and *may be dangerous*. Intravenous sodium bicarbonate, especially given as a bolus to a poorly ventilated asphyxiated acidotic infant, may exacerbate hypercarbia and intracellular acidosis whilst lowering blood pressure via its vasodilator and negative inotropic actions.

Resuscitation difficulty

If the resuscitative measures discussed above fail or are inadequate, then consideration should be given to the following diagnosis:

Meconium aspiration syndrome (pages 32 and 87)
Diaphragmatic hernia (pages 34 and 178)
Pneumothorax/pneumomediastinum (page 88)
Pleural/pericardial effusion (page 89
Congenital pneumonia/sepsis (page 88)
Pulmonary oedema/haemorrhage (page 88)
Pulmonary hypoplasia (page 90)
Congenital heart disease (page 117)
Persistent fetal circulation (page 121)
Hypovolaemia due to blood loss (page 225)
Cerebrospinal trauma/hypoxia/malformation (page 144)
Cerebral depression from drugs (page 8)
Severe metabolic disturbance (page 192)
Extreme prematurity (page 57)
Malformation of the respiratory tract (page 90), such as congenital
   lobar emphysema

Consideration of some of these special problems may be found later
in this section or elsewhere as indicated.

Failed resuscitation

If, in spite of persistent resuscitative efforts for 30 min, the infant
remains profoundly depressed and unresponsive, consideration must
be given to the appropriateness of continuing intensive care. The
critical question is whether the infant has suffered irreversible damage or has a severely handicapping congenital anomaly. *The most
senior paediatrician available should be summoned or informed and
the situation discussed fully with the parents. If there is any doubt
about the prognosis, intensive care efforts should be continued.* If
resuscitation is to be discontinued, the parents may wish the baby to
be baptized first. They may then wish to be left with their child during
the final minutes.

Summoning assistance

Neonatal resuscitation may present challenges requiring great experience. *Junior members of the staff should never hesitate to summon
the assistance of senior colleagues (sooner rather than later).* When the
problem occurs or may be anticipated in a GP maternity unit or at
home, then the neonatal transfer team should be called without
delay.

Some DO NOTS of neonatal resuscitation
(1) DO NOT let the baby get cold.
(2) DO NOT blindly and repeatedly aspirate the pharynx with a
   suction catheter.

(3) DO NOT persist with unsuccessful attempts at intubation (stop, and give the baby IPPV bag and mask).
(4) DO NOT over-flex or over-extend the infant's neck.
(5) DO NOT give NaHCO$_3$.
(6) DO NOT leave an open ETT in place.
(7) DO NOT delay calling for assistance if in difficulty.
(8) DO NOT place the infant head down.

Special resuscitation problems

Meconium aspiration

Inhalation of meconium may lead to severe respiratory distress. Partial airway obstruction by sticky meconium ('ball–valve effect') leads to patchy atelectasis and over-inflation of the lungs, which combined with the chemical pneumonitis caused by meconium and the commonly associated persistent fetal circulation, makes this a *very* difficult condition to treat and leads to substantial mortality and long-term morbidity, with a high risk of pneumothorax (see Chapter 8).

SYMPTOMATIC MECONIUM ASPIRATION SYNDROME IS A CONDITION LARGELY PREVENTABLE BY CORRECT DELIVERY ROOM MANAGEMENT, as detailed below:

Paediatric staff should attend *all* deliveries with meconium-staining of the liquor. A competent assistant is needed.

NB   Apparent meconium staining may be due to vomited bile or to infection with listeria.

Delivery room procedure

(1) Briefly outline to the parents what is to be done (preferably before the baby is born).
(2) After delivery of the face, before delivery of the chest, gently clear meconium from nose and mouth using an oral mucus extractor.
(3) If thick meconium is present gentle chest compression by the assistant after delivery of the trunk *may* delay the first gasp and prevent aspiration during initial suctioning.
(4) Quickly dry and wrap the infant.
(5) Gently suck meconium out of the mouth, pharynx and nose. Use a laryngoscope to see the vocal cords and suck out the posterior pharynx and larynx under direct vision. This may be performed on the delivery bed before cutting the cord to reduce the risk of early gasping.

(6) If meconium is present in the posterior pharynx or larynx transfer the child to the resuscitation trolley and intubate. Apply gentle suction to the ETT whilst removing the tube. If a plug of meconium is removed with the ETT, repeat the process. *We can no longer recommend mouth suction because of the risk of HIV.*
(7) Resuscitate the infant with bag-and-mask ventilation or endotracheal IPPV.

NB   Do not use IPPV before clearing the airway: meconium may be forced into the bronchial tree. If the infant cries vigorously before the trachea has been intubated and suctioned, abandon the attempt. A forced intubation may injure the infant's mouth and airways.

Tracheal lavage with saline is *not* recommended and has been shown to worsen the outcome.

With practice the process of clearing the airways should not greatly delay resuscitation.

All babies from whom meconium is aspirated from below the cords should be kept under close observation for 4–6 hours. If no respiratory signs (e.g. tachypnoea, grunting, temperature instability, hypoglycaemia, cyanosis) develop within 6 hours the infant may go to a normal postnatal ward with its mother but should be kept under observation for 24 hours, as pneumothorax and infection can occur later. If any respiratory signs develop, transfer to SCBU or NICU, X-ray the chest and manage as described in Chapter 8.

Hypovolaemia due to fetal blood loss (see page 225)

The infant presents with 'white asphyxia', is pale, hypotensive, apnoeic and has a weak pulse that may be slow or rapid. If the infant does not respond to IPPV, give a rapid transfusion (10–20 ml/kg over 5–10 min) of unmatched fresh O Rh-negative blood (or blood cross-matched against the mother's blood) and reassess. A second similar transfusion may be necessary (see Chapter 15). Use Apt's test to distinguish fetal from adult blood (see page 225).

Hydrops fetalis

Generalized oedema, ascites, pleural effusions, anaemia and hepatosplenomegaly may occur with severe fetal anaemia (e.g. Rh disease, Chapter 18; thalassaemia, Chapter 15), congenital infections (syphilis, toxoplasma, CMV, Chapter 14), maternal diabetes (Chapter 5), cardiac failure (Chapter 9), hypoproteinaemia (e.g.

congenital hepatitis or nephrotic syndrome), or twin-to-twin transfusion.

Initial problems are similar, whatever the cause:

Respiration

Sustained IPPV through an ETT is always needed (with frequent suction to clear pulmonary fluid). Drain ascites $\pm$ pleural effusions immediately if they are embarrassing respiration (Chapter 26).

Anaemia and hypoproteinaemia

Correct the anaemia *slowly* with repeated small exchange transfusions of packed red cells (20–40 ml/kg) to avoid major fluid shifts and pulmonary oedema from a rapid rise in oncotic pressure.

Haemorrhage

Risk is decreased by giving 1 mg i.v. vitamin K_1 immediately after birth (Chapter 15), and by exchange transfusion with fresh blood (Chapter 18, page 265 and Chapter 26, page 354).

Cardiac failure and poor urine output

Give frusemide, 1–2 mg/kg, 12-hourly $\pm$ digoxin (see Chapter 9). Create a fluid deficit (10–20 ml/kg) during exchange transfusion (see Chapter 18, page 265).

Hypoglycaemia

Monitor capillary blood sugar 2–4 hourly. Give 10–15 % glucose i.v. at 6–10 mg/kg/min (see Chapter 13, page 192).

Investigation

(a) Examine the placenta carefully.
(b) Take blood from the placenta for blood group, Coombs' test, haemoglobin (Hb) and packed cell volume (PCV), bilirubin (direct and total), serum proteins, transaminase levels and congenital infection screening (see Chapter 14).

Diaphragmatic hernia (see Chapter 12, page 178)

The suggestive clues include a history of maternal hydramnios (50%), signs of mediastinal shift, a difference in air entry between the two sides of the chest, and a relatively 'empty' abdomen. When this diagnosis is suspected it is especially important to position the infant tilted head-up, and to avoid bag-and-mask resuscitation.

Caesarean delivery of preterm infants

These infants are at considerably increased risk of maladaptation to extrauterine life and to respiratory distress syndrome, compared with infants delivered vaginally. Adaptation to extrauterine life depends on the achievement of adequate alveolar ventilation, followed closely by a greatly increased pulmonary blood flow and other profound changes in the circulation. The key to successful adaptation is the replacement by air of the lung fluid which fills the alveoli prior to delivery. Evacuation of the lung fluid is partially achieved during labour by the surge in fetal catecholamines, by thoracic compression during the second stage of labour and, after birth, by pulmonary lymphatic drainage. The latter requires the 'milking' action of respiration and also a low central venous pressure.

Clearance of lung fluid is often inadequate when a preterm infant is delivered by Caesarean section (particularly when the latter is elective). *Firstly*, the fetus is deprived of the surge in catecholamines. *Secondly*, there is no vaginal squeeze to the thorax during delivery. *Thirdly*, respiratory movements may be absent or weak because of such factors as maternal anaesthesia, compliant rib cage, increased airway resistance etc. *Fourthly*, cord clamping at delivery of vigorously pulsating umbilical vessels cuts off the low-resistance placental circulation and causes a sharp rise in systemic blood pressure. In the presence of a continuing high pulmonary vascular resistance, both sides of the heart may exhibit transitory 'failure' with raised venous pressures in the pulmonary as well as the central veins. A raised pulmonary venous pressure may lead to pulmonary oedema and the passage of plasma proteins into the lungs, causing hyaline membrane formation and inactivating or displacing surfactant. Meanwhile, a raised central venous pressure (CVP) will impede lymphatic drainage. Resuscitation in the head-down position will raise the CVP even more and may increase the risk of periventricular haemorrhage. The following technique was devised to counteract the above problems.

Paediatric management of the preterm Caesarean section (Dunn, 1973)

(a) Two members of the paediatric staff attend the delivery; one of them 'scrubs up', and with sterile mucus catheter and warmed towel, stands by the obstetrician.

(b) The obstetrician delivers the baby's head and then pauses while the anaesthetist injects an oxytocic agent into the mother's arm vein. The uterus normally contracts in response to this injection after a delay of 50 sec.

(c) 30 sec after the injection the obstetrician completes the delivery of the baby who is wrapped in the warmed towel and laid flat on the mother's legs. The paediatrician gently clears the nose and mouth.

(d) As the uterus starts to contract the obstetrician eases the placenta out of the incision with minimum handling or pulling on the umbilical cord. (If the placenta is damaged, the cord is then clamped and divided as near the placenta as possible.)

(e) The placenta is placed inside the warmed towel *alongside* the baby and, with intact umbilical circulation, the whole feto-placental unit is transferred to the resuscitation platform where the baby is placed on a head-up slope.

(f) The status of the infant is then assessed. The interval since delivery is usually 1–2 min.

(g) If the infant is breathing vigorously, is pink, shows no evidence of inspiratory retraction, has good alveolar air entry, and cord pulsation has ceased at the umbilicus, then the cord may be clamped and divided and the infant transferred to the SCBU or transitional ward.

(h) If the above conditions are not satisfied, the infant is intubated and IPPV instituted and maintained usually for at least 10–20 min. Most infants of gestation <30 weeks require intubation and IPPV. It is important to use the minimum positive pressure sufficient to bring about a steady improvement. Fluid is incompressible and use of high pressure is liable to cause alveolar rupture. A main purpose of the IPPV is to milk alveolar fluid steadily through the lymphatics to the central venous pool.

(i) Meanwhile, the placenta lies alongside the infant (unless the latter is thought to be hypovolaemic, in which case the placenta may be raised above the baby). Note that any rise in central venous pressure may be discharged backwards down the umbilical vein (which has no valves) to the placenta.

(j) When the conditions mentioned in (g) above have been achieved and the cord is white and non-pulsatile, it may be clamped and divided in the usual way.

Aftercare in the delivery room

After resuscitation

Following successful resuscitation and the establishment of respiration, the infant should be examined for other problems, then wrapped in a warm towel and handed without delay to the mother and father with an explanation for the need for resuscitation. If the infant is very small or sick, or has suffered from 'white asphyxia', he or she should be shown to and held briefly by the parents before being placed in the transport incubator and transferred to the special care baby unit (see Chapter 17 and 5).

The placenta

(a) This should be weighed and examined carefully for abnormalities such as vasa praevia, clots, infarction, amnion nodosum, single umbilical artery etc. In multiple births it is particularly important to examine the membranes for zygosity and the placental vessels for evidence of twin-to-twin transfusion. A placenta weighing >25% infants' birthweight is suggestive of congenital nephrotic syndrome (see page 243).

(b) It is sensible practice to conserve a 5–10 ml sample of clotted blood from each placenta in a labelled test tube. This should be kept for five days in the labour suite fridge in case it is required as a source for investigation. If the mother is rhesus negative or has blood group iso-immunization, blood should be sent to the laboratory at once for grouping, Coomb's test, and for haemoglobin and serum bilirubin estimations.

The records

The details of resuscitation and examination should be recorded at once in the infant's notes together, when necessary, with instructions for further investigation and care in the nursery or SCBU. In particular watch for signs of hypoglycaemia, hypothermia and cerebral dysfunction in the postasphyxiated infant (see Chapter 10). Order *immediate* antibiotic therapy if infection is suspected. *All infants* should receive vitamin K_1, 0.5–1.0 mg, i.m. or orally soon after birth.

Transfer to the SCBU/NICU (see Chapter 5)

All infants who still require respiratory support and are being transferred to the SCBU/NICU should be accompanied by a doctor or nurse. Never transfer an intubated infant without IPPV or continuous positive airway pressure (CPAP) (4–5 cm H_2O). Every precaution should be taken to prevent hypothermia or hypoxaemia during transport (see Chapter 7).

The parents

If it is necessary to transfer the baby to SCBU/NICU, the parents should be given a full explanation and arrangements made for them to visit. When it is not possible for the mother to visit, a Polaroid photograph of her baby should be made available (see Chapter 20).

Bibliography

Bersin, R. M. and Arieff, A. I. (1987). Recent advances in the therapy of lactic acidosis. *Intensive Care World*, **4**, 128–33.

Cooke, R. W. I. (1983). *A Guide to Resuscitation of the Newborn Infant*. Basingstoke: Vickers Medical.

Dunn, P. M. (1973). Caesarean section and the prevention of respiratory distress syndrome of the newborn. In: *Perinatal Medicine*, pp. 138–45. (3rd European Congress of Perinatal Medicine, Lausanne, 1972). Eds J. Bossart, J. M. Cruz, A. Huber, L. S. Prod'hom and J. Sistek. Bern: Hans Huber.

Dunn, P. M. (1989). Perinatal factors influencing adaptation to extrauterine life. In: *Advances in Gynaecology and Obstetrics*, Chapter 5, *Pregnancy and Labour*. Ed. P. Belfort, J. A. Pinotti, and T. K. A. B. Eskes. **5**, pp. 119–23, Carnforth, Lancs: Parthenon Press.

Freeman, J. M. and Nelson, K. B. (1988). Intrapartum asphyxia and cerebral palsy. *Pediatrics*, **82**, 240–9.

Klaus, M. H. and Fanaroff, A. A. (1987). *Care of the High-Risk Neonate*, 3rd edn. Philadelphia: W. B. Saunders.

Milner, A. D. and Vyas, H. (1982). Lung expansion at birth. *J. Pediatr.*, **101**, 879–86.

Olver, R. E. (1981). Of labour and the lungs. *Arch. Dis. Child.*, **56**, 659–62.

Ritter, J. M., Doktor, H. S. and Benjamin, N. (1990). Paradoxical effect of bicarbonate on cytoplasmic pH. *Lancet*, **i**, 1243–6.

Strang, L. B. (1977). *Neonatal Respiration: Physiological and Clinical Studies*. Oxford: Blackwell Scientific.

Sykes, G. S., Molley, P. M., Johnson, P. *et al.* (1982). Do Apgar scores indicate asphyxia? *Lancet*, **i**, 494–6.

Thibeault, D. W. and Gregory, G. A. (1979). *Neonatal Pulmonary Care*. Menlo Park, Cal.: Addison-Wesley Publ. Co.

3

Birth trauma

Obstetric events predisposing to birth trauma
Injuries to the scalp and skull
Injuries to the face
Brachial plexus injuries
Fracture of the clavicle
Fracture of the cervical spine
Fractures of the long bones of the limbs
Visceral intra-abdominal trauma
Trauma to external genitalia
Generalized bruising

All newborn infants should be examined carefully at birth for evidence of birth injury. *Any findings, even minor ones, should be shown to and discussed with the parents with appropriate explanation and reassurance.*

Obstetric events predisposing to birth trauma

The following obstetric events are particularly likely to be associated with birth trauma to the baby:

Fetomaternal disproportion:
   Dystocia with head, shoulders or abdomen
Malpresentation:
   Breech, brow, face
Instrumental delivery or manual extraction, especially Kielland's forceps
Preterm delivery
Precipitate delivery

In association with fetal distress causing cerebral venous congestion and rapid obstetric delivery

Twins:
   Vaginal delivery of second, larger twin; use of oxytocic agent before delivery of undiagnosed second twin

Caesarean delivery:
   Scalpel incision

The influence of fetal presentation at vaginal delivery on the incidence of certain birth traumas among 4754 infants born in the Birmingham Maternity Hospital, 1960–1961 (Dunn, 1981) is shown below.

Type of birth trauma*	Breech rate per 1000 births (Br)	Vertex rate per 1000 births (Vx)	Ratio of Br/Vx
Cephalhaematoma	2.8	9.9	0.3
'Cerebral' signs	27.9	8.3	3.4
Cerebral trauma death	8.4	1.1	6.0
Facial nerve palsy	2.8	2.8	1.0
Erb's palsy	2.8	0.8	3.5
Fractured bones	14.0	0.5	28.0
Testicular trauma	30.7	0.0	'100+'

* With improved obstetric practice during the last 20 years these incidences would now be much lower. From Dunn, P. M., in *Outcomes of Obstetric Intervention in Britain*. Royal College of Obstetricians and Gynaecologists.

It is particularly important that infants showing evidence of birth trauma should receive vitamin K_1, 1 mg i.m., following delivery.

Injuries to the scalp and skull

Caput succedaneum

The boggy appearance of the 'presenting' scalp quickly subsides. No treatment required.

'Chignon'

This is the oedematous part of the scalp that has been sucked into a vacuum extractor. There may be haemorrhage and necrosis of the skin. Local toilet may be required. Scars may result occasionally.

Subaponeurotic haemorrhage

Very considerable haemorrhage may occur beneath the epicranial aponeurosis with little to show except for a boggy feel to the scalp. The infant may suffer from haemorrhagic shock, anaemia, and later from jaundice. Negro infants and infants delivered by ventouse extraction are particularly at risk. Treatment is as for acute haemorrhage (see page 228).

Lesions due to scalp electrode clips or scalp blood sampling

These small lesions usually require local toilet at the most. Occasionally they may lead to infection and abscess formation. They should not be confused with cutis aplasia (congenital scalp defects) (see page 67).

Cephalhaematoma

These subperiosteal haemorrhages usually occur over one or other of the parietal bones, and less frequently over the occipital bone. They occur in about 1% of infants, especially at and after term. Frequently there is an associated hairline fracture of the outer table of the bone, while the extent of the haemorrhage is limited by the suture lines. The swelling usually becomes obvious and fluctuant on the second day. A hard, calcified rim around the edge gives the false impression of a hole in the skull. Cephalhaematoma may cause anaemia and jaundice especially when multiple. Associated intracranial trauma is rare and no treatment is required for the actual haematoma. Aspiration should never be undertaken.

Depressed fractures of the skull

These are very rare. Surgical advice should be sought.

Intracranial haemorrhage and traumatic brain damage

(See Chapter 10, page 137.)

Injuries to the face

Traumatic cyanosis

Cyanosis, bruising and petechial haemorrhages of the face may follow pressure on the neck from the cervix or umbilical cord during delivery. The pinkness of the rest of the body rules out cyanotic heart disease. No treatment is needed, though jaundice may develop.

Superficial injuries

Fat necrosis over the zygoma and facial paralysis, may be caused by forceps. Subconjunctival haemorrhages and bruising of the face may be associated with face and brow presentations. All resolve rapidly. No specific treatment is needed.

Scalpel incisions

Incisions occurring accidentally during Caesarean delivery may affect any part of the body and may require suturing. When they are on the face, it is wise to obtain the help of a plastic surgeon. A photographic record should be made.

Facial nerve palsy

Some cases are caused by pressure on the nerve during forceps delivery. The paralysis is usually unilateral. When the infant cries, the eye on the affected side remains open and the mouth is drawn to the opposite side. No treatment is required except perhaps the use of artificial tears for the open eye. Differential diagnosis includes intrauterine pressure neuropraxia and congenital defects of the 7th nerve (often bilateral). Recovery is usually complete within days or weeks.

Brachial plexus injuries

The brachial plexus may be injured during lateral flexion of the neck or traction on the arms while trying to deliver the shoulders with vertex presentation or the arms and head during breech delivery. The injuries may be associated with fracture of the clavicle, or with phrenic nerve damage causing unilateral diaphragmatic paralysis, or with damage to the cervical sympathetic nerves leading to Horner's syndrome (myosis, ptosis, and enophthalmos), or more rarely with fracture dislocation of the shoulder.

Injuries to the brachial plexus may be very varied but are usually divided into those affecting the upper plexus (Erb's palsy) and those affecting the lower plexus (Kulmpke's paralysis).

Erb's palsy, involving mainly the C5 and C6 nerve roots, accounts for most cases of brachial plexus injury. The arm is maintained limply alongside the body with the forearm pronated ('waiter's tip' position). There is loss of movement.

In **Klumpke's paralysis**, involving mainly the C8 and T1 nerve roots, the small muscles of the hand and the wrist flexors are affected causing a 'claw hand'. Besides the signs of the lower motor neuron paralysis, there may be loss of sensation and sweating.

X-ray of the spine, shoulder and arm should be undertaken to exclude fracture. Electromyelography and myelogram may be indicated in severe cases. Treatment consists mainly of gentle full-range passive movement of the affected joints several times a day. This may be taught to the parents. Splinting is of little value and may delay recovery. Recovery occurs spontaneously in two-thirds of cases, usually commencing within six weeks. Improvement may continue for 12 or more months.

Neuropraxia of facial, radial, sciatic and obturator nerves, sterno-mastoid torticollis and other deformities due to intrauterine pressure are mentioned in Chapter 6.

Fracture of the clavicle

This is usually associated with shoulder dystocia or with delivery of the arms in breech presentation. It may be detected by palpation of the break and crepitus and by pseudoparalysis of the arm on that side, and should be distinguished from pseudoarthrosis of the clavicle in which there is no pain, tenderness or callus formation. Confirm the diagnosis by X-ray. Minimal treatment is required except for gentle handling. A gauze pad in the axilla and a crepe figure-of-eight bandage may relieve discomfort during the two to three weeks required for the fracture to unite.

Fracture of the cervical spine

This rare injury is usually associated with breech extraction. Typically there is a fracture dislocation in the C6–8 region with damage to the cord. Diaphragmatic breathing is maintained through the phrenic nerves. There is a flaccid quadriplegia and urinary retention. The prognosis is gloomy.

Fractures of the long bones of the limbs

These are usually of the mid-shaft and sustained during manipulation of the arms or legs in breech delivery; twisting manipulations may cause avulsion of the lower epiphyses of either femur or tibia. Diagnosis is made because of angulation or shortening, through palpation or because of pseudoparalysis. Diagnosis should be confirmed by X-ray. Treatment consists of light splinting in good alignment. When the infant has been lying *in utero* as a breech presentation with extended legs, then alignment of the femur may be best achieved by bandaging legs over abdomen; but do not obstruct respiration. Union is usually achieved within three weeks or so. The bones of the newborn exhibit a great capacity for remodelling.

Visceral intra-abdominal trauma

Birth trauma to the liver, the spleen, or to some other abdominal organ is rare. Typically, it is associated with breech extraction or with abdominal dystocia due to hepatosplenomegaly, but may occur spontaneously in infants of mothers on anticonvulsants (see Chapter 1, page 4). The signs of haemorrhagic shock may be delayed for two to three days until a subcapsular haematoma ruptures. A primary or secondary coagulopathy may be present. Always give vitamin K_1, 1 mg i.m. Manage as for acute haemorrhage (see page 228). Surgery may be indicated.

Trauma to external genitalia
Testicular birth trauma

Significant scrotal bruising and testicular enlargement may be found in approximately 10% of male infants delivered by the breech. Typically the infant is a large singleton born at or after term. The external genitalia are very tender and severe cases with haemorrhagic infarction may lead to testicular hypoplasia and sterility. It is inadvisable to discuss this remote possibility with the parents. Discrete examination of the testicles at follow-up is recommended. At birth no treatment is required except perhaps analgesia in severe cases and minimal handling.

Differential diagnosis

Congenital torsion of the testicle. Usually delivery by the vertex; minimal scrotal bruising; unilateral stony hard testicular enlargement; typically painless unless of recent origin, in which case urgent surgery is indicated.

Vulval haematoma

Female breech-born infants may suffer bruising and haematoma of the vulva. Spontaneous recovery may be expected within a few days.

Generalized bruising

This is particularly likely to occur following breech delivery of the very low birthweight infant. There is also often extensive associated haemorrhage into the muscles. Hypovolaemic shock, oliguria, anaemia and jaundice are complications to be anticipated.

Bibliography

Avery, G. B. (1981). *Neonatology: Pathophysiology and Management of the Newborn*, 2nd edn. Philadelphia: J. B. Lippincott.

Avery, M. E. and Taeusch, W. (1984). *Diseases of the Newborn*, 5th edn. Philadelphia: W. B. Saunders.

Dunn, P. M. (1981). Breech delivery: a paediatric view. In: *Outcomes of Obstetric Intervention in Britain*, pp. 63–79. Eds R. W. Beard and D. B. Paintin. (Proceeding of the RCOG Scientific Meeting). London: Royal College of Obstetricians and Gynaecologists.

Sharrad, W. J. W. (1979). *Paediatric Orthopaedics and Fractures*, 2nd edn. Oxford: Blackwell Scientific.

4

Routine care of the newborn infant

In the delivery room
On the postnatal ward
Routine nursing care

In the delivery room (see Chapter 2)

Ensure delivery rooms are warm (23–28° C) and free of draughts.
Carefully dry baby after delivery and wipe secretions etc., from face, then wrap in warmed towel or blanket and hand him/her to the mother, with appropriate reassurance.
Most babies should be put to the breast within a few minutes of delivery.
Mother's body heat will keep the baby warm if he/she is directly against the mother's skin.
Avoid cold stress; use a radiant warmer if the baby is exposed.
Give vitamin K_1, 1 mg orally, to all infants (0.5 mg i.m. to high-risk infants).

On the postnatal ward

Routine examination

A rapid examination of all infants in the delivery room is important but the infant must not be cold stressed or unnecessarily separated from his/her parents.

All babies must be fully examined by a doctor within 24 hours of birth (Tables 4.1 and 4.2) preferably in the presence of the mother, so that her questions can be answered and any problems discussed.

Table 4.1 Routine first-day assessment of the newborn infant: history

Mother
Family history
Previous medical conditions (e.g. diabetes, thyrotoxicosis, drug abuse)
Known social problems
Past obstetric history (e.g. preterm delivery, perinatal deaths)
This pregnancy
  Dates (certain?)
  Complications (e.g. infections, blood pressure, proteinuria)
Blood group (and known antibody status)
Labour and delivery
  Onset (spontaneous/induced)
  Presentation
  Fetal distress (type ?)
  Type of delivery
  Membrane rupture-to-delivery interval
  Maternal pyrexia ?
  Liquor offensive ?

Baby
Birthweight
Apgar score at 1 and 5 min
Resuscitation
Temperature
Feeding – breast or bottle – any problems?
Passed stools/urine yet?
Dextrostix (if birth asphyxia, low birthweight, cold or tachypnoeic or if
  >4 kg)
Any problems noted already?

Routine nursing care (see Chapter 21)

Feeding

Advice on breast feeding should start in the antenatal clinic.

Mothers may need help and advice on the techniques of feeding and breast care (see Chapter 11, page 152).

The more frequently a baby is put to the breast the sooner will feeding be established and the lower will be the risk of sore nipples (most babies will feed 8–12 times a day in the first 48 hours).

Test weighing is inaccurate and likely to increase maternal anxiety (see Chapter 11, page 155).

If the baby is passing urine once every 3–4 hours, fluid intake is adequate. If necessary assess hydration by checking urine specific gravity (if <1.010, hydration is likely to be adequate).

Bottle feeding (see Chapter 11, page 158).

Table 4.2   Routine first-day assessment of the newborn infant: examination

Age at time of examination	Cardiovascular system (heart sounds, murmurs, femoral pulses, liver size)
Weight, length and head circumference (and plot on centile chart)	Abdomen (liver, spleen, kidney, umbilicus–number of vessels)
Gestation (by dates and by examination) (see page 272)	Genitalia
Posture	Anus (site, tone)
Colour (cyanosis, pallor, plethora, jaundice)	Spine (dimple, hairy patches, lipoma, scoliosis)
Skin (dry, peeling, vernix, any naevi?)	Arms and hands (including palmar creases)
Nutrition (subcutaneous tissue, well or poorly nourished)	Hips (full movements, not dislocatable or dislocated) (see Chapter 6, page 75)
Oedema (and site)	Legs and feet
Skull (moulding, cephalhaematoma, sutures, fontanelle)	Behaviour and activity (including response to handling)
Facies (anomalies, asymmetry)	Muscle tone
Ears (size, shape, low-set)	Movements (asymmetry)
Eyes (and epicanthic folds)	Cry
Nose/nasal airway	Reflexes (suck, grasp, Gallant, step, place, Moro. NB Plantar reflex is down-going in normal infant)
Mouth and palate (NB feel for posterior palatal spine)	
Neck (and clavicles, sternomastoid contracture)	*Assessment*
Chest (shape, respiratory pattern and effort, auscultation)	? Normal healthy infant
	? Appropriate size for gestation
	Discuss any problems with the mother and reassure her if all is well.

Prevention of infection (see Chapter 21)

Careful cleaning of equipment and scrupulous hand washing by *all* staff is essential. There is no evidence that the use of gowns or masks reduces infection risk and no evidence that visiting by healthy adults or other children increases it.

Weighing

Alternate day weighing is sufficient for most normal infants. Normal infants may lose up to 10% of birthweight in the first week and not regain birthweight until 10–14 days.

Temperature

Avoid cold stress (see Chapter 5). Axillary temperature should be routinely checked on admission to the postnatal ward and again at

6–12 and 18–24 hours. Always use a low-reading thermometer, and warm the baby if axillary temperature is <36°C, or if the extremities feel cold.

NB (a) Temperature instability may be a very important sign of sepsis.
   (b) Check capillary blood sugar (e.g. Dextrostix, BM stix) in all cold infants.

Passage of urine and meconium

Approximately 25% of infants pass urine in the delivery room and this may not be noted. Infants who have not passed urine by 24 hours old should be examined for palpable bladder or kidneys.

Ninety-nine per cent of infants pass urine by 48 hours

Failure to do so may be due to obstruction to urine flow (enlarged bladder: e.g. meatal obstruction, urethral valves, neurogenic bladder, ureterocele) or to decreased urine production (bladder not enlarged: e.g. hypovolaemia, dehydration, renal agenesis, acute tubular necrosis, renal venous thrombosis, acute cortical necrosis, inappropriate antidiuretic hormone (ADH) secretion) (see Chapter 16).

Eighty per cent of infants pass meconium in the first 24 hours and 99% by 48 hours

Low birthweight infants, especially if they are sick and not being fed, may have delayed passage of meconium. Infants who have not passed meconium by 48 hours should be examined for evidence of bowel obstruction (vomiting, abdominal distension) or anorectal abnormalities (e.g. imperforate anus, ectopic anus). An erect X-ray of the abdomen may show evidence of bowel obstruction (Chapter 12). Gentle digital examination of the rectum may provoke passage of meconium, or a plug of white mucus ('meconium plug') followed by meconium.

Infants with delayed passage of meconium (>48 hours) and a meconium plug should be investigated for possible cystic fibrosis (serum immunoreactive trypsin level, stool tryptic activity and/or sweat test). Also consider the possibility of Hirschsprung's disease (see Chapter 12).

Baths

Early bathing of babies (i.e. <48 hours of age) is a major cold stress and may increase infection risk. Babies should not be routinely bathed in hospital. The main value of bathing a normal infant in hospital is to teach the mother how to do it.

Discharge examination

This is as for the first-day examination (see Table 4.2) but in addition the following specific points must be checked:

(1) *Feeding and weight* Ensure feeding is established and there has not been excessive weight loss.
(2) *Jaundice* Significant jaundice must be investigated (Chapter 17). Babies should not go home until the bilirubin level is stable or falling.
(3) *Arrangements for follow-up* Ensure the parents know who to contact if any problems develop and whether any follow-up is needed. In addition the parents must be reassured and their questions answered.
(4) *Advice* should be given to the parents on keeping the baby warm, on the use of vitamins, and on the need for immunization.
(5) Complete the discharge record (copies to obstetric and neonatal records and to the primary health-care team).

Bibliography

McMilan, J. A., Stockman, J. A. and Oski, F. A. (Eds) (1977, 1979, 1982). *The Whole Pediatrician Catalog*, Volumes 1, 2 and 3. London: W. B. Saunders.
Vulliamy, D. G., Johnston P. (1987). *The Newborn Child*, 6th edn. Edinburgh: Churchill Livingstone.

5

Care of the high-risk infant

Definition of 'special' and 'intensive' care of the newborn
Thermal care
Feeding
Monitoring
Minimal handling
Problems of the preterm infant
The small-for-gestational-age (SGA) infant
The large-for-gestational-age infant

Definition of 'special' and 'intensive' care of the newborn

Both special and intensive care units should include adequate facilities for resuscitation and delivery room care of normal and high-risk infants. **Intensive care** includes assisted ventilation, intravenous feeding, and the management of babies with severe cardio-respiratory, metabolic or infectious illnesses, plus postoperative care. The nurse-to-patient ratio should be 5 to 1 (BPA/RCOG, 1984). **Special care** includes the care of infants with less severe or more transient problems and the care of infants no longer needing intensive care. The nurse-to-patient ratio should be 1.5 to 1 (BPA/RCOG, 1984). Most units in the UK have a mixture of neonatal intensive care- and special care-designated cots. Most infants requiring special care can be satisfactorily cared for with their mothers, on transitional care wards, provided adequate trained nursing staff levels can be maintained (see also Chapter 29). For indications for admission to special care baby units (SCBU) and neonatal intensive care units (NICU) see Table 5.1 and 5.2.

Table 5.1 Indications for admission to SCBU (or transitional care ward) for close observation. (NB   see Table 5.2 for babies needing intensive care.)

(A)	**All infants with the following problems**
	Gestation <36 weeks
	Birthweight <2200 g
	Major malformations
	Respiratory distress
	Tachypnoea (>70/min)
	Grunting any 2 at >1 hour of age or
	Cyanosis at any age if need >30%
	Indrawing oxygen to abolish cyanosis
	Severe birth asphyxia
	Apgar score <3 at 1 min
	<5 at 5 min
	Symptomatic hypoglycaemia (see page 193)
	Symptomatic polycythaemia (see page 234)
	Symptomatic anaemia (see page 234)
	NB Almost all infants who require intubation and IPPV for birth asphyxia should be admitted to SCBU/transitional care ward for observation for 12–24 hours
(B)	**Most of the following infants** (NB All require careful observation/monitoring)
	Infants in whom meconium was found below the cords (see Chapter 2)
	Infants of narcotic-addicted mothers
	Infants born through offensive smelling liquor
	Rh iso-immunization
(C)	**Some of the following infants** (NB Review 2–4 hourly for 24 hours)
	Mother given opiate analgesic and infant needing naloxone to reverse early respiratory depression
	Infants born after prolonged (>24 hours) rupture of membranes or after maternal pyrexia during labour (NB Screen for infection, see Chapter 14)

Thermal care

Thermal care is by far the most important part of the care of the high-risk infant. Even mild cold stress results in significantly reduced survival. The adverse effects of cold stress are listed in Table 5.3. Table 5.4 lists routes of heat loss and ways to reduce them.

Significant cold stress may be present with a normal rectal temperature as this falls only when the normal compensatory mechanisms fail. Cold stress can be minimized by monitoring both core temperature (axillary is preferable to rectal) plus peripheral temperature (e.g. big toe or shin) and maintaining the latter in the range 35–36°C.

The neutral thermal environment is the ambient temperature range which leads to minimum oxygen consumption. It is especially

Table 5.2 Indication for admission to NICU (or transfer to a hospital with NICU facilities)

Gestation <32 weeks
Birthweight <1500 g
Moderate or severe respiratory distress
  Apnoea
  PaO_2 <50 mm Hg in 40% oxygen
  pH < 7.20
  $PaCO_2$ > 60 mm Hg
Complications of respiratory distress
  Shock
  Air leak
    Pneumothorax
    Pneumomediastinum
    Marked interstitial emphysema
Symptomatic meconium aspiration
  Meconium found below cords and infant needs >40% oxygen to abolish
    cyanosis
Congenital heart disease
  Cyanosis   } In the neonatal
  Cardiac failure } period
Major malformations, e.g.
  Diaphragmatic hernia
  Oesophageal atresia/tracheo-oesophageal fistula (TOF)
  Exomphalos/gastroschisis
  Lobar emphysema
Hydrops fetalis or severe Rh iso-immunization
Convulsions
Bleeding problems
Major trauma

Table 5.3 Adverse effects of cold stress

Increased oxygen consumption
Increased energy expenditure
  Hypoxia and acidosis
  Hypoglycaemia
  Increased early weight loss
  Slow or delayed weight gain
Pulmonary hypertension or persistent fetal circulation
Increased risk of sepsis and haemorrhage
Increased capillary permeability
  Hypovolaemia and increased blood viscosity
General impairment of enzyme efficiency
Decreased surfactant production
Neonatal cold injury
Increased mortality

Table 5.4 Heat loss and its prevention in the newborn infant

Type of heat loss	Prevention
Evaporation	Carefully dry babies after delivery or after washing
	Maintain high relative humidity (60–80%) in the nursery
	Humidify incubators for all infants <1500 g or <30 weeks gestation
	Use incubators rather than open cots with radiant overhead heaters
	Wrap very small infants in clingfilm or smear skin with petroleum jelly
Conduction	Warm all bedding, clothes, surfaces etc. before the infant comes into contact with them
	Nurse babies clothed rather than naked
Convection	Keep infants out of draughts
	Close one end of heat shields in incubators (to reduce velocity of air-flow past baby)
	Nurse babies clothed rather than naked
	Avoid the use of cold, unhumidified oxygen or air for resuscitation
Radiation	Use heat shield within the incubator
	Cover the infant's head with a woollen bonnet
	Nurse babies clothed rather than naked
	Maintain nursery temperature 24–25°C
	Do not place incubators close to outside windows

important to minimize oxygen consumption in infants with cardiac or respiratory disease (who may have limited ability to take up oxygen), preterm infants (who may not be able to sustain high respiratory work rates) and infants with nutritional or gastrointestinal problems (i.e. substrate deficiency). Cold stress also results in a reduction of oxygen delivery to vital organs, particularly the brain and heart. Neutral thermal ranges for infants of different birthweights and ages are shown in Fig. 5.1.

Feeding

Small or sick infants urgently need calorie intake to minimize catabolism and maintain growth (especially brain growth). Preterm infants (<34 weeks) are unlikely to achieve safe breast or bottle feeding in the first 2–3 days. If there is no respiratory distress or gastrointestinal problem they should be given orogastric or transpyloric feeds initially. Infants with respiratory or gastrointestinal problems, and all infants <30 weeks gestation should be given only intravenous fluids for the first 48 hours at least.

Monitoring

The type and complexity of monitoring needed depends on the size, gestation and condition of the infant, and the following are intended as guidelines.

Apnoea monitors

Mattress type or abdominal pressure sensor (Graseby). All infants <35 weeks should be on an apnoea monitor (or respiratory monitor) for at least the first week. Set the delay to 20 sec and ensure the monitor is 'triggering' with each breath.

Cardiorespiratory monitors (e.g. ECG and transthoracic impedance pneumograph)

These should be used for all infants with significant respiratory distress, all infants <30 weeks gestation and all acutely ill infants. Heart rate alarm limits are usually set at 90–100 (low alarm) and 160–180 (high alarm).

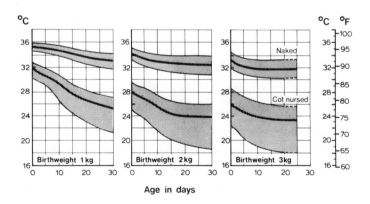

Fig. 5.1 Neutral thermal ranges for infants of different birthweights and ages. (From Hey, 1971, *Recent Advances in Paediatrics*, with permission from Churchill Livingstone)

Temperature

Monitor core temperature (axilla) and peripheral temperature (skin of shin or big toe) continuously in all sick infants.

Blood pressure

Measure 2–6 hourly in all sick infants, using a Doppler device (manual or automatic), or continuously from indwelling arterial cannula. NB Automatic oscillometric devices commonly overestimate blood pressure in small sick babies (e.g. Dynamap, Sentry). CAS (Medical Systems, Inc.) type may be more reliable.

Blood glucose

Capillary blood glucose (Dextrostix; BM stix) should be checked 4 hourly in all high-risk infants, and maintained between 2.5 and 7 mmol/l.

Blood gases

Check arterial blood gases 4–6 hourly in all infants with respiratory distress.

Oxygen saturation monitors (pulse oxymeters) or transcutaneous ($TcPO_2$) monitors?   Because of the shape of the haemoglobin dissociation curve (see Fig. 8.2, page 93) saturation (Sa) monitors may increase the risk of hyperoxia (a rise in SaO_2 from 90 to 98% may represent a rise in PaO_2 of more than 50 mm Hg). $TcPO_2$ is safer in the acute phase of care of small sick infants whilst SaO_2 is of particular value in the older infant, particularly the baby with significant chronic lung disease. SaO_2 may be of value in the rapid assessment of the response to changes in ventilator setting in the very sick infant with persisting hypoxaemia.

Both $TcPO_2$ and SaO_2 should be regularly checked against PO_2 measured on arterial samples of blood (see Chapter 8).

Inspired oxygen concentration

Monitor continuously in all infants receiving extra oxygen; aim to keep PaO_2 in the range 50–70 mm Hg (see Chapter 8).

Blood tests in all sick infants

Urea, Na, K, Cl, Ca
    Check daily
Bilirubin

Check daily for the first 5–6 days at least
Haemoglobin or packed cell volume (PCV)
   Check daily (record whether capillary or venous)
White blood cells (WBC) and platelets
   Check on admission, and then if there is any suspicion of sepsis:

Urine testing

Check urine for blood, protein, sugar (dipstick tests) daily-monitor urine output and measure specific gravity every 6–24 hours.

Weighing

Daily weight is the best measure of fluid balance in a sick infant (but remember minimal handling).

Surveillance for infection

Nose, rectal and umbilical swabs should be sent for culture twice weekly.

Minimal handling (see Chapter 21)

Sick babies do not like being handled. Even minor procedures may cause severe hypoxaemia. Use the monitors and do not disturb the baby to carry out observations (e.g. counting the heart rate) which can be obtained from the monitor. Allow the baby rest periods with *no* handling whenever possible. Keep noxious procedures (vene-punctures, heel pricks, arterial stabs, endotracheal or pharyngeal suctioning, X-rays) to a minimum. Monitor the infant's conditions (ECG, respiration, TcPO$_2$) throughout the procedure, and *stop* if there is hypoxaemia, bradycardia or apnoea. Keep extraneous noise to a minimum. Try to establish diurnal variation in lighting levels.

Problems of the preterm infant
(see Chapter 2 for delivery room management)

Thermal care

See page 53, Tables 5.3 and 5.4 and Fig. 5.1.

Respiratory difficulties

Respiratory distress syndrome (Chapter 8)

Apnoea (Chapter 8)
Aspiration pneumonia (because of immaturity of pharyngeal co-ordination and protective reflexes)
Oxygen toxicity and retinopathy of prematurity (ROP) (Chapters 8 and 23)

Neurological problems

Immaturity of sucking and swallowing
Immaturity of control of respiration leading to apnoea (Chapter 8)
Subependymal and intraventricular haemorrhage (Chapters 8 and 10)

Gastrointestinal problems

Feeding may cause abdominal distension because of poor gut motility; abdominal distension may compromise respiration
Poor absorption of fat (and thus fat-soluble vitamins)
Poor nutritional reserve (fat, glycogen, iron, fat-soluble vitamins) (see Chapter 11)
Risk of necrotizing enterocolitis (see Chapter 11)

Jaundice

Hepatic immaturity leads to increased jaundice; immaturity of blood–brain barrier may increase the risk of kernicterus at lower levels than in term infants (see Chapter 18)

Haemorrhage

Low levels of vitamin K may lead to defective blood clotting (see Chapter 15)
Anaemia (see Chapter 15)

Renal problems

Low glomerular filtration rate (GFR) and poor tubular function lead to inability to excrete large water or solute load, and poor ability to conserve water or sodium (see Chapters 17 and 18)

Metabolic problems

Hypocalcaemia (see Chapter 13)
Hypoglycaemia (see Chapter 13)

Infections

Increased susceptibility to infection (especially group B streptococci, *Escherichia coli, Staphylococcus epidermidis, Pseudomonas aeruginosa, Serratia marcescens*)

Cardiovascular problems

Patent ductus arteriosus (see Chapter 9).

Social problems

Separation of mother and baby (see Chapter 20).

The small-for-gestational-age (SGA) infant

'Symmetric' low weight, length and head size for gestation suggests early onset of intrauterine growth retardation (IUGR), e.g. early intrauterine infection (CMV, toxoplasmosis, rubella), chromosomal abnormality (see Chapter 6), severe placental insufficiency or severe maternal disease (e.g. diabetes, renal disease, hypertension, alcohol) (see Chapter 1).

'Asymmetric' low weight with relative 'sparing' of length and head size (fetal malnutrition), suggests onset of growth retardation in last few weeks of pregnancy, e.g. placental insufficiency, pre-eclampsia, maternal smoking, or less severe maternal disease (e.g. renal disease, hypertension) (see Chapter 1).

Problems of SGA infants

Hypoglycaemia

Hypoglycaemia occurs because of low glycogen stores. Check capillary glucose 4 hourly (see Chapter 13).

Birth asphyxia

Mild intrapartum asphyxia may cause severe effects because of the poor fat and glycogen stores (and thus poor ability to maintain anaerobic metabolism). Meconium aspiration is a particular risk (see Chapter 2).

Thermal care

Mild cold stress may cause or exacerbate hypoglycaemia.

Polycythaemia

Polycythaemia may exacerbate respiratory problems and hypoglycaemia (see Chapter 15).

The large-for-gestational-age infant

Causes

Maternal diabetes (which may not be clinically apparent).
Constitutional large size (often familial).
Beckwith's syndrome.
Hyperinsulism (see Chapter 13)

Problems of the infant of a diabetic mother (IDM)

Good diabetic control during pregnancy reduces the risk of most of the problems of the IDM but has not been shown to reduce the risk of malformations.

Birth injury

Injury may occur because of large size (see Chapter 3)

Hypoglycaemia

This may develop in the first 1–2 hours and persist or recur for 24–48 hours (see Chapter 13).

Respiratory distress syndrome (RDS) (especially after elective Caesarean section)

Surfactant is relatively deficient in phosphatidyl glycerol (PG) and RDS may develop even in the presence of a normal amniotic lecithin: sphingomyelin ratio. To assess the risk of RDS either measure amniotic fluid PG levels or 'surfactant profile' before planning elective delivery.

Jaundice (see Chapter 18)

Hypocalcaemia (see Chapter 13)

Polycythaemia (see Chapter 15)

Immaturity of sucking and swallowing reflexes

This may necessitate orogastric tube feeds (see Chapter 11).

Cardiomyopathy

This leads to congestive cardiac failure ± left ventricular outflow
obstruction
Diagnose by echocardiogram
Treat with propranolol rather than digoxin

Small left colon syndrome

This leads to temporary bowel obstruction (± meconium plug)
possibly due to immaturity of the myenteric plexus
Clinical and radiological features are similar to Hirschsprung's disease (see Chapter 12).
It resolves spontaneously

Congenital malformations

Up to 13% of IDM have congenital malformations, especially neural
tube defects, ventricular septal defects, transposition of the great
vessels, coarctation of the aorta, vertebral anomalies, sacral
agenesis, anorectal anomalies

Renal vein thrombosis

This may lead to transient or permanent renal impairment with
haematuria (microscopic or macroscopic) (see Chapter 16)

Management of the IDM

Blood sugar monitoring

Check capillary glucose within the first hour, then 2–4 hourly for
24–48 hours or until blood sugar is consistently >4 mmol/l. (See
Chapter 13 for management of hypoglycaemia.)

Early feeding

If there is no respiratory distress, start feeds by 2–3 hours of age. If
tachypnoea (>60 breaths/min) precludes feeding, commence i.v.
glucose 10% at a rate of 60–80 ml/kg/day initially (see Chapter 13).

Other problems

For example, respiratory distress, polycythaemia, jaundice; these should be managed as for any other infant.

Bibliography

British Paediatric Association/British Association of Perinatal Medicine (1985). Categories of babies requiring neonatal care. *Arch. Dis. Child.*, **60**, 599–600.

Cowett, R. M. and Schwartz, R. (1982). The infant of the diabetic mother. *Pediat. Clin. N. Amer.*, **29**, 1213–32.

Goodwin, J. W., Godden, J. O. and Chance, G. W. (Eds) (1976). *Perinatal Medicine*. Toronto: Longman.

Hey, E. N. (1971). The care of babies in incubators. In: *Recent Advances in Paediatrics*. Ed. D. Gairdner and D. Hull. Edinburgh: Churchill Livingstone.

Klaus, M. H. and Fanaroff, A.A. (Eds) (1987). *Care of the High-Risk Neonate*, 3rd edn. London: W. B. Saunders.

Roberton, N. R. C. (1986). *A Manual of Neonatal Intensive Care*, 2nd edn. London: Edward Arnold.

Swyer, P. R. (1975). *The Intensive Care of the Newly Born*. Basel: S. Karger.

Vidyassagar, D. (Ed.) (1986). The tiny baby. *Clin. Perinatol.*, **13**, 233–490.

Whitelaw, A., Cooke, R. W. I. (eds) (1988). The very immature infant. *British Medical Bulletin*, **44**, 4. Edinburgh: Churchill. Livingstone.

6

Congenital abnormalities

Introduction
Malformations
Deformations

Introduction

Definitions

Birth defect

Some imperfection, impairment or disorder of the body, intellect, or personality present or arising at birth.

Congenital anomaly

A morphological defect present at birth (and included in the chapter on congenital anomalies in the *International Classification of Disease*, ICD-9, 1979).

Congenital malformation

A primary error in morphogenesis arising during the embryonic period of prenatal life.

Congenital deformation

An alteration in the morphology of a previously normally formed part of the body arising during the fetal period.

Incidence

This varies between different geographical areas and populations but, on average, approximately 5% of infants are found to have a congenital anomaly at birth, in the proportion three malformed infants to two with deformation.

Examination

Because of the high incidence of anomalies all infants should be examined carefully using the usual methods of inspection, palpation, percussion, auscultation and manipulation (e.g. the hips). Clinical examination may be supplemented when appropriate by trans-illumination, ultrasound, radiological examination, chromosome culture techniques, and other haematological and biochemical investigations.

Malformations

Certain history factors are associated with an increased likelihood of congenital malformation, and may help to elucidate aetiology:

Family history of genetically determined malformation
Previous sibling malformed
High maternal age
Pregnancy exposure to radiation, infection (e.g. rubella) or drugs
Polyhydramnios or oligohydramnios
Intrauterine growth retardation of the fetus
Prenatal suspicion of malformation (e.g. high maternal serum alpha-fetoprotein (AFP) or ultrasound examination)
Malpresentation of the fetus
Multiple pregnancy

After birth suspicion of malformation is increased in the following circumstances:

Small-for-dates infant
Presence of any other anomaly including:
    Single umbilical artery (present in 1% of all babies; ⅕ babies have associated anomalies)
    Single palmar crease (⅕ have associated anomaly)
    Unusual facies.

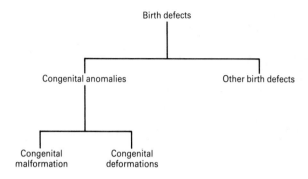

Deformations

The great majority of congenital deformations affect the musculoskeletal system and are referred to as 'congenital postural deformities' (see Fig. 6.1). Their incidence is increased by the following factors:

First pregnancies   Maternal hypertension
Maternal uterine anomaly   Oligohydramnios
Breech presentation   Intrauterine growth retardation
Multiple pregnancy

If one deformity is present, then a most careful search should be made for others, as multiple deformities are present in a third of cases.

Deformations may also occur secondary to certain malformations, especially those that cause oligohydramnios (such as those involving the urinary tract), or those that involve the neuromuscular system (e.g. myotonia dystrophia or spina bifida).

Some of the characteristics of malformations and deformations are contrasted in Table 6.1.

Photographic record

It is most important that all congenital anomalies are well documented. All of any significance that are visible should be photographed. This is particularly important in cases where therapy will alter appearance (as in cleft lip or talipes), or when the infant is likely to die. Apart from the medical and legal reasons for having a photographic record, parents often wish to have a photograph to

Table 6.1 Some contrasting characteristics of congenital malformations and congenital postural deformities

	Malformation		*Deformation (postural)*
Incidence before 20th week	Approximately	5.0%	0.1%
Incidence after 28th week		3.7%	2.0%
Perinatal mortality	41/1000		6/1000
Structural changes	Usual		Rare
Spontaneous correction	Very rare		Usual
Correction by posture	Not possible		Usually possible

keep themselves, even when the child may appear most unattractive to others.

Malformations

Congenital anomalies of the skin (see also Chapter 22)

Haemangiomata

Naevus flammeus ('stork mark')   Fine non-raised capillary naevus, usually in midline (upper lip, forehead–upper nose, nape of neck) that tends to fade in the early months of life. No treatment is required.

Port wine stain   Darker capillary naevus that persists and may be cosmetically disfiguring, especially on the face. When the naevus is over the distribution of the ophthalmic division of the trigeminal nerve, there may be an associated intracranial haemangioma which may give rise to cerebral complications (Sturge–Weber syndrome).

Cavernous haemangioma   Raised naevus that may extend into the subcutaneous tissues. They may be present at birth or appear as small bright red spots after 1–2 weeks ('strawberry naevi'). They often enlarge for weeks or months and then regress spontaneously. Usually they disappear within a few years. No treatment is required unless very large, and associated with thrombocytopenia (see Chapter 15, page 225) or on the face leading to complications such as occlusion of an eye. In such cases a short course of high-dose prednisolone may be effective in shrinking the lesion.

Pigmented naevus

Small pigmented congenital naevi require no treatment. Large hairy 'bathing trunk' or 'forequarter' naevi have a risk of later malignancy and may require plastic surgery.

Epidermal naevus

A velvety or warty lesion, pink or yellowish brown in colour, which may be localized or extensive. Whorled and linear patterns occur. When widespread there can be associated skeletal and CNS abnormalities.

Sebaceous naevus

Pinkish yellow or orange plaques, usually on the scalp or hair margin. They may evolve into basal cell carcinoma later in life, so should be removed during childhood.

Aplasia cutis

A localized absence of skin, most commonly on the scalp, presenting as a glistening red area. Most heal spontaneously leaving a bald patch. Injury from a fetal scalp electrode and epidermolysis bullosa may need to be excluded. Also seen in trisomy 13.

Cystic hygroma

These cystic lymphangiomas are usually located in the neck (where they may cause respiratory embarrassment) or axilla. They transilluminate well and may grow slowly or rapidly. Treatment is usually surgical.

Dermal sinuses

These may be found most commonly in the sacral area (pilonidal sinus), on the side of the front of the neck (branchial sinus), or in front of the ear (pre-auricular sinus). The main complication is infection. Treatment is by surgical excision. (NB Sacral sinuses may rarely communicate with the spinal canal.)

Anomalies of the face

Craniostenosis

Premature closure of one or more of the cranial sutures may give rise to a variety of cranial and facial deformities, since growth is arrested in a direction perpendicular to the affected suture. The incidence is about 1 in 5000. Associated anomalies may occur giving rise to a variety of syndromes that may be genetically determined (e.g. Crouzon, Apert, Carpenter). The diagnosis may be confirmed radiologically. If unilateral or involving only one suture, no treatment is usually necessary, but surgery may be required to prevent pressure effects on the brain or cranial nerves.

Choanal atresia

This is due to a bony or membranous obstruction between the nasal cavity and the nasopharynx. It may be unilateral or bilateral. As most newborn infants are preferential nose breathers in the early weeks of life, the clinical presentation is that of airway obstruction and cyanosis that is relieved by crying or opening of the mouth. The diagnosis is confirmed by failing to pass a nasal catheter, or by X-ray. Initial treatment consists of inserting an oral airway. This is followed by early surgical correction. The incidence is about 1 in 10 000.

Anomalies of the ears

Ensure the patency of the auditory meatus. If this is absent, tomographic studies of the middle and inner ear should be undertaken, with auditory evoked responses. An ENT opinion should be sought. Accessory auricles require surgical removal.

Anomalies of the eyes (Chapter 23)

If microphthalmia, coloboma, glaucoma, corneal opacities, cataract or strabismus are present, it is essential to examine the retina. Aetiology includes chromosomal and genetic factors, prenatal infection (Chapter 14) and inborn errors of metabolism (Chapter 13). Seek an ophthalmic opinion.

Macroglossia

Congenital macroglossia may occur in association with Down's syndrome, hypothyroidism, or as part of the Beckwith–Widemann syndrome (which typically includes associated omphalocele, gigantism and hypoglycaemia). It may also be due to haemangiomatous or lymphangiomatous infiltration or simply due to muscle fibre hypertrophy. The size of the tongue may interfere with feeding and require surgical recession for this or for cosmetic reasons.

Tongue tie

This is caused by a congenitally short frenulum extending to the tip of the tongue, binding it to the floor of the mouth, and interfering with normal sustained sucking (and later speech). The tongue presents a V-shaped confirmation. The incidence is about 1 in 1000. Surgical treatment is occasionally necessary (see page 155).

Ranula

This is a mucus gland retention cyst under the tongue. It has a bluish appearance. Often it will rupture and disappear spontaneously. Surgical resection may rarely be necessary. The incidence is about 1 in 5000.

Congenital teeth

Teeth, usually lower incisors, may be present at birth. The incidence is 1 in 2000. If they are supernumerary or very loose, they should be removed to avoid possible inhalation.

Cleft lip and cleft palate

Cleft lip may be unilateral or bilateral, occur on its own or, more usually, in association with cleft palate. The incidence is approximately 1 in 700 births. Other malformations may be present in 1 in 7 cases. There may be a family history in which case the chance of recurrence may be increased to about 1 in 20. Because the appearance may be very unattractive it is important to show the parents 'before' and 'after' photographs of similar babies who have undergone repair. Early management should include oral surgical/orthodontic collaboration. The malformation should be photographed and 'dental' impressions made. A plate may be fitted in cases of cleft palate. If breast or bottle feeding is difficult, a long, soft teat with a large hole may be used, or alternatively spoon or tube feeding undertaken. Early complications include middle-ear infections and aspiration pneumonia. Late complications include middle-ear hearing problems, speech difficulty and orthodontic problems. Repair of the lip is usually undertaken by 3 months (commonly in the first 1–2 weeks) and of the palate at 6 months so as to complete surgery before speech develops. Multidisciplinary follow-up, including speech therapy, orthodontic and hearing assessment, needs to be continued throughout childhood (see Chapter 20, page 286 for details of the Cleft Lip and Palate Association, CLAPA).

Pierre Robin syndrome

The combination of retrognathia, glossoptosis and respiratory difficulty, with or without midline posterior cleft palate, is known as the

Pierre Robin syndrome. The incidence is about 1 in 3000. There is evidence to suggest that the retrognathia may be due to acute flexion of the head and chin onto the front of the chest in early fetal life. This leads to backwards and upwards displacement of the tongue which may impede fusion of the lateral palatal arches. The syndrome is not infrequently found in association with other congenital anomalies, especially of the heart and musculo-skeletal system. In general the complications and management are similar to that for cleft palate (see above). The main specific problem is that of respiratory tract obstruction by the tongue. It is essential to ensure a clear airway by nursing the infant prone or by using, if necessary, an oropharyngeal airway or other device. Pulse oxymetry may be valuable (see page 56). Occasionally endotracheal intubation is required. The retrognathia tends to disappear over the first 2–3 years.

Anomalies of the gastrointestinal tract (see Chapter 12)

Anomalies of the CNS (see Chapter 10)

Anomalies of the CVS (see Chapter 9)

Anomalies of the respiratory system (see Chapter 8)

Anomalies associated with chronic fetal infection (see Chapter 14)

Urogenital tract anomalies (see Chapter 16)

Potters syndrome

This syndrome is caused by oligohydramnios because of fetal anuria or oliguria (due to renal agenesis or malformation, or to obstructive uropathy), or may occur after prolonged leakage of amniotic fluid (see below). The incidence is around 1 in 2000 births, and usually involves male infants. The baby has a compressed appearance, with multiple postural deformities affecting all parts of the body, and a typical facies including a squashed nose, pouches under the eyes and low-set abnormal ears flattened against the side of the head. Amnion nodosum may be found on the fetal surface of the placenta. Resuscitation problems and respiratory insufficiency due to pulmonary hypoplasia and secondary pneumothorax are the rule and usually lead to death within hours of birth. Genetic advice varies according to the cause of oligohydramnios.

WARNING   When the syndrome follows premature rupture of the membranes and prolonged leakage of amniotic fluid, the urinary tract is normal and such infants may be potentially viable (see Chapter 1).

Hypospadias (see Chapter 16, page 241)

Ambiguous genitalia (see Chapter 13, page 200)

Epispadias (see Chapter 16, page 241)

Imperforate hymen

This may be readily diagnosed at birth if, on examination, the labia are separated. Hormone-induced secretions cause the hymen to bulge outwards. The condition should be differentiated from the more common mucus-retention cysts. These are rounded and white and usually more laterally placed. They disappear after spontaneous or artificial rupture. Occasionally, an imperforate hymen may lead to congenital hydrometrocolpos, with enormous distension of the uterus by retained secretions. Treatment is surgical.

Cryptorchidism (see Chapter 16, page 241)

Hydrocele

This is not a congenital anomaly but will be discussed briefly here. Usually hydroceles are bilateral, of little significance unless associated with inguinal herniae, and disappear spontaneously over a period of weeks or months. Occasionally they may form part of a more general condition such as hydrops fetalis, or Milroy's oedema. If unilateral, consider associated pathology such as torsion of the testis. If the hydrocele is very large, tense and persistent, a surgical opinion should be sought.

Inguinal hernia (see Chapter 12)

Malformations of the musculoskeletal system

Limb malformations

The limb(s) may be absent ('amelia'), hypoplastic, or show various deficiencies affecting the proximal segment of the limb ('phocomelia'), the distal segment ('hemimelia'), or a lateral segment (e.g. radial hypoplasia). The later may be associated with thrombocytopenia. Management usually includes orthopaedic or plastic surgery and may require the fitting of prostheses. Photographic and radiological records should be made. (NB See Chapter 20, pages 289–90 for parents' support groups: 'Reach' and 'Steps'.)

Malformation of the digits

Extra digits (polydactyly) are especially common among Negro babies (dominant inheritance). Usually a tiny finger is attached to the ulnar side of the hand by a fine pedicle. It may be removed either surgically or by using a silk ligature. Fused digits (syndactyly) may require plastic surgery and may be associated with other malformations (e.g. Apert's syndrome: coronal synostosis and syndactyly).

Arthrogryposis multiplex congenita

This condition of multiple contractures of the joints may be due to primary disease of the neuromuscular system or to severe prolonged prenatal constraint or paralysis of the fetus. In the former case there is usually a history of polyhydramnios and the prognosis is poor. When the cause is oligohydramnios due to premature rupture of the membranes or to other non-renal causes, steady improvement may occur. Management usually involves orthopaedic surgery and physiotherapy. The incidence is about 1 in 5000.

Small stature or dwarfism

This may be 'constitutional'. The infant is normally formed but of small size and grows more slowly than normal. Some cases are associated with severe, prolonged intrauterine growth retardation. A second group is made up of the *primordial* dwarfs of which there are a great variety including the Russel-Silver, Cornelia de Lange, Seckel's bird-head dwarf etc. There is no especial shortening of the limbs. The third group consists of the *chondrodystrophic* dwarfs which have disproportionately short limbs. The most common subgroups are achondroplasia, thanatophoric dwarfism and osteogrenesis imperfecta. Late pregnancy in this group is often complicated by polyhydramnios. For further details concerning the later two groups, consult Jones (1988).

Chromosomal syndromes

Perhaps 1 in 300 liveborn infants has a chromosomal anomaly. Only four of the most common syndromes will be considered here. (See Chapter 24 on Clinical Genetics).

Trisomy 21 (Down's syndrome or Mongolism)

The incidence rises from 1 in 1500 among young mothers to 1 in 110 at 40 years at age. The overall incidence is 1 in 650.

Features include small-for-dates, characteristic facies with upward slanting eyes, Brushfield's spots, small ears, protruding tongue, flat occiput, open 3rd fontanelle, general hypotonia, stubby hands with short incurving 5th finger, single palmar creases, distal palmar triradius, gap between 1st and 2nd toes, congenital heart disease (50%) and duodenal atresia (10%). Mental development is delayed. The infants are prone to infection. Survival depends on associated malformations.

Ninety-five per cent are due to non-dysjunction (low recurrence) and 5% to translocation (high recurrence). Clinical diagnosis should be confirmed with urgent chromosome studies. Management of parents (breaking news and support) demands great skill and sensitivity. Families need continued support (see Chapter 20, page *282* for details of the Down's Syndrome Association).

Trisomy 18 (Edward's syndrome)

The *incidence* is 1 in 8000.

Features include small-for-dates, prominent occiput, narrow bifrontal diameter, microcephaly, metopic suture, low-set malformed auricles, short palpebral fissures, small mouth, narrow palatal arch, micrognathia, clenched hands with inner fingers overlapped by outer ones, short hallux, rocker-bottom feet, hypertonia, congenital heart disease, cryptorchidism, renal and many other malformations, single umbilical artery and mental retardation. Almost all die soon after birth.

Trisomy 13–15 (Patau's syndrome)

The *incidence* is 1 in 14000

Features include small-for-dates, large 'onion' nose, cleft lip/palate, microphthalmia, colobomata, abnormal ears, capillary haemangiomata, scalp skin defects, microcephaly, polydactyly, cryptorchidism, single umbilical artery, congenital heart disease and severe mental retardation. Almost all die in the neonatal period.

XO syndrome (Turner's syndrome)

The *incidence* is 1 in 2500 girls.

Features include small-for-dates, 'shield-like' chest, webbed-neck, cubitus valgus, lymphoedema of feet and coarctation of the aorta. Survival is normal except when there are severe associated anomalies. Intelligence is normal.

Table 6.2   Musculoskeletal deformations of mechanical origin present at birth

Site	Deformation
Skull	Dolichocephaly; plagiocephaly; depressions in skull
Face	Potter's facies; nasal and oral deformities; mandibular asymmetry; retrognathia; mid-line cleft palate; facial nerve neurapraxia
Neck	Sternomastoid contracture, 'tumour' and torticollis
Upper limbs	Dislocation of the shoulder; club-hand; compressed arm and hand (in Potter's syndrome); radial nerve neurapraxia
Body	Pigeon chest; pectus excavatum; postural scoliosis
Lower limbs	Dislocation of the hips; bowing of the long bones; genu recurvatum; various deformities of the feet including talipes equinovarus, calcaneovalgus, and metatarsus varus; sciatic and obturator nerve neurapraxias
Whole body	Arthrogryposis multiplex congenita, general compression (as in Potter's syndrome)

Note: Not all cases of some of the conditions noted here are due to mechanical factors (e.g. cleft palate and arthrogryposis).

Deformations

The various congenital postural deformities are listed in Table 6.2. Only a few of the main ones will be considered here. Their importance stems from the fact that they are common and, with early treatment, are usually easily correctable, because growth is proceeding rapidly and the tissues are still relatively plastic.

Congenital sternomastoid torticollis

This occurs in approximately 1 in 300 births. The condition is unilateral. Often there is associated plagiocephaly and invariably the jaw is tilted away from the affected side. Contracture of the sternomastoid is present at birth and may be demonstrated by turning the chin towards the shoulder on the affected side. Normally the head may be rotated so that the chin points over the back of the shoulder. When significant contracture is present the chin will not turn as far as the front of the shoulder. As granulation forms in the damaged muscle, a tumour develops. This is usually first palpable at about 2 weeks of age. As stretching of the damaged muscle is painful and may cause further haemorrhage, treatment, consisting of passive gentle stretchings which the mother may be taught to do, should not be commenced until 6 weeks of age. Very occasionally a tenotomy and neck collar may be required later in the first 1–2 years.

Congenital postural scoliosis

The incidence is approximately 1 in 1000 births. There is a single, gentle curve, which is not to be confused with the usually more angular scoliosis due to malformation of the spine. If the spine is not examined routinely for lateral flexion, the condition is easily missed until the infant sits. Examination is best carried out by lifting the laterally lying infant from the bed with a hand under the baby's side just under the rib cage. This is then repeated on the other side. In suspected cases an X-ray should be taken in full lateral flexion to the right and to the left. Orthopaedic advice and careful follow-up are required.

Congenital dislocation of the hip (CDH)

Approximately 1.5% of all newborn infants have either dislocation of the hip (10%) or dislocatable hips (90%) at birth. While many of these hips will stabilize without treatment, some will not and others may destabilize or become dysplastic later in infancy. Early diagnosis and treatment of all cases offers the safest and most satisfactory outcome. Therefore it is most important that the hips are examined on the first day of life and again before discharge from hospital (or on the 10th day). Thereafter the hips should be carefully examined at 6–12 weeks and at regular intervals until the child has a stable gait at 18–24 months. If the initial screening for CDH is being undertaken by a relatively inexperienced examiner, it is essential that suspect hips be checked again on the same day by a more experienced colleague. Note that CDH is four times more common in girls than boys, and 10 times more common in association with breech presentation. Examination should also be particularly careful if there is a family history of CDH or if other deformities such as talipes are apparent.

Examination

This should be gentle. Preferably the examiner's hands should be warm and the infant relaxed. The baby is placed on its back with legs towards the examiner.

First, examine for asymmetry, wide spacing of the thighs, and limited abduction of the hips. These signs are rare at birth but are increasingly common after the first 2–3 months.

Second, manipulate the hips to determine whether they are unstable using Ortolani and Barlow's manoeuvres: The examiner grasps the baby's legs as in Fig. 6.2a placing the middle finger of each hand over the greater trochanter; the flexed leg is contained in the

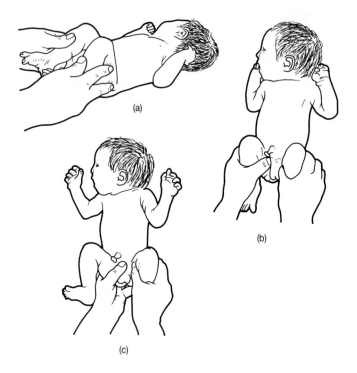

Fig. 6.2   Examination for CDH (see text)

palm of the hand, with the thumb on the inner side of the thigh opposite the lesser trochanter (Fig. 6.2b). Alternatively, the pelvis may be held and steadied by one hand while the other manipulates one hip at a time (Fig. 6.2c). With the thighs in flexion and slight abduction an attempt is now made to move each femoral head in turn gently forward into or backwards out of the acetabulum. If the head of the femur is *dislocated*, then it may be felt to reduce forwards into the joint with anteriorly directed pressure. If, on applying backwards pressure the hip is felt to displace out of the acetabulum but returns spontaneously when the pressure is released, then it is *dislocatable*. These movements are of the order of 0.5 cm in extent and are termed 'clunks'. Ligamentous 'clicks' *without* movement out of or into the acetabulum may be elicited in 5–10% of hip joints and are usually of no significance. Experience in hip examination may be acquired through use of a teaching simulator such as the 'Baby Hippy' produced by Medical Plastics Laboratory (PO Box 38, Gatesville, Texas 76528).

Static and dynamic ultrasound examination of the hips offers a useful adjunct to diagnosis and follow-up surveillance during the first six months. It may also be used for back-up screening of infants at high risk of CDH. With further experience it may prove safe to

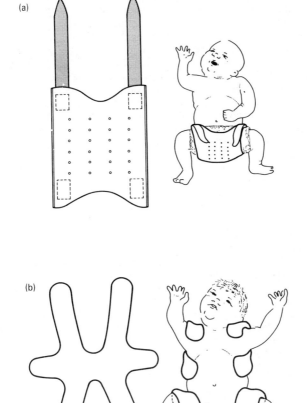

Fig. 6.3 (a) the Aberdeen splint; (b) the von Rosen splint (see text)

observe without splinting a proportion of newborn infants with hip instability whose static ultrasound morphology falls within normal limits. Radiological examination is of limited value in the first 3 months of life but then becomes progressively more useful.

Management

Dislocatable hips are usually cured by 6 weeks' treatment in a plastic over-nappy abduction splint (the Aberdeen splint), which may be removed by the mother when changing the nappies (Fig. 6.3a). If the hip is still unstable at 6 weeks, continue treatment until 12 weeks.

Dislocated hips should be treated for 6 weeks in a metal abduction splint such as a von Rosen splint (Fig. 6.3b), followed by a similar period in an Aberdeen splint. Pressure should **never** be used to achieve abduction because tension of the adductor muscle may lead to ischaemic necrosis of the femoral head. Abduction should not exceed 80°. If there is a limitation of abduction, seek orthopaedic advice. If the hip is still unstable at 3 months, X-ray (single adducted A–P film of hips) and seek orthopaedic advice. All cases should be followed up with clinical and radiological examination at 6 months and 1 year. Occasional cases will require a longer period of surveillance.

Informing the parents

Explain that the hip joint is lax because the baby has been tightly curled up in the womb, and the ligaments softened by pregnancy hormones. Explain this is quite a common finding, that the baby is *not* abnormally formed in any way, is not in pain, and that, with early treatment with the legs kept wide for a few weeks, full recovery is the rule; and that there will be no reason why the child should not be an athlete in due course. It is essential to ensure that the parents are not unnecessarily worried or distressed and also that they know how to handle the baby and splint.

Congenital talipes

Deformities of the feet affect approximately 1 in 250 babies. The commonest variety is *talipes calcaneovalgus* which is not uncommonly associated with CDH. Next comes *talipes equinovarus* or 'clubfoot', followed by metatarsus varus. (This last deformity may also be acquired during the early weeks of life if the infant is nursed prone with the weight of the leg resting on the forefoot. This must be avoided as the deformity is often difficult to treat and tends to give rise to problems when shoes are worn.) If the deformity is mild, the infant can move its foot into the neutral position, and the deformity can be over-corrected by gentle manipulation; treatment is then unlikely to be required. In more serious cases treatment should be instituted *at once*. This may range from passive exercises, to strapping or splinting in over-correction, to the need for surgical correction. All severe cases should be photographed and referred *at once* to an orthopaedic surgeon as the ligaments of the feet tend to tighten up within a day or two of birth, making correction more difficult.

Neurapraxias

These are temporary lower motor neurone paralyses due to pressure on a peripheral nerve *in utero* (in contract to trauma as in Erb's palsy). The most common neurapraxias affect the facial nerve causing unilateral facial palsy (which may be associated with tilted mandible and contracture of the sternomastoid muscle), the radial nerve causing wrist drop (which may be bilateral), and the sciatic and obturator nerves (usually associated with breech presentation). The muscle weakness seldom lasts more than days or weeks. Treatment, if any, is confined to physiotherapy.

Bibliography

Report of the SMAC/SNMAC Working Party (1986). Screening for the detection of congenital dislocation of the hip. *Arch. Dis. Child.*, **61**, 921–6.

Graham, J. M. (1988). *Smith's Recognisable Patterns of Human Deformation* (ed.), 2nd edn. Philadelphia: W. B. Saunders.

Harper, P. S. (1974). *Practical Genetic Counselling*, 2nd edn. Bristol: John Wright and Sons.

McKusick, V. A. (1972). *Heritable Disorders of Connective Tissue*, 4th edn. St Louis: C. V. Mosby Co.

Sharrard, W. J. W. (1979). *Paediatric Orthopaedics and Fractures*, 2nd edn. Oxford: Blackwell Scientific.

Jones, K. L. (1988). *Smith's Recognisable Patterns of Human Deformation* (ed.), 4th edition. Philadelphia: W. B. Saunders.

Warkany, J. (1971). *Congenital Malformations*. Chicago: Year Book Medical Publ.

Williams, P. F. (1982). *Orthopaedic Management in Childhood*. Oxford: Blackwell Scientific.

World Health Organisation (1977). *International Classification of Diseases*, Volume I, Chapter 14, pp. 417–37, 9th revision. Geneva: World Health Organization.

7

Transport of the sick newborn infant

Organization of a neonatal transport service
Stabilization of the infant before transport
Care of the infant during transport
Transport of infants with special problems

Whenever possible infants likely to need special or intensive care should be transported *in utero* to a hospital with appropriate facilities. Transport of mothers who are ill, bleeding, or in preterm labour may carry risks to the *mother* and should be avoided. Despite careful antenatal selection some infants born at home or in obstetric units without neonatal special or intensive care do become sick and require transfer to a hospital with a special care baby unit (see page 52) or a neonatal intensive care unit (see page 53). In hospitals with good transitional care wards many infants who would otherwise require SCBU admission can be nursed with their mothers.

Organization of a neonatal transport service

(a) **Doctor in referring hospital should:**
   Request transfer of sick infants *early*, and give a clear history to the staff at the referral centre
   Ask for telephone advice if needed before the arrival of the transport team
   Prevent cold stress, hypoxia and hypoglycaemia in the infant until the transport team arrive
   Take appropriate samples for culture (see page 213) and commence antibiotics if sepsis seems likely
   Explain to the parents what is happening

Table 7.1 Necessary equipment for the transport of sick newborn infants

Transport incubator	With heater (able to work independently of ambulance)
	With internal light
	With oxygen cylinder and air cylinder or compressor
	With thermometer
Transport ventilator	Able to work without mains/ambulance power supply
	With adjustable FiO_2 and oxygen analyser
	With facilities for CPAP, IPPV, PEEP and IMV
Monitors	Temperature (2 probes). Thermometer (low reading)
	Transcutaneous PO_2
	Blood pressure (either automatic BP recorder of anaeroid sphygmomanometer + Doppler apparatus) + selection of cuff sizes
	Stethoscope
Resuscitation equipment	Bag + selection of masks
	Two laryngoscopes (neonatal plus preterm size) + selection of endotracheal tubes (2.5, 3.0 and 3.5 mm) + fixation equipment and connectors
	Magill's forceps
	Suction apparatus and oral suction mucus traps
	Pneumothorax drains and Heimlich valves
Intravenous infusion equipment	Syringes, tubing, cannulae, tape, taps, needles
	Battery syringe infusion pump (safer and easier to regulate in transit than drips)
Other equipment	Polaroid camera
	Set of maps
	Dextrostix or BM stix (fresh)
	Lancets
	Sample bottles (for clotted blood, cultures etc.)
Drugs	Dried salt-poor albumin
	Calcium gluconate 10% solution
	Dextrose 10% infusion 500 ml

Table 7.1   *Continued*

Dextrose 50% injection
Digoxin injection
Frusemide injection
Gentamicin or netilmicin injection
Heparinized saline (10 units/ml) (for arterial lines)
Naloxone
Pancuronium injection
Penicillin G injection
Phenobarbitone injection
Phenytoin injection
Prostaglandin E_2 injection
Vitamin K_1 injection
Water for injections

Ensure notes, X-rays and a sample of mother's blood (plus cord blood if possible) are available for the transport team

Obtain written consent from parents for any planned surgical procedure.

(b) Neonatal transport team (an experienced doctor and experienced nurse) should:

Travel to the referring hospital as quickly as possible

Be fully equipped to institute and to maintain intensive care of sick infants during transport (Table 7.1)

Spend as long as necessary (sometimes several hours) at the referring hospital stabilizing the infant's condition

Give a full explanation to the infant's parents, show them the infant, leave a Polaroid photograph, and ensure they know the telephone number of the referral centre

Obtain notes, X-rays, consent forms and a sample of mother's blood

Explain to the ambulance crew the need for the above procedures, and ensure the ambulance is warm (25°C) and has windows closed

Ensure details on baby's identification band are correct

Travel back to the referral centre smoothly rather than rapidly

Stabilization of the infant before transport

Thermal care

If rectal temperature is below 36°C then rewarm baby rapidly before transport (check blood pressure frequently during rewarming).

Respiratory care

Intubate infants with significant respiratory distress (do not leave an 'open' endotracheal tube in place: always connect to a continuous positive airway pressure (CPAP) of >3 cm H_2O or intermittent positive-pressure ventilation (IPPV) with positive end-expiratory pressure (PEEP) >2 cm H_2O).

Insert intercostal drain if pneumothorax is present and connect a Heimlich 'flutter' valve.

Give adequate oxygen and respiratory support to prevent cyanosis. (If possible check blood gases before transport.)

Blood sugar

Check heel-prick blood sugar (Dextrostix or BM stix).

Commence i.v. infusion of 10–15% dextrose at 80–100 ml/kg/day (to give 6–10 mg/kg/min of dextrose).

Maintain infusion with syringe pump during transport.

Blood pressure

If the blood pressure is low (see pages 416–17) or falls during stabilization, give plasma or albumin solution 10–15 ml/kg i.v. over half to one hour.

Empty the stomach

Aspiration of gastric contents is a major risk, especially after bag-and-mask resuscitation.

Leave an open gastric tube in place for transport.

Care of the infant during transport

Thermal care

Keep the ambulance warm (25°C) and minimize draughts.

Wrap baby in silver swaddler, bubble plastic or cling film and cover with a blanket.

Avoid opening the incubator if possible.

Maintain incubator temperature in thermoneutral range (page 55).

Monitoring

Monitor the skin and axillary or rectal temperature; ECG; transcutaneous PO_2; respiration; and fractional inspired oxygen concentration (FiO_2).

Ensure the lighting is adequate to detect colour changes and to see respiratory movements.

Transport of infants with special problems

Gastroschisis or omphalocele

Minimize evaporative heat and water loss by placing the whole trunk and legs (up to axillae) in a plastic bag.

Intravenous fluids are needed (100–150 ml/kg/day) (see Chapter 12, page 183).

Oesophageal atresia/tracheo-oesophageal fistula

Nurse flat or head *up*.

Keep upper oesophagus clear by frequent suction on indwelling tube (see Chapter 12, page 184).

Diaphragmatic hernia

Intubate and transport on IPPV.

Sedate or paralyse if fighting ventilator (morphine 0.05 mg/kg i.v. ± pancuronium 0.05 mg/kg).

Keep stomach empty by very frequent aspiration of gastric tube (see Chapter 12, page 179).

Convulsions

Check capillary blood glucose and CSF microscopy before transport.
Treat with i.v. phenobarbitone 10–20 mg/kg (see page 136).

Bibliography

Chance, G. W., Mathew, J. D., Gash, J. *et al.* (1978). Neonatal transport: A controlled study of skilled assistance. *J. Pediatr.*, **93**, 662–6.

Greene, W. T. (1980). Organisation of neonatal transport services in support of a regional referral center. *Clin. Perinatol.*, **7**, 187–95.

Modanlou, H. D. and Dorchester, W. L. (1979). Effectiveness of neonatal transport. *J. Pediatr.*, **94**, 682–3.

Roy, R. N. and Kitchen, W. H. (1977). NETS: A new system for neonatal transport. *Med. J. Austral.*, **2**, 855–8.

Segal, S. (Ed.) (1972). *Manual for the Transport of High-risk Newborn Infants: Principles, Policies, Equipment, Techniques.* Vancouver: Canadian Pediatric Society.

8

Neonatal respiratory problems

Causes of respiratory distress
Care of the baby with respiratory symptoms
Continuous positive airway pressure
Mechanical ventilation
Chronic lung disease
Recurrent apnoea

Many neonatal cardiac and respiratory disorders present with the same clinical signs of tachypnoea, grunting, retraction of the chest wall and cyanosis. Although the supportive care of the various disorders is basically the same, it is essential to make a definitive diagnosis so that more specific treatment can be given.

Causes of respiratory distress

Table 8.1 gives a detailed list of conditions presenting with 'respiratory distress' (not to be confused with respiratory distress syndrome). It is usually not difficult to distinguish between the different conditions, based upon the history, clinical examination and chest X-ray appearances.

Some relevant features of the more important disorders are given below.

Respiratory distress syndrome (RDS)

Preterm delivery, lecithin: sphyngomyelin ratio in amniotic fluid <2 (surfactant deficiency) or <3 in the infant of a diabetic mother. Commoner following Caesarean section, birth asphyxia and hypothermia, abruptio placenta and maternal sedation. Onset of

Table 8.1 Causes of respiratory distress

Disorders presenting with one or more of the physical signs of tachypnoea, grunting, retraction of the chest wall, cyanosis. (Some of these conditions may also present with shock, hypoventilation or apnoea.)

Respiratory distress syndrome (surfactant deficiency)	Diaphragmatic hernia
Transient tachypnoea/wet lung	Choanal atresia
Meconium aspiration	Congenital heart defects
Other aspiration syndromes (amniotic fluid, blood, milk)	Cardiac failure
	Myocarditis
Pneumothorax	Persistent fetal circulation
Pneumomediastinum	Polycythaemia
Interstitial emphysema	Anaemia
Pneumonia (especially Group B streptococcal infection)	Hypoglycaemia
	Hypothermia
Pulmonary haemorrhage	Septicaemia/meningitis
Atelectasis	Drugs (e.g. diazepam, opiates etc.) given to mother in labour
Wilson–Mikity syndrome	Birth asphyxia, cerebral oedema / haemorrhage / trauma
Pulmonary hypoplasia, (e.g. Potter's syndrome)	Neuromuscular disorder (myasthenia gravis, myotonic dystrophy)
Lung anomalies (e.g. cysts, sequestered lobe, adenomatous malformation)	

grunting, retraction and tachypnoea within an hour or birth. There may be reduced breath sounds or bronchial breathing on auscultation. The babies are usually oedematous. Signs persist beyond 24 hours of age, but the natural history is for recovery to start within 96 hours. Chest X-ray shows a reticulogranular appearance with an air bronchogram. Pneumothorax and pneumonia are common complications.

Transient tachypnoea of newborn (TTN)

Usually a term infant with mature lungs but delayed clearing of lung fluid. Transient tachypnoea of newborn commonly occurs after delivery by elective Caesarean section. Onset of tachypnoea and mild grunting within two to three hours of birth. Chest X-ray shows coarse streaking and fluid in the fissures, the 'wet lung' appearance. Usually responds to 30–40% FiO_2 but may persist for 3 or 4 days.

Meconium aspiration syndrome

Usually term or post-term with fetal distress and meconium-stained liquor. Inhalation of this liquor causes the syndrome, which may be largely prevented by pharyngeal and tracheal suction immediately on delivery (see Chapter 2). There is early onset of respiratory distress, which may be severe. Chest X-ray shows hyperinflated lungs with coarse streaking and patchy consolidation. Alveolar rupture and pneumonia are common complications. Similar disorder may be caused by inhalation of normal amniotic fluid, blood (following antepartum haemorrhage) or milk. Baby may also show clinical features of asphyxia.

Air leaks (alveolar rupture)

Pneumothorax, pneumomediastinum or interstitial emphysema may be spontaneous but more often follow active resuscitation, artificial ventilation or continuous positive airway pressure (CPAP), and also occurs in babies with aspiration syndromes, RDS, or pulmonary hypoplasia. A small air leak may give minimal respiratory symptoms but a tension pneumothorax usually causes severe cardiorespiratory collapse. Diagnosis is aided by transillumination of the chest with a powerful cold-light source: the pneumothorax shows as increased transillumination. Confirm by X-ray, including a shoot-through lateral view. In an emergency 'needle' both sides of the chest (see Chapter 21, page 353).

Congenital pneumonia

May occur at any gestation. Commonly but not always after prolonged rupture of membranes. Usually due to group B streptococcus, which mimics RDS, and may have identical chest X-ray appearances. Onset of respiratory symptoms is usually within 3 hours of birth but may be delayed for 24–48 hours. Patients may have severe shock and apnoea. Organisms seen in gastric aspirate and found on blood culture. Survival depends on intensive support and early administration of penicillin $\pm$ an aminoglycoside (e.g. netilmicin, gentamicin). Because this condition can mimic other respiratory disorders we give all babies with 'RDS' penicillin until cultures are known to be negative.

Pulmonary haemorrhage

Usually a haemorrhagic pulmonary oedema presenting as frothy, blood-stained fluid coming out of the trachea or welling up the endotracheal tube in babies ill with some other disorder. Associated with asphyxia, hypothermia, infection, congenital heart disease, severe rhesus disease and haemorrhagic states such as disseminated intravascular coagulation (DIC).

Primary atelectasis

Failure of alveolar expansion at birth usually in the very preterm baby (<27 weeks) due to pulmonary immaturity. Clinical features are those of RDS but X-ray shows 'white out' appearance.

Wilson–Mikity syndrome

Gradual onset of respiratory distress towards end of first week in babies below 1.5 kg birthweight. Also known as pulmonary dysmaturity. Chest X-ray shows diffuse coarse streaking, becoming confluent and later cystic. Often confused with bronchopulmonary dysplasia but does not follow treatment with mechanical ventilation or oxygen.

Pleural effusion

Uncommon. If unilateral, there may be a mediastinal shift and reduced breath sounds. X-ray shows opaque lung field. Causes include chylothorax, hydrops fetalis, pneumonia or cardiac failure. Diagnosis confirmed by pleural tap. May be diagnosed antenatally on ultrasound scan.

Diaphragmatic hernia

Respiratory symptoms vary from severe to none. There may be a history of hydramnios. May present at birth or after several hours. Usually left sided in which case the mediastinum is shifted to the right. The abdomen is commonly scaphoid and audible bowel sounds in the chest are a late and unreliable sign. Right-sided hernias are more difficult to diagnose as the mediastinal shift is not so obvious. Chest X-ray shows bowel pattern in the thoracic cavity and absent diaphragmatic shadow. Pneumothorax is a common complication (see Chapter 12, page 178).

Cystic adenomatoid malformation

A rare malformation of the lung, presenting as a large cystic mass most commonly in the upper and middle lobes and nearly always unilateral. There are three types depending on the size of the cysts: (1) Multiple large cysts resembling lobar emphysema on X-ray. (2) Medium cysts often associated with other malformations such as hydranencephaly or prune belly syndrome. (3) Small cysts appearing as a solid mass on X-ray. Half the babies are preterm and hydramnios or fetal hydrops occur in 30%. Presents with respiratory distress from birth and may be confused with diaphragmatic hernia. Treatment is by lobectomy.

Congenital lobar emphysema

Over-expansion of part of a lung due to external bronchial compression by cysts, tumours or aberrant vessels, or internal bronchial obstruction by plugs, mucosal folds or stenosis. Usually only a single lobe is involved, 50% left upper, 28% right middle, 20% right upper. Half the cases are symptomatic in the neonatal period. Chest X-ray may show a solid area on day 1 due to retained lung fluid, but then becomes hyperexpanded with emphysema and mediastinal shift. Bronchoscopy may help diagnose and clear plugs but treatment is usually surgical. Insertion of a 'pneumothorax' drain is dangerous and is not recommended. Fifteen per cent may have co-existing cardiac defect.

Acquired lobar emphysema

Localized cystic emphysema is usually found in preterm babies with RDS complicated by interstitial emphysema, though the onset may be delayed for several weeks. Most often it affects the right lung. Chest X-ray shows a large cystic area and mediastinal shift. Management is conservative. Occasionally, bronchial lavage to remove plugs may be needed. Selective bronchial intubation to collapse the hyperinflated lung for 2–3 days may be tried in severe or progressive cases. Surgery is rarely indicated. Do not insert a 'pneumothorax' drain.

Pulmonary hypoplasia

Associated with oligohydramnios of any cause, e.g. renal agenesis or dysplasia, obstructive uropathy or prolonged rupture of the membranes. Also found in association with diaphragmatic hernia, pleural effusion, skeletal dysplasias affecting the rib cage and neuromuscular disorders. Respiratory failure, which is often severe, pneumothorax and persistent fetal circulation occur commonly in these babies.

Persistent fetal circulation (see Chapter 9)

Persistent pulmonary hypertension causes right-to-left shunting through the foramen ovale and ductus arteriosus, with severe hypoxia. It may occur as a primary disorder when the lungs appear normal or even oligaemic on X-ray. It also occurs in RDS, meconium aspiration syndrome, polycythaemia and diaphragmatic hernia. It is easily confused with cyanotic congenital heart disease. The severe hypoxia is not usually accompanied by hypercapnoea, and there is little response to ventilation and high FiO_2. After correction of acidosis and systemic hypotension many cases respond to infusion of tolazoline which can be used as a diagnostic/therapeutic test (1 mg/kg i.v. as a slow bolus dose, followed by an infusion of 0.1–1 mg/kg/hour). This is a general vasodilator and may cause systemic hypotension which should be corrected by infusion of plasma. Tolazoline can also cause gastrointestinal bleeding.

Care of the baby with respiratory symptoms

In the delivery room

Prompt effective resuscitation will reduce the severity of subsequent respiratory distress (see Chapter 2).

In the special care baby unit

A suitable *supporting environment* is an essential background to more active measures.

Thermoneutral environment   Nurse in an incubator set to maintain skin temperature at 36.5°C (see Chapter 5, Table 5.4).

Give *humidified oxygen* via a headbox. Use a transcutaneous O_2 monitor to start with, before inserting an arterial line (see page 346). Do not feed enterally, start a peripheral *intravenous infusion* of 10% dextrose at 60–80 ml/kg/day. Avoid using the umbilical vein if possible (see Chapters 5 and 11).

Minimal handling   Any disturbance of a sick baby may cause apnoea or a fall in a PaO_2 or blood pressure. Use electronic monitors to record heart rate, respiration, temperature and PaO_2 or $TcPO_2$. *Nurse in the prone position* as this improves oxygenation, reduces the work of breathing, heat loss and gastro-oesophageal reflux.

Send *blood for culture*. Start intravenous penicillin. This can be stopped in 48 hours if cultures are negative (see Chapter 14). Do an Antero Posterior supine *chest X-ray* and an abdominal X-ray to confirm position of umbilical catheter if used (see Chapter 21).

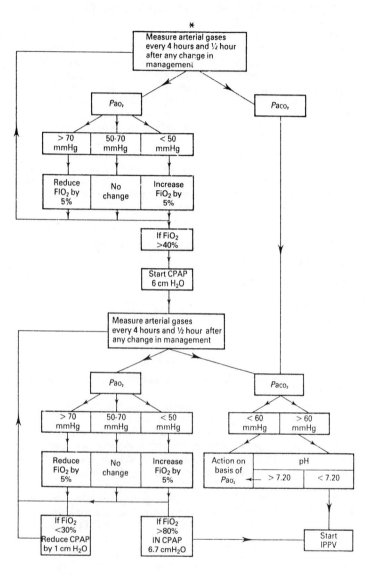

Fig. 8.1   Flow chart for respiratory management of infants with RDS. Start at point marked *, with infant in 40 per cent oxygen by headbox. To convert blood gas tensions in mmHg to kPa, multiply by 0.13.

Measure *blood pressure* regularly. If low (see page 417) give i.v. plasma 10–15 ml/kg over 1 hour depending on severity of the hypotension. Oscillometric blood pressure monitors consistently over-read in sick, very low birthweight babies and consequently hypotension may be missed. Continuous intra-arterial monitoring is more reliable.

Blood gas and pH measurements

An arterial line, either peripheral or umbilical, should be inserted if the baby is given more than 40% oxygen or the respiratory signs persist beyond the age of 4 hours. Intermittent puncture of peripheral arteries can itself cause a fall in PaO_2 and give misleading results. Continuous PaO_2 recording using an intra-arterial PO_2 electrode or a transcutaneous PO_2 electrode is very valuable. But no matter which

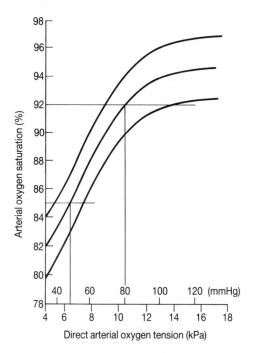

Fig. 8.2 Comparison of 125 paired measurements of transcutaneous arterial oxygen saturation and arterial oxygen tension. The fitted mean curve ± 2 S.D. is shown. Adapted from Wasanna, A., Whitelaw, A. G. L. (1987). *Arch. Dis. Childh.* **62**; 957–71.

technique is used PaO_2, $PaCO_2$ and pH should be measured every 4–6 hours and 0.5 hour after any change in management (see flowchart in Fig. 8.1).

The measurement of oxygen saturation using a pulse oxymeter can be a helpful adjunct to the above but may lead to unrecognized hyperoxia or hypoxia (see Fig. 8.2). Saturation should be kept between 85 and 92%.

Other investigations

Haemogloblin, white blood cell count, packed cell volume, platelets	At birth and every 2–3 days
Urea, electrolytes, creatinine	Daily
Capillary blood sugar (BM stix)	4–6 hourly
Blood culture	At birth and as indicated
Nose, throat swabs for culture	At birth and as indicated

Babies on CPAP or IPPV should have a tracheal or pharyngeal aspirate sent for culture every 2 days.

Keep a flow chart at the cotside on which are recorded nursing observations of vital signs, FiO_2, ventilator settings and blood gas results. Keep a cumulative record of the volume of blood taken from the baby for all investigations.

Respiratory management

See the flowchart in Fig. 8.1. Start at the top with the baby in 40% oxygen in a head box and manage according to blood gas results.

Continuous positive airway pressure (CPAP)

Indications

Respiratory distress syndrome

Continuous positive airway pressure of 6–8 cm H_2O should be started if the PaO_2 is below 50 mm Hg (6.5 KPa) in FiO_2 40% or more. *Early use of CPAP, preferably within the first 4 hours of birth, may reduce the severity of subsequent respiratory problems.*

Recurrent apnoeic attacks

Continuous positive airway pressure of 3–4 cm H_2O is an effective way to reduce or abolish apnoeic attacks in immature babies.

Weaning off mechanical ventilation (see page 102)

Methods of applying continuous positive airway pressure

Figure 8.3 shows the circuit diagram of a system suitable for delivering CPAP using nasal cannula, endotracheal tube (ETT) or face mask. Continuous positive airway pressure can also be administered using any ventilator with an IMV circuit.

Nasal continuous positive airway pressure

For treating RDS use Portex twin prongs sizes 2.5 or 3.0. Start with an FiO_2 of 50% and a CPAP of 6 cm H_2O. *For apnoeic attacks* a single prong using an ETT passed to the upper pharynx is usually effective; start with a CPAP of 3–4 cm H_2O in air. Insert a size 6FG orogastric tube to prevent gastric distension, leave the end open and aspirate 1–2 hourly.

Endotracheal continuous positive airway pressure

Endotracheal CPAP should be administered using a ventilator, because CPAP alone down an ETT may cause progressive atelectasis. To prevent this use slow IMV of 2–5 breaths per minute. *Never* leave an 'open' ETT in place without CPAP/IMV.

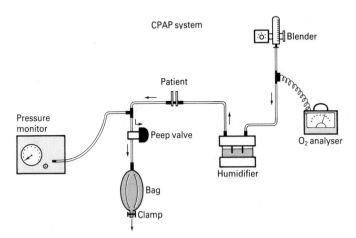

Fig. 8.3 Diagrammatic representation of CPAP circuit. Suitable for applying CPAP by nasal prong, endotracheal tube or face mask. (NB. The pressure monitor should be attached to the flow circuit as close as possible to the baby).

Face mask continuous positive airway pressure

Use a face mask of appropriate size for the baby held in place with a netelast helmet. Complications include nasal obstruction, corneal ulceration and a higher incidence of pneumothorax.

Management of the baby on continuous positive airway pressure

Measure blood gases within 0.5 hour of starting CPAP and 4–6 hourly thereafter according to Fig. 8.1.

If the PaO_2 falls below 45 mm Hg in CPAP 7–8 cm H_2O and FiO_2 80%, start ventilation.

The main complication of CPAP is tension pneumothorax and this should always be suspected if the baby's condition deteriorates.

As the baby's respiratory status improves, gradually reduce the FiO_2 and CPAP in stages. When CPAP has been stopped watch for apnoeic attacks. If these become frequent it may be necessary to restart CPAP and prescribe aminophylline. Do not feed enterally for 24 hours after stopping CPAP or if the respiratory rate is above 60/min.

Mechanical ventilation

Indications

Try to anticipate the need for ventilation rather than let the baby deteriorate to the state where it becomes an emergency procedure. The indications will usually be obvious, for example, apnoea. In the management of RDS or recurrent apnoeic attacks CPAP should be tried first. If the PaO_2 is below 40 mm Hg (5.2 kPa) in spite of a CPAP 7–8 cm H_2P and FiO_2 80% or the $PaCO_2$ is over 60 mm Hg (7.8 kPa) and the pH <7.20 the infant should be ventilated (see Fig. 8.1).

General principles of neonatal ventilation

There are many different types of ventilator available and this description will be confined to techniques using time cycled, pressure-limited ventilation with machines capable of applying a positive end expiratory pressure (PEEP) and intermittent mandatory ventilation (IMV).

There are many different ways of ventilating babies involving various manipulations of ventilator rate, inspired : expired (*I–E*) ratio and pressures, and it is certain that no one style of ventilation is suitable for all babies. When setting up the ventilator it is essential to bear in mind the baby's gestation, size and diagnosis.

The initial settings will almost certainly need to be adjusted to those which best suit the individual baby and will need to be further modified as the baby's condition changes, particularly if complications such as emphysema or pneumothorax develop. There are, however, certain basic principles to be considered.

Mean airway pressure (MAP)

Oxygenation is closely related to MAP which is calculated from the equation:

$$MAP = (PIP-PEEP)\,(T_i/(T_i + T_e)) + PEEP$$

MAP can therefore be altered by changes in peak inspiratory pressure (PIP) or end expiratory pressure (PEEP) and in $I{:}E$ ratio. When changing ventilator settings it is important to stop and think about how those changes will alter MAP (see Fig. 8.4).

Peak inspiratory pressure

An increase in PIP will improve oxygenation by increasing MAP. It will also increase tidal volume and reduce $PaCO_2$. But high PIP

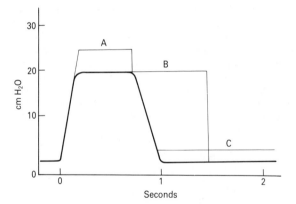

Fig. 8.4 Airway pressure wave-form generated by a time-cycled, pressure-limited constant-flow-generating ventilator (see text). Mean airway pressure (and hence oxygenation may be increased by (A) increasing peak inspiratory pressure, (B) prolonging inspiratory time or (C) increasing PEEP. Adapted from Reynolds, E.O.R. (1974) In *Neonatal and Pediatric Ventilation*. Ed. D. H. Keuskamp. Boston: Little, Brown and Co.

causes barotrauma with risk of pneumothorax and bronchopulmonary dysplasia (BPA). Try to keep PIP <25 cm H_2O if possible and rarely use a pressure >30 cm H_2O.

Positive end expiratory pressure

An increase in PEEP will improve oxygenation by increasing MAP. It may also reduce tidal volume and hence increase $PaCO_2$. The optimal PEEP for infants with RDS is usually 5–6 cm H_2O; higher levels may not improve oxygenation but will significantly reduce tidal volume with CO_2 retention.

I:E ratio

A prolonged inspiratory time (T_i) will improve oxygenation by increasing MAP, but is not as effective as increases in PIP or PEEP. Normally a ratio of 1:1 is used, but ratios of up to 1.5:1 or even 2:1 may be used in severe RDS with slow ventilator rates (<40bpm). It is, however, better to consider the actual inspiratory and expiratory times rather than ratios, and T_i is usually kept in the range 0.5 to 1.0 sec.

Rate

If the $I:E$ ratio is unchanged, an increase in rate should not alter MAP. Prolonged T_i and PEEP appear to be most effective at rates of 30–40/min. It has been suggested that rates of 60–120/min may reduce the incidence of pneumothorax by entraining the baby to breath in synchrony with the ventilator. Higher rates may also be associated with improved oxygenation particularly in the presence of severe pulmonary interstitial emphysema (PIE), though there is little evidence that rates over 60/min are beneficial. The benefits of fast ventilation (>100/min) appear to be confined to spontaneously breathing infants and are not usually seen in babies who have been given muscle relaxants.

Minute ventilation may fall at rates over 75–80/min. If a very short expiratory time (T_e) is used at fast rates there is a risk of incomplete expiration and gas trapping known as 'inadvertant PEEP'.

Inadvertant positive end-expiratory pressure

Inadvertant PEEP occurs when alveolar pressure is higher than the proximal airway pressure because T_e is too short. The expiratory times necessary for 95% exhalation depend on the baby's size and lung disease; for example, for a normal term infant: 0.45/sec; for a preterm infant with RDS: 0.1/sec; for a term baby with meconium aspiration: 1.0 sec. Inadvertant PEEP does not appear on the ventilator pressure gauge but is additive to applied PEEP and may have the same effect on improving oxygenation. This may explain why some babies with RDS improve with faster rate ventilation. Inadvertant PEEP may cause gas trapping especially during recovery from RDS. This will cause CO_2 retention which paradoxically may be corrected by reducing the rate. Barotrauma, pneumothorax and compromised pulmonary circulation are also possible. When using fast rates with short T_e, it is advisable to reduce applied PEEP to only 2 cm H_2O. It is also *essential* to know the characteristics of your ventilator expiratory valve as this may not be able to cope with fast rates and hence further increase inadvertant PEEP.

Oxygen

High FiO_2 >80% causes resorption atelectasis and increased right-to-left shunting even in babies on ventilation. This will lead to a fall in oxygenation and a need for higher ventilator settings. An FiO_2 >50% may cause decreased ciliary activity and increased capillary leakage in the airways, thus increasing the risk of atelectasis and ETT blockage. Try to improve oxygenation by better ventilation rather than turning up the FiO_2 above 80%; though sometimes this is unavoidable.

Surfactant

Several preparations of replacement surfactant are now available in the UK from artificial (Alec, Exosurf) or animal sources (Curosurf), usually as part of extensive clinical trials. There is firm evidence that surfactant improves the clinical course of babies with RDS in terms of mortality and morbidity. Trials are presently establishing optimal dose, timing and frequency of administration.

Initial ventilator settings

These will depend on the disorder for which the baby is to be ventilated and the gestation. Settings should be individualized for each baby; for example, a high PEEP and prolonged inspiratory time would be detrimental to a baby with normal lungs being ventilated for apnoea, meconium aspiration syndrome or alveolar rupture. A suggested range of initial settings is given below:

(1) FiO_2 40–50%
(2) Inspiratory time 0.8–0.6 sec ⎫ *I:E* ratio 1:1
(3) Expiratory time 0.8–0.6 sec ⎭ Rate 37–50/min

(4) Inspiratory pressure (PIP) 18–20 cm H_2O
(5) Expiratory pressure (PEEP) 4 cm H_2O
(6) Flow 8 l/min

Example   Pressure 20/4 cm H_2O
rate 50/min
$T_i = T_e = 0.6$ sec.
$MAP = (20 - 4)(0.6)/(1.2) + 4$
     $= 12$ cm H_2O

Measure blood gases 0.5 hour after starting ventilation and adjust the settings to manipulate MAP so that you aim to keep PaO_2 in the range 50–80 mm Hg (6.5 – 10.4 kPa) and $PaCO_2$ 35–50 mm Hg (4.5 – 6.5 kPa). **It is not necessary to have perfect blood gases and there is evidence that vigorous ventilation intended to keep $PaCO_2$ in the normal range is associated with an increased incidence of BPD.**

Deterioration during ventilation

(1) Sudden clinical deterioration

This is usually accompanied by a fall in PaO_2 ± a rise in $PaCO_2$.

Action: Disconnect ventilator and use a manual inflation bag.

(a) *Baby's condition improves*: presume the deterioration was due to a ventilator problem.

Possible causes: mechanical or electrical ventilator failure; disconnected tube or leaking connection; excess condensation in tubing; fall in FiO_2.

Action: Correct fault.

(b) *Baby's condition remains poor with manual inflation bag*: presume a baby problem.

Possible causes: ETT displaced, blocked or down main bronchus; pneumothorax.

Action: Suck ETT, check air entry bilaterally, if no improvement – reintubate at once.
Transilluminate the chest, take antero-posterior and lateral

chest X-ray. If condition is critical, needle pleural spaces to relieve possible tension pneumothorax (see Chapter 21).

(2) Gradual deterioration

This is usually accompanied by a slow fall in PaO_2 and/or rise in $PaCO_2$. This may also be due to a displaced or blocked ETT or alveolar leak and these should be excluded first.

Other possible causes:

Inappropriate ventilator settings

(a) Due to progressive deterioration in disease state:
   consider increasing peak inflation pressure, inspiratory time, rate or FiO_2.
(b) due to improvement in disease state: consider reduction in peak inflation pressure, PEEP or inspiratory time.

Baby 'fighting' against ventilator   Reconsider the need for ventilation. If IPPV is essential then use a muscle relaxant ± morphine. NB The ventilator settings may need to be significantly increased when the baby is sedated or given muscle relaxants as its own efforts are no longer contributing to gas exchange. Raising the ventilator rate to 80–100 breaths per minute may cause the baby's efforts to synchronize with the ventilatory breaths, thus avoiding the need for sedation or muscle relaxants, but see page 102.

Intraventricular haemorrhage   Check PCV for sudden fall. If available do an ultrasound brain scan.

Patent ducts arteriosus   (see Chapter 9).

Infection   Do a full septic screen and chest X-ray. Consider antibiotic therapy (see Chapter 11).

Hypotension   Check BP and if low (see pages 416–17) give plasma (10–15 ml/kg).

Anaemia   Check PCV and Hb. If PCV <40% or HB <12 g/dl, transfuse.

Metabolic imbalance   Check blood urea, electrolytes, calcium, glucose and bilirubin.

Poor environmental support   Avoid excessive handling. Ensure the baby is in a thermoneutral environment (see Chapter 5, page 52).

(3) Refractory hypoxia

If the PaO_2 remains below 40 mm Hg (5.2 kPa) despite apparent adequate ventilation and $FiO_2 > 80\%$, this may be due to the baby 'fighting' or breathing out of synchrony with the ventilator or due to increased intrapulmonary shunting caused by progressive atelectasis or to pulmonary hypertension with shunting through the foramen ovale and/or ductus arteriosus.

Try the effect of:

(a) Increasing the ventilator rate to 60–80/min.
(b) Sedation with morphine and/or muscle relaxation with pancuronium:

Possible benefits: Better gas exchange
Less barotrauma and BPD
Less risk of pneumothorax
More stable PaO_2
Less risk of IVH

Possible dangers: Worse gas exchange
Increased ventilation requirements
Tachycardia/hypotension
Fluid retention and oedema
Jaundice
Drug interaction (gentamicin + pancuronium)

(c) Increase FiO_2 to 90–100%
Increase PIP to 35 cm H_2O
Increase PEEP to 5–6 cm H_2O
(d) Bolus i.v. injection of tolazoline, 1 mg/kg. This may cause severe hypotension so monitor blood pressure and have plasma immediately available to correct hypotension. If PaO_2 improves with tolazoline start a continuous i.v. infusion of 0.1 mg/kg/hour, which may be increased to 1 mg/kg/hour if necessary.

Weaning off the ventilator

When the baby's condition has improved as shown by a consistent PaO_2 over 70 mm Hg (9.1 kPa) and $PaCO_2$ below 45–50 mm Hg (5.85–6.5 kPa), start to reduce the PIP and FiO_2 gradually in alternate steps. When FiO_2 is <50% and PIP <20 cm H_2O stop giving sedation and muscle relaxants and allow their effects to wear off. Reduce T_i gradually to 0.5 sec, at the same time maintain or reduce rate by increasing T_e.

Keep T_i at 0.5 sec; reduce PIP to 16–18 cm H_2O; reduce FiO_2. Consider use of aminophylline.

When the rate is 5/min, FiO_2 <35%, pressure 16/3–4, extubate to either headbox oxygen or nasal CPAP.

Do not feed enterally for 24 hours after extubation.

Take chest X-ray after 12–24 hours.

Chronic lung disease

Causes of chronic ventilator dependency and/or need for prolonged increase in FiO_2

(1) **Congenital pulmonary hypoplasia**, e.g. associated with diaphragmatic hernia, Potter's syndrome and other causes of oligohydramnios.
(2) **Bronchopulmonary dysplasia** (BPD) associated with positive pressure ventilation and high FiO_2.
(3) **Wilson–Mikity syndrome** of pulmonary dysmaturity.
(4) **Chronic pulmonary insufficiency of prematurity.** Secondary atelectasis probably due to chronic hypoventilation in the very immature baby.
(5) **Pulmonary interstitial emphysema**.
(6) Chronic lung disorder may also be associated with **patent ductus arteriosus (PDA)**, **pulmonary haemorrhage, infection, inspissated secretions, milk aspiration and osteopenia of prematurity**.

There is considerable overlap in the clinical and radiological signs of all these conditions, but particularly between BPD and Wilson–Mikity syndrome.

These babies may require prolonged IPPV or IMV and are usually difficult to wean off ventilation. They may then have a dependency on increased FiO_2 for many weeks.

Management

(1) Give aminophylline to aid weaning from ventilation.
(2) Provide adequate nutrition, if possible enterally using gastric or transpyloric route, but if necessary i.v.
(3) Treat any intercurrent infections.
(4) Treat heart failure which may be due to PDA, or right heart failure associated with chronic lung disorder.
(5) Many babies with chronic lung disease, even in the absence of right heart failure, benefit from regular low-dose diuretic treatment. Chlorthiazide and a potassium-sparing diuretic (spironolactone) are preferred to frusemide because of reduced risk of

nephrocalinosis and decreased urinary losses of Ca^{2+}, K^+ and Na^+. This may improve pulmonary compliance, reduce the work of breathing, and recent evidence shows improved survival. (NB Monitor blood electrolytes weekly.)

(6) X-ray chest and a wrist; measure alkaline phosphatase (see page 405).

(7) Transfuse to keep Hb above 12.0 g/dl.

(8) Monitor PaO_2 and $PaCO_2$. Transcutaneous PO_2 monitoring should be done for several hours each day, but tends to under-read in the older baby. Recording of saturation using a pulse oxymeter is particularly useful in this group of patients (see page 94). Give sufficient oxygen to maintain Tc$PO_2 >$ 50 mm Hg or saturation 85–92%.

(9) Reduce increased FiO_2 levels very slowly. This may take many weeks and the requirement may only be for 22–30% oxygen. This can be provided in an incubator using a headbox, but once the baby is big enough to be nursed in a cot the oxygen can be provided using a low flow system, which facilitates bottle or breast feeding.

(10) In the infant with severe chronic lung disease who is still ventilator dependent, there is good evidence that steroid treatment may improve lung function and facilitate weaning from ventilator.

Give dexamethasone, 0.2 mg/kg, 8 hourly for 7 days. Improvement may occur rapidly and frequent blood gas analysis and reduction in ventilator settings may be necessary. Deterioration may occur on stopping treatment and a further reducing course of steroids over 1–2 weeks may be required. The main concern with this treatment is serious infection. Less commonly cardiac failure or fluid and electrolyte disturbances may occur.

Low-flow oxygen

Use a flow meter graduated in 100 ml/min, connected to an un-humidified oxygen source and infant nasal oxygen cannula (Salter Labs). Alternatively, cut two small side holes in a feeding tube and tape this across the baby's upper lip so that the holes are below the nostrils, close the end hole with a piece of tape and connect the other end to the flow meter. Start at 200 ml/min and monitor TcPO_2 (or saturation) confirmed by arterial PO_2 measurement. Alter flow rate (100–500 ml/min) according to the baby's needs. The flow rate often needs to be increased at the time of feeds. This system facilitates nursing and can be used in the home.

Recurrent apnoea

It is normal for the preterm infant to have periodic breathing. Apnoeic attacks are repeated episodes of absent breathing for 10–30 sec or shorter episodes of apnoea associated with bradycardia and/or colour change (pallor or cyanosis). PaO_2 and $TcPO_2$ will normally fall during an apnoeic attack. Apnoeic attacks are very common in the very low birthweight baby and such infants must have continuous cardiorespiratory monitoring for the first two weeks at least.

Causes

Lung disease ± hypoxia
Airway obstruction
Cardiac disorder (especially PDA)
Cerebral oedema/haemorrhage (in some infants apnoeic attacks may be the only manifestation of convulsions)
Infection
Anaemia
Metabolic imbalance (hypoglycaemia, hypocalcaemia, hyponatraemia, acidosis)
Drugs (e.g. maternal sedation/analgesia in labour)
Unstable environmental temperature (apnoea commonly occurs as the environmental temperature rises)
REM sleep
Intolerance of enteral feeds
'Apnoea of prematurity'

Investigations

Review history, description and timing of attacks
Physical examination, especially cardiorespiratory system, neurological behaviour, evidence of infection. Measure BP.
Review feeding – volume and route. Remember that a *naso*gastric tube will obstruct 50% of the airway.
Haemoglobin (Hb) packed cell volume (PCV)
White blood cell count (WBC)
Blood glucose
   Urea, electrolytes
   Calcium, magnesium
   Albumin
Blood pH, gases, HCO_3
Infection screen to include
   Blood culture

Urine culture
CSF microscopy and culture
Nose, umbilical, rectal swabs
Chest X-ray
Ultrasound brain scan

Management

(a) Continuous monitoring of:

Heart rate
Breathing
TcPO_2/saturation
Skin and environmental temperatures

(b) Treat any underlying cause:

Antibiotics for infection
Remove any airway obstruction, e.g. a nasogastric tube
Temporarily reduce volume of enteral feeds (orogastric/trans-
    pyloric)
Treat cardiac failure with diuretic
Transfuse if Hb is <12 g/dl
Correct hypotension by transfusion of blood or plasma
Correct low glucose, calcium, sodium or albumin levels
Stabilize the thermoneutral environment
Nurse the baby prone to reduce the work of breathing and improve
    the effectiveness of diaphragmatic activity

(c) Treatment and prevention of attacks

Many apnoeic attacks are self-correcting or respond to tactile stimulation. Babies <35 weeks' gestation who have frequent apnoeas
should be commenced on aminophylline (see below). If more vigorous resuscitation is needed (e.g. bag-and-mask ventilation) or the
apnoeic attacks occur more often than every 3–4 hours then specific
treatment should be started.

(1) Start nasal CPAP (single- or double-prong), 2–4 cm H_2O
    pressure in air.
(2) FiO_2 may need to be increased slightly to prevent hypoxia but
    can cause hyperoxia in between attacks and these babies have a
    high risk of retinopathy of prematurity (ROP). Hyperoxia may
    also lead to less frequent but more severe apnoea. Monitor blood
    gases and keep PaO_2 in the range 50–70 mm Hg (6.5–9.1 kPa).
(3) Start aminophylline, 6 mg/kg i.v. loading dose, followed by 2

mg/kg 12 hourly. Monitor levels and adjust the dose to keep in the range 28–55 micromol/l. It may be necessary to increase the frequency to 8 hourly.

(4) If the attacks persist try IMV at a peak pressure of 10–15 cm H_2O at a rate of 5–15 breaths per minute down the nasal prongs.

(5) If all else fails, intubate and start IPPV at a rate of 10–20 breaths per minute. Pressures of 16 cm H_2O and PEEP of 3 cm H_2O with an inspiratory time of 0.5 sec.

(6) Doxapram may be helpful in the management of refractory apnoea (Barring *et al. J. Pediatr.*, 1986, **108:** 125–129.

Bibliography

Avery, M. E., Fletcher, B. D. and Williams, R. G. (1981). *The Lung and its Disorders in the Newborn Infant*, 4th edn. Philadelphia: W. B. Saunders.

Capitanio, M. A. and Kirkpatric, J. A. (1969). Roentgen examination in the evaluation of the newborn infant with respiratory distress. *J. Pediatr.*, **75**, 896–908.

Roberton, N. R. C. (1983). The care of neonates with respiratory failure. In: *Recent Advances in Perinatal Medicine*, Volume 1, Chapter 10. Edinburgh: Churchill Livingstone.

Ramsden, C. A. and Reynolds, E. O. R. (1987). Ventilator settings for newborn infants. Controversy and commentaries. *Arch. Dis. Child.*, **62**, 529–38.

Yu, V. H. (1986). Respiratory disorders in the newborn. *Current Reviews in Paediatrics*, Volume 2. Edinburgh: Churchill Livingstone.

9

Cardiac problems

Incidence
Assessment of the infant with suspected heart disease
The cyanosed infant
The infant with heart failure
Asymptomatic heart murmurs
Neonatal arrhythmias

Incidence

Congenital heart disease (CHD) is found in approximately 7 per 1000
live births. It may occur as an isolated defect but is frequently found
in association with other malformations such as oesophageal atresia,
ano-rectal anomalies, exomphalos and skeletal defects. Congenital
heart disease is particularly common in chromosal defects and in
some maternal disorders:

	CHD frequency (%)	Common malformations
Chromosomal disorders		
Down's syndrome	40–60	Atrioventricular septal defect ventricular septal defect (VSD), atrial septal defect (ASD), patent ductus arteriosus (PDA)
Trisomy 18	90	VSD, PDA
Trisomy 13	80	ASD, VSD Atrial isomerism
Turner's syndrome	10–20	Coarctation Aortic and mitral valve abnormalities

	CHD frequency (%)	Common malformations
Maternal factors		
Rubella infection	35	PDA Pulmonary stenosis VSD, ASD
Diabetes mellitus	3–5	Transposition VSD Coarctation
Phenylketonuria	25–50	Tetralogy of Fallot
Fetal alcohol syndrome	25	VSD, ASD
Phenytoin	2–3	Pulmonary and aortic stenosis
Systemic lupus erythematosus (SLE)	30–40	Complete heart block

Assessment of the infant with suspected heart disease

History

Birth details (? peripartum asphyxia)
Maternal illness or drug ingestion
Family history
Symptoms in baby:
    Cyanosis
    Poor feeding
    Breathlessness
    Excess weight gain

Examination

Colour (cyanosis or pallor)
Respiratory rate, respiratory distress
Heart rate
Peripheral pulses: ? Inequality of volume between right and left brachial pulses
              ? Weak femoral pulses
              ? Pulses weak or bounding
Apex beat (RV or LV prominence)
Heart sounds: ? S2 single, widely split, or loud
             ? Gallop or ejection click
Murmur: nature, duration, loudness, site and radiation
Hepatomegaly

Lesion	Cyanosis	Heart failure	Heart shape	Pulmonary vascularity	Electrocardiogram
Pulmonary atresia with VSD	Severe	None	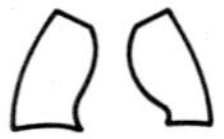 Hollow pulmonary arc; uptilted apex	Reduced	RAD RVH
Pulmonary atresia with intact septum	Severe	Occurs when RV very small	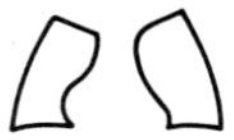 RA+	Reduced	Normal axis LVH or decreased right ventricular activity for age
Tricuspid atresia	Severe	None	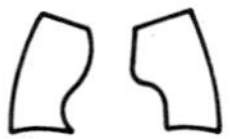 Square heart. RA+ Pulmonary arc hollow	Reduced	LAD LVH RAH
Tricuspid atresia with high pulmonary flow	Slight or moderate	Frequently	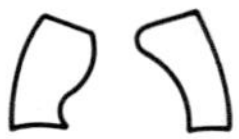 RA + Pulmonary arc +	Increased	LAD LVH RAH

Fig. 9.1 From Jordan S. C. and Scott O. (1981) *Heart Disease in Paediatrics*, 2nd Edit. London; Butterworth and Co. with permission

Condition	Cyanosis	Heart failure	Heart shape/size	Pulmonary vasculature	ECG
Severe pulmonary stenosis with VSD	Slight initially, gradually increasing	Rare in first month		Reduced	RAH++ RVH
Ebstein's disease	Moderate	rare in first month	Large RA	Reduced	RAH Right bundle branch block
Transposition with intact septum	Rapidly becomes severe	Second to fourth week	Large RA — Narrow pedicle, Egg-shaped heart	Normal or increased	RVH
Total anomalous PVD with obstruction	Rapidly becomes severe	Liver enlarged if drainage below diaphragm	Normal size	Pulmonary venous congestion	RAH RVH
Hypoplasia of left heart	Slight at first, increasing by third day	First few days of life and is severe	General enlargement	Increased + pulmonary venous congestion	RVH RAD

Fig. 9.1 (continued)

Lesion	Cyanosis	Heart failure	Heart shape	Pulmonary vascularity	Electrocardiogram
Coarctation of aorta	Slight	In first week; left heart failure frequent	General enlargement	Increased + pulmonary venous congestion	RVH RAD
Truncus	Slight or moderate	In first few weeks	Pulmonary arteries high up or not seen	Increased	RVH but may be LVH or combination of RV + LV
Atrioventricular canal	None	In first few weeks	RA + PA + RV + LV +	Increased	LAD, rsR pattern in $V_3R + V_1$. Usually combined ventricular hypertrophy
Normal heart with enlarged thymus	None	None	Broad pedicle	Normal	Normal

Fig. 9.1 (continued)

Oedema
Peripheral perfusion and temperature
Blood pressure in all four limbs

Investigation

Chest X-ray
ECG
Arterial blood gas
Hyperoxia test if hypoxaemic
Echocardiogram

Chest X-ray interpretation (see Fig. 9.1)

Heart size, shape and position. Do not be confused by the thymic
    shadow which is very variable in size and shape
Pulmonary vascularity: ? Oligaemic or plethoric
Pulmonary oedema, fluid in horizontal fissure
Position of aortic arch: ? Left or right sided
Position of liver and gastric bubble: ? Abnormal situs
Skeletal abnormality

ECG interpretation (see Fig. 9.1)

QRS axis (see Fig. 9.2)

(1) Use leads 1 and aVF or 1 and 11.
(2) Measure the height of R and subtract depth of S in lead 1, plot
    $(R-S)$ along axis of lead 1.
(3) Repeat the above procedure for lead aVF (or 11) and plot along
    axis of aVF (or 11).
(4) Draw lines perpendicular to the lead axes through the plotted
    points. Joint the point of intersection of the perpendicular lines
    to the origin, this is the **QRS** axis.

The normal neonatal **QRS** axis is 60°–160° (mean 130°). The axis
moves to the left during the first months of life and is 5°–105° (mean
60°) by 6 months of age.
    Left axis deviation (0–90°) in a cyanotic infant suggests tricuspid
atresia and in a non-cyanotic infant suggests an atrioventricular
septal defect.

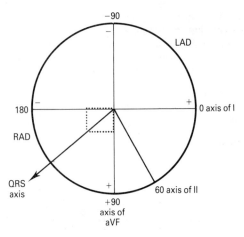

Fig. 9.2   Calculation of QRS axis of ECG (see text).

P wave

$P > 3$ mm in any lead = right atrial hypertrophy.
Biphasic *P* or terminal *P* inversion in lead V1 > 1 mm = left atrial hypertrophy.

PR interval

Normal range: 0.07–0.16 sec.
Prolonged in first degree heart block. Shortened in Wolff–Parkinson–White syndrome and junctional rhythm.

Q wave

$Q > 4$ mm in V6 = septal hypertrophy.
$Q > 0.03$ sec is pathological, e.g. in myocardial infarction associated with anomalous origin of the left coronary artery.

T wave

During the first 3 days the *T* wave may be inverted in leads I, aVL and V6 and upright in V1. After the 3rd day the *T* wave axis changes and becomes upright in I, II, aVF and V6 and inverted in V1.

Right ventricular hypertrophy

QR pattern in V1 (need to look carefully to exclude a small initial positive deflection).

$R > 30$ mm in V1, S in V6 > 10 mm.
Upright T in V1 after 48 hours of age.
Right ventricular hypoplasia as seen in tricuspid atresia or pulmonary atresia with intact ventricular septum may be suspected if there are low right-sided voltages, e.g. R in V1 $< S$ in V1.

Left ventricular hypertrophy

S in V1 > 22 mm
R in V6 > 16 mm

***ST* segment**

Elevation seen in pericarditis, myocarditis and myocardial infarction. Depression suggests myocardial ischaemia (e.g. peripartum asphyxia), 'ventricular strain' or digoxin treatment.

Hyperoxia test

Suspected cyanosis must always be confirmed by measurement of the PaO_2 on blood obtained from the right radial artery. The hyperoxia test requires measurement of the PaO_2 (or $TcPO_2$ from preductal skin) in air and after breathing 100% oxygen for 10 min. If the PaO_2 fails to exceed 150 mm Hg (19.5 kPa) a right-to-left shunt due to CHD or severe respiratory disease is present.

Echocardiography

Cross-sectional and Doppler echocardiography has facilitated the rapid and accurate diagnosis of CHD. Many neonatal units have ultrasound scanners suitable for screening patients with suspected heart disease but, even in specialized units, conditions such as anomalous pulmonary venous connection may be difficult to diagnose. If in doubt it is better to seek cardiological opinion early.

The normal echocardiographic views are shown in Fig. 9.3.

Presentation of infants with heart disease

Presentation is usually with cyanosis, heart failure, cardiac murmur or any combination of these.

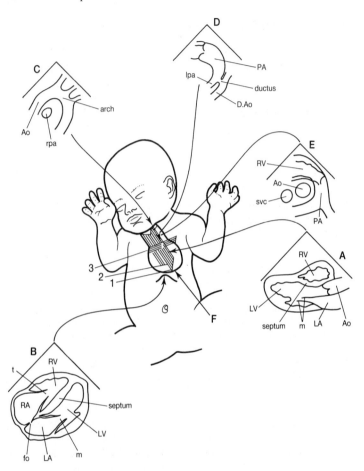

Fig. 9.3 Diagram illustrating echocardiographic cross-sectional planes (2D). *1*: Long axis plane (approximately sagittal); *2*: Four chambers plane (approximately frontal): *3:* Short axis plane (approximately transverse).

Transducer sites and planes obtainable are indicated as follows: A. Left parasternal (long axis plane – also short axis and parasternal four chambers, obtained by rotating and angling transducer. B. Subxiphoid (Four chambers – also long axis by rotating transducer). C. High parasternal and transternal (High short axis or long axis parasagittal – 'ductus' cut). F. Apex (four chambers or long axis). D, E. Suprasternal (semi-long axis for aortic arch).

A, B, C, D, E, F. Diagrammatic representations of normal cross-sectional views.

A. 'Long axis' cut as seen with transducer in left parasternal position.

The cyanosed infant

Common causes of cyanosis

Transposition of the great arteries; Pulmonary atresia ± VSD;
Tetralogy of Fallot; Tricuspid atresia; Total anomalous
pulmonary venous connection; Ebstein's malformation.
Persistent pulmonary hypertension (persistent fetal circulation)
Severe lung disease

Transposition of the great arteries

The most frequent cyanotic defect in the neonatal period. The aorta
arises from the right ventricle and lies anterior to the pulmonary
artery arising from the left ventricle. Depth of cyanosis is dependent
on the degree of mixing between the two parts of the circulation,
either via the foramen ovale, PDA or VSD when present. Cyanosis is
present from birth and usually increases over the first 24–48 hours in
the absence of a significant VSD. Signs of heart failure may develop
after 2 or 3 weeks if there is a large PDA or VSD. Murmur is absent
unless VSD or pulmonary stenosis is present.

The ECG shows right ventricular hypertrophy (RVH) but may
appear normal initially.

Chest X-ray is frequently normal but may show pulmonary
plethora or 'egg on side' cardiac shadow with a narrow superior
mediastinum.

Echocardiography confirms the diagnosis.

Treatment   Maintain ductal patency with a prostaglandin infusion
(see page 122). Balloon atrial septostomy (Rashkind) is performed to

---

B. 'Four chambers' cut as seen from sub-xiphoid view.
C. Semi-long axis cut of aortic arch as obtained from the supernatural view.
D. High long axis para-sagittal view to show ductus arteriosus.
E. Short axis cut through the great arteries just above the heart.
Abbreviations: RV = Right ventricle. LV = Left ventricle. Ao = Aorta.
m = Mitral valve leaflets. t = Tricuspid valve leaflets. fo = Foramen ovale.
rpa = Right pulmonary artery. lpa = Left pulmonary artery. PA =
Pulmonary artery. D. Ao = Descending aorta. svc = Superior vena cava.
LA = Left atrium. RA = Right atrium.

From Roberton, N. R. C. *Textbook of Neonatology*. Churchill
Livingstone, London 1986 with permission.

create a large ASD to allow intracardiac mixing. Corrective surgery using the arterial switch operation may be performed in the first or second week.

Pulmonary atresia

There is no direct connection between the right ventricle and the pulmonary artery, so pulmonary blood flow depends on the PDA and severe cyanosis develops when the duct closes. The commonest type of atresia occurs with VSD. The degree of development of the pulmonary arteries is very variable; in a few cases the pulmonary arteries may be absent and pulmonary flow is dependent on collateral arteries.

Murmurs are frequent and usually originate from the PDA or collateral arteries. Single second heart sound is present.

The ECG shows RVH initially, later biventricular hypertrophy may be seen.

Chest X-ray shows pulmonary oligaemia with a hollow pulmonary arc and an uptilted apex.

Echocardiography shows the VSD with aortic over-ride and the atretic pulmonary valve. The hypoplastic pulmonary arteries and PDA can usually be seen.

Treatment   Maintain ductal patency with prostaglandin infusion (page 122). Urgent palliative surgery is usually required.

Pulmonary atresia with intact interventricular septum

This presents in a similar way. In the absence of a VSD the right ventricle is hypoplastic.

The ECG shows left ventricular dominance with reduced RV voltages.

There may be significant tricuspid regurgitation resulting in a murmur.

Right atrial dilatation is seen on the chest X-ray.

The echocardiogram shows a small cavity right ventricle with thickened walls and pulmonary atresia.

Treatment   As for pulmonary atresia with VSD.

Critical pulmonary stenosis

This presents in a similar manner to pulmonary atresia with intact ventricular septum, but the right ventricle tends to be less hypoplastic and may even be hypertrophied. There is usually a harsh pulmonary ejection murmur and ejection click.

Echocardiography shows the stenosed pulmonary valve.

Treatment Maintain ductal patency (page 122) until either surgical valvotomy or balloon valvoplasty can be performed.

Tetralogy of Fallot

This usually presents outside the neonatal period, but is often diagnosed early because of echocardiographic screening of infants with a cardiac murmur.

It is characterized by a malalignment VSD with an over-riding aorta and narrowing of the right ventricular outflow tract, pulmonary valve and pulmonary arteries. Cyanosis in the neonatal period is usually associated with severe infundibular stenosis and pulmonary artery hypoplasia. Less severe forms tend to present with a harsh pulmonary ejection murmur, single second sound and mild cyanosis.

The ECG shows RVH.

The chest X-ray shows pulmonary oligaemia and sometimes a hollow pulmonary arc and uptilted apex. The aortic arch is right sided in 30% of cases.

Echocardiography demonstrates the typical anatomy and the side of the aortic arch.

Treatment Infants with hypoxaemia may require a prostaglandin infusion and subsequent systemic-to-pulmonary shunt operation. The typical cyanotic spells seen in older children are rare during the neonatal period.

Tricuspid atresia

There is either complete absence or imperforate tricuspid valve with an obligatory right-to-left shunt via the foramen ovale. Pulmonary blood flow is duct dependent when there is associated pulmonary atresia. Usually there is a VSD with narrowing of the right ventricular outflow and pulmonary valve. Depth of cyanosis depends on the size of the VSD and the degree of pulmonary stenosis. In 20% of cases there is transposition of the great arteries. This group has a high pulmonary flow and a poor long-term prognosis.

There is often a murmur at the lower left sternal border and a single second sound.

The ECG shows left axis deviation and left ventricular dominance.

Chest X-ray may show pulmonary oligaemia and a prominent right atrium.

Echocardiography reveals the right ventricular hypoplasia, the absent or imperforate tricuspid valve and the size of the VSD and degree of pulmonary stenosis.

Treatment   Prostaglandin infusion may be required if severe cyanosis occurs. Severe cyanosis after the ductus has closed requires a systemic-to-pulmonary shunt operation.

Total anomalous pulmonary venous connection

The pulmonary veins form a confluence behind the left atrium and thence connect either to the superior vena cava via an ascending vein (supracardiac) or to the portal vein via a descending vein (infracardiac) or directly to the right atrium or coronary sinus (intracardiac). Obstruction to pulmonary venous flow is commonly seen with the infracardiac and supracardiac forms. With severe obstruction the infant will be very ill soon after birth. Cyanosis is severe and is associated with respiratory failure from the pulmonary oedema. Hepatomegaly may be present. There is usually no murmur and this disorder is often confused with severe respiratory disease.

The ECG may be normal at first, but later shows RVH and right atrial hypertrophy (RAH).

Chest X-ray in obstruction may show a normal heart size with severe pulmonary venous congestion and pulmonary oedema. It may appear similar to RDS.

Echocardiography can usually demonstrate the presence and site of the anomalous pulmonary venous connection. The left ventricle and left atrium appear small with a dilated right atrium and ventricle. When the pulmonary flow is low it may be less easy to recognize and cardiac catheterization may be necessary.

Treatment   Surgical repair is required (urgent if obstructed). Prostaglandin infusion may be deleterious.

Ebstein's malformation

The posterior and septal leaflets of the tricuspid valve are attached nearer the right ventricular apex than normal. This results in a small right ventricular cavity and a variable degree of tricuspid regurgitation. Anatomically more severe defects present soon after birth with moderate cyanosis and heart failure. Cyanosis usually improves during the first month as the pulmonary vascular resistance falls.

Large 'v' waves and a pulsatile liver may be seen when regurgitation is severe.

The ECG may appear normal initially but later usually shows RAH, right bundle branch block and first degree heart block.

Chest X-ray shows gross cardiomegaly due to right atrial dilatation and pulmonary oligaemia.

Echocardiography demonstrates the tricuspid anatomy and right atrial dilatation.

Treatment Heart failure may require the use of diuretics. Surgical treatment in infancy has poor results and supportive therapy is the best option as spontaneous improvement is likely. Less severe forms carry a much better prognosis.

Persistent pulmonary hypertension (persistent fetal circulation)

This may occur as a primary disorder or be associated with RDS, asphyxia, meconium aspiration, polycythaemia or diaphragmatic hernia. Cyanosis occurs soon after birth. The heart is structurally normal but there is right-to-left shunting at atrial and ductal levels because of high pulmonary vascular resistance. Murmurs or signs of cardiac failure are not usually a feature. The ECG likely to be normal.

Chest X-ray may show pulmonary oligaemia and a normal heart size. There may be evidence of meconium aspiration or RDS.

Echocardiography will reveal a normal heart with a large PDA. The main difficulty is differentiating from obstructed total anomalous pulmonary venous connection, and a careful examination of the pulmonary veins is required.

Treatment Correct polycythaemia and hypotension. Mechanical ventilation is often required. Tolazoline, 0.5–1 mg/kg, i.v. as a bolus followed by an infusion of 0.1–1.0 mg/kg/hour is the treatment of choice. This is a general vasodilator, not a selective pulmonary vasodilator, and systemic hypotension may need correction by plasma infusion. Epoprostanol (prostacyclin) can be used as an alternative by infusion at 5–10 ng/kg/min.

Management of cyanotic heart disease

All patients with suspected cyanotic CHD require referral for paediatric cardiological assessment. The major difficulties are to differentiate heart disease from persistent pulmonary hypertension, RDS or transient tachypnoea.

Prostaglandin E$_1$ therapy

Maintenance of ductal patency is important in the majority of the cyanotic defects and in certain obstructive lesions on the left side of the heart (see page 117). This can be achieved by iv. or oral prostaglandin therapy. An intravenous infusion is the preferred route for sick infants and the usual dose is 10–20 ng/kg/min, although occasionally up to 50 ng/kg/min may be used. To prepare an i.v. infusion put 500 microg of prostaglandin E$_1$ in 500 ml of 5% glucose to make a solution of 1 microg/ml. This can be run at 1 ml/kg/hour to achieve an infusion rate of 16 ng/kg/min. The oral dose is 62.5 microg 1–3 hourly. The side-effects include apnoea, usually with the higher doses, pyrexia and jitteriness. It may also predispose to necrotizing enterocolitis.

Prostaglandin therapy is generally well tolerated and can dramatically improve sick infants. If the diagnosis of a duct-dependent lesion is incorrect, it is unlikely to cause harm (but see above: Total anomalous pulmonary venous connection).

Treatment of metabolic acidosis   Maintain thermoneutral environment and consider IPPV, particularly if there is a respiratory component to the acidosis. If hypotensive give plasma and/or positive inotropic support using a dopamine infusion (5–10 microg/kg/min). Heart failure may need treating with diuretics.

The infant with heart failure

Clinical signs of neonatal heart failure

Tachycardia >200/min at rest
Tachypnoea >60/min; 'respiratory distress' and/or apnoea in the preterm infant
Hepatomegaly >1.5 cm below the costal margin (most specific sign)
Gallop rhythm
Peripheral oedema and excessive weight gain
Hypotension and poor peripheral perfusion is a later sign

Causes of neonatal heart failure

Cardiac failure has many causes and is not always due to a structural heart abnormality.

(1) Congenital heart defects

(a) Left heart obstructive lesions:
Hypoplastic left heart syndrome
Coarctation of the aorta
Interrupted aortic arch
Aortic stenosis
Cor triatriatum

(b) Left-to-right shunts:
Patent ductus arteriosus
Ventricular septal defect
Atrioventricular septal defects
Common arterial trunk (truncus arteriosus)
Complex lesions with high pulmonary blood flow (e.g. double inlet left ventricle)

(c) Primary myocardial failure:
Endocardial fibro-elastosis
Hypertrophic cardiomyopathy (infant of diabetic mother, glycogen storage disease or familial)
Myocarditis
Myocardial ischaemia secondary to birth asphyxia
Anomalous origin of the left coronary artery from the pulmonary trunk

(d) Arrhythmias:
Supraventricular tachycardia
Complete heart block

(2) Other causes
Anaemia
Polycythaemia
Sepsis
Hypoglycaemia
Hypocalcaemia
Hypo- or hyperthyroidism
Arterio-venous malformation (usually cerebral or hepatic)
Fluid overload

Hypoplastic left heart syndrome

Comprises hypoplasia of the ascending aorta and left ventricle (unless VSD is also present), associated with either hypoplasia or atresia of the aortic and mitral values. Systemic circulation is supplied via a large PDA. Infants may appear normal at first but rapidly become ill when the PDA starts to close (usually after 12–72 hours). They appear pale and cyanosed with weak pulses. Severe heart failure ensues. There is often a soft ejection murmur at the left sternal border, and the second sound appears loud and single.

The ECG shows RVH with reduced left ventricular voltages.

Chest X-ray shows cardiomegaly with pulmonary plethora and oedema. Occasionally, the heart size is normal with intense pulmonary oedema similar to obstructed total anomalous pulmonary venous connection.

Echocardiography demonstrates the aortic hypoplasia (diameter usually <4 mm), left ventricular hypoplasia and aortic and mitral valve atresia.

Coarctation and interruption of the aorta

This includes spectrum of aortic arch abnormalities varying from the discrete narrowing below the left subclavian artery to complete interruption of the aortic arch. Associated lesions are common; usually aortic valve stenosis or VSD. Systemic flow to the lower part of the body is dependent on a PDA.

Presentation with heart failure occurs from 1–10 days of age. Femoral pulses will be weak or absent when the PDA has started to close. Inequality of the volume of the brachial pulses may be present in interruption or if the left subclavian artery is involved in the area of coarctation. A blood pressure difference of >20 mm Hg between the upper and lower limbs is a valuable sign. There will be an ejection murmur and gallop rhythm in many cases.

The ECG usually shows RVH, but it may be normal.

Chest X-ray reveals cardiomegaly with pulmonary plethora.

The anatomy of the aortic arch can usually be seen from the suprasternal of high parasternal echocardiographic views.

Treatment   Give diuretics for heart failure; in sick infants assisted ventilation and dopamine infusion may be necessary. Dramatic improvement is often seen with prostaglandin therapy. Urgent surgical repair is required.

Aortic valve stenosis

Severe aortic valve stenosis causes heart failure during the first few days of life. The peripheral pulses are weak or impalpable. There is an aortic stenotic murmur, sometimes with an ejection click.

The ECG shows LVH with variable T wave changes. Chest X-ray shows cardiomegaly. Echocardiography will reveal a thickened narrow valve, and hypertrophied and often poorly functioning left ventricle.

Treatment Medical treatment is required as for coarctation, and surgical or balloon valvotomy at the time of cardiac catheterization.

Cor triatriatum

This is a rare condition where a membrane divides the left atrium into two chambers and restricts flow from the pulmonary veins into the left ventricle.

Presentation, ECG and radiographic features are similar to obstructed total anomalous pulmonary venous connection. The main difference is the absence of cyanosis. The left atrial membrane can be seen well by echocardiography.

Treatment Surgical excision of the membrane is curative.

Patent ductus arteriosus

This is an important cause of heart failure in the preterm infant (see page 127).

Ventricular septal defect

A large VSD may cause increasing heart failure from the 2nd to 3rd week, as the pulmonary vascular resistance starts to fall and the left-to-right shunt increases. There is a harsh murmur at the left sternal border and a mitral diastolic murmur at the apex.

The ECG shows biventricular hypertrophy.

Chest X-ray shows cardiomegaly with pulmonary plethora.

Echocardiography can identify the site and size of the defect. Doppler echocardiography can predict the degree of pulmonary hypertension.

Treatment Use medical therapy at first with diuretics, but surgical closure is required for infants who fail to thrive or have severe pulmonary hypertension after 6 months of age.

Atrioventricular septal defect

This is commonly seen in Down's syndrome. There is a common atrioventricular valve rather than separate mitral and tricuspid valves. Presentation is similar to VSD. The infant may have pan-systolic murmur of atrioventricular valve regurgitation.

The ECG shows left axis deviation and biventricular hypertrophy.
Chest X-ray shows cardiomegaly and pulmonary plethora.

Echocardiography demonstrates the typical anatomy of the defect and any associated lesions (e.g. PDA).

Treatment　As for VSD.

Common arterial trunk (truncus arteriosus)

There is a single main artery leaving the heart with varible origin of the pulmonary arteries from it. A VSD is present and the common arterial valve over-rides the ventricular septum. Cyanosis is mild, with high volume peripheral pulses, an ejection systolic (and sometimes early diastolic) murmur, ejection click and single second sound.

The ECG shows biventricular hypertrophy $\pm$ LV strain pattern.

Chest X-ray shows cardiomegaly and pulmonary plethora.

Echocardiography identifies the abnormal truncal valve overriding the ventricular septum.

Treatment　Surgical correction in infancy.

Anomalous origin of the left coronary artery from the pulmonary trunk

This is a rare condition causing heart failure at 1–4 months of age.

The ECG is often diagnostic showing deep, wide Q waves and T wave inversion in the left-sided chest leads.

The anomalous origin of the left coronary artery can be seen on echocardiogram and the degree of left ventricular dysfunction assessed.

Treatment　Usually treatment is surgical with re-implantation or reduction of the left coronary artery.

Treatment of heart failure

Supportive treatment consists of oxygen therapy, temperature maintenance and respiratory support as necessary.

Fluid restriction to 75% of maintenance requirements and diuretic therapy (frusemide, 1–2 mg/kg, 12 hourly) are the mainstays of treatment. Additional benefit may be obtained using vasodilator therapy, e.g. captopril or hydrallazine.

Digoxin probably has little effect in conditions with a large left-to-right shunt but may be useful if there is any left ventricular dysfunction. Digoxin dose is 8 microg/kg/day for preterm infants and 10 microg/kg/day for term infants, both in two divided doses. Great caution is required in the presence of renal impairment and frequent monitoring of serum levels is recommended.

In the presence of systemic hypotension and peripheral hypoperfusion, give dopamine, 5 microg/kg/min by i.v. infusion.

If the above measures fail to control the heart failure then surgical correction should be considered.

Patent ductus arteriosus in the preterm infant

Clinically apparent PDA occurs in about 75% of infants of <1.0 kg and in 10–15% of those of 1.5–2.0 kg. The lower the gestational age and sicker the infant, the less likely it is that the PDA will close.

Clinical features

High volume peripheral pulses.
Systolic murmur peaking towards the second heart sound, maximal upper left sternal border and radiates to the back. Continuous murmur sometimes.
Need for increased or prolonged respiratory support without evidence of increased lung disease.
Pulmonary plethora and cardiomegaly on chest X-ray.

Management

(1) Restrict fluid to 75% of basal requirement.
(2) Avoid hypoxia as this will tend to keep ductus open.
(3) Maintain haemoglobin (Hb) >12 g/dl by small volume blood transfusions.
(4) Diuretic therapy (frusemide, 1–2 mg/kg, 12 hourly).
(5) If the above measures do not succeed consider indomethacin therapy (see below).
(6) If indomethacin fails or is contraindicated and symptoms persist consider surgical ligation.

Indomethacin therapy

Indomethacin is a prostaglandin synthetase inhibitor which can be used to close the duct but has many side-effects including:

Transient renal failure: oliguria, rising blood urea and creatinine (see p. 235)
Hyponatraemia
Gastrointestinal and intracranial bleeding
Decreased platelet aggregation
Displacement of bound bilirubin

Its use is therefore contraindicated in babies with bleeding disorders (including Intraventricular haemorrhage), thrombocytopenia, necrotizing enterocolitis, bilirubin over 200 micromol/l, a creatinine over 100 micromol/l or urea over 5 mmol/l.

Dose   Two regimens are in use:

(1) 0.2 mg/kg/24 hours i.v. or oral, once daily for a maximum of three doses.
(2) 0.1 mg/kg/24 hours i.v. or oral, once daily for a maximum of six doses.

Measure urea, creatinine, electrolytes, FBC, platelets and urine output before treatment and then daily, i.e. before next dose and for three days after treatment.

Asymptomatic heart murmurs

Murmurs are common in the neonatal period and are often innocent, but the diagnosis of an innocent murmur should be made with caution. The murmur of a PDA is often present during the first 24 hours but should disappear subsequently.

The most common murmur encountered is a mid-systolic murmur at the left sternal border often radiating to the back. This is frequently innocent but is difficult to differentiate from mild pulmonary or aortic stenosis.

The murmur of significant pulmonary or aortic stenosis will be present on the first day and is usually associated with an ejection click.

Ventricular septal defects usually produce a harsh pansystolic murmur after the first 24 hours, as the pulmonary vascular resistance falls.

Management

All babies with a murmur must have a full examination and if the murmur persists beyond the age of 36–48 hours the following should be carried out:

Chest X-ray
ECG
Regular observations of heart rate, respiratory rate, feeding and
daily weight
Examine daily until discharge at 7 days
Follow-up in 4 weeks

Neonatal arrhythmias

Supraventricular tachycardia (SVT)

Paroxysmal episodes of heart rate 200–300/min occur. These usually
start and stop abruptly. The heart is commonly structurally normal,
but occasionally it is associated with Ebstein's malformation.

The infant presents with pallor, sweating, rapid breathing and
difficulty with feeding. Tachycardia is often well tolerated despite a
heart rate of 300/min. Diagnosis is made from an ECG where a
tachycardia with a narrow *QRS* complex is seen. *P* waves may be seen
between *QRS* complexes (best seen in V1). About 30% of cases have
Wolff–Parkinson–White syndrome and following return to sinus
rhythm this should be looked for (short *PR* interval with a delta wave
on the upstroke of the *QRS* complex).

Management

If attacks are short lived and infrequent then no drug treatment will
be necessary. Prolonged episodes may cause heart failure but rarely
cause death.

(1) Vagal stimulation by carotid sinus massage or a facial ice pack
    can be used first.
(2) Give three doses of digoxin, 10 microg/kg/i.m. 8 hourly followed
    by the standard maintenance dose. Great caution required in the
    presence of renal impairment when it is best to give a single dose
    and then check the serum level.
(3) If the infant is sick, synchronized D.C. cardioversion should be
    tried. Start with 5 joules, but this can be increased to 3–4
    joules/kg if necessary.
(4) Drug therapy can be used for regaining sinus rhythm. Pro-
    pranolol, 1 mg/kg, 8 hourly can be given orally. Caution is
    required when giving this i.v. (dose, 0.01–0.1 mg/kg, slowly).
    Verapamil should be avoided in infants as it may cause acute
    cardiovascular collapse and death. Flecainide (1–2 mg/kg, i.v.
    over 20 min) and disopyramide (0.5–2 mg/kg, i.v., slowly)

appear relatively safe and are particularly effective in Wolff –Parkinson–White syndrome.

Many infants with SVT have only a single episode. If recurrence occurs maintenance treatment with oral digoxin is required for 12 months.

Congenital heart block

This is often diagnosed antenatally because of persistent fetal brady-cardia. The heart rate is usually <80/min. Fifty per cent of infants have structural heart defects, usually 'congenitally corrected' trans-position or left atrial isomerism with atrioventricular septal defect. Many of those without structural abnormalities are associated with maternal anti-Ro antibodies as seen in systemic lupus erythematosus.

Presentation is with a persistent bradycardia (40–60/min). Heart failure may occur in a small proportion.

The ECG shows dissociation between the atrial and ventricular activity (3rd degree block).

Treatment Frequently no treatment is required. If there is a structural heart abnormality, heart failure, wide *QRS* complex, persistent bradycardia <55/min or frequent ventricular ectopy car-diac pacing should be considered. In sick infants with severe brady-cardia isoprenaline infusion can be used to increase the heart rate.

Bibliography

Anderson, R. H., Macartney, F. J., Shinebourne, E. A. and Tynan, M. (1987). *Paediatric Cardiology*. London: Churchill Livingstone.

Davignon, A., Rautaharju, P., Boisselle, E. *et al.*, (1979). Normal ECG standards for infants and children. *Pediatr. Cardiol.*, **1**, 123–31.

Jordan, S. C. and Scott, O. (1989). *Heart Disease in Paediatrics, 3rd edn*. Guildford: Butterworth Scientific.

Gersony, W. M., Peckham, G. J., Ellison, R. C. *et al.* (1983). Effects of indomethacin in premature infants with patent ductus arteriosus: results of a national collaborative study. *J. Paediatr.*, **102**, 895–906.

10

Neurological disorders

Neurological assessment
Neonatal convulsions
Haemorrhagic and ischaemic brain lesions
Hydrocephalus
Perinatal asphyxia and cerebral intensive care
The floppy infant
Spina bifida and meningomyelocele
Other developmental defects

The newborn infant is susceptible to a wide range of neurological disorders, both congenitally determined and acquired during ante-natal, perinatal and postnatal life. Longer term neurological integrity is perhaps the most important factor in determining the quality of life for the child and parents. Careful and appropriate medical intervention is thus essential.

Neurological assessment

Neonatal neurological assessment is particularly sensitive to external influences (Table 10.1) which may make interpretation difficult. Always record the child's behavioural state (asleep, quiet and awake, irritable etc.). Neurological assessment may form part of gestational assessment (see Chapter 18). A fuller protocol is found in Dubowitz and Dubowitz (1979).

Head circumference (HC)

Measure carefully and plot on a centile chart (see Fig. 19.1 and 19.2, pages 273–4). Hold the end of the tape over the flat temporal region

Table 10.1   Factors which may influence neurological assessment

Drugs
(Direct administration or via placenta or breast milk)
   Drugs of abuse/alcohol
   Antihypertensives
   Analgesics/sedatives/anaesthetics
   Anticonvulsants (especially benzodiazepines/phenobarbitone)

Systemic illness
   Infection, RDS, hypothermia

Short gestation
   See Chapter 18

Behavioural state
   Initially alert but somnolescence from 48 hours

Hunger
   Irritable before feeds

Maternal illness
   Diabetes, toxaemia

Perinatal history

Family history

for greatest reproducibility. The HC may change by 5–6 mm as moulding resolves in the first few days and subsequently increases by 5–8 mm/week. Review HC before discharge if >97th centile; early ultrasound scan will show presence or absence of hydrocephalus. The commonest cause of a large HC is constitutional or familial; check parents' HC (97th centile: adult men 58.5 cm; adult women 58 cm). If the HC is below the 3rd centile look for evidence of congenital infection (Chapter 14) or dysmorphic features (Chapter 6).

Neurological examination

Assess posture, movement, limb and truncal tone, reflexes and neurobehaviour.

Posture   Check degree of limb flexion when supine.

Movement   Note frequency of spontaneous movement, tremors, hand clenching, thumb adduction, rhythmic mouthing and 'cycling' or 'swimming' movements of limbs.

Limb tone: Look for asymmetry. Assess by degree of elbow and knee flexion during arm and leg traction, respectively. Note also degree and speed of recoil on release.

Neck and truncal tone: Assess extensor and flexor muscles separately – better extensor control suggests abnormally high extensor tone or compensation for upper airways obstruction. Head control is assessed by the ability to return the head to vertical after allowing it to fall forwards and then back when held in the sitting position. Then compare the head posture in ventral suspension with head lag during traction to sitting posture.

Reflexes: Check tendon reflexes – there should be a wide range of normal reflex activity. Primitive reflexes, e.g. palmar, plantar, rooting, Moro response (useful if asymmetrical but otherwise only measure of degree of responsiveness) may be present in anencephalic infants.

Neurobehaviour: Check auditory response – startle or stilling to rattle at 10 cm, from 28 weeks' gestation.

Check visual response – light reactive pupils, blinking to flashes, fixation on an object at 20 cm. Some neonates may follow laterally and vertically.

Also assess *alertness, irritability* and *consolability* when crying.

Skin signs and neurological problems

Signs	*Association*
Jaundice	Kernicterus
Café-au-lait spots	Neurofibromatosis
Depigmented patches	Tuberous sclerosis
Trigeminal port-wine stain	Sturge–Weber syndrome
Giant pigmented lesions of the head	Meningeal naevi: convulsions and hydrocephalus

Neonatal convulsions

Neonatal convulsions are common and underdiagnosed because of the relative rarity of classic tonic/clonic signs.

Categories of convulsions

Subtle: The most common type. Look for tonic deviation of the eyes, fluttering of the eyelids, sucking and chewing, 'cycling' of the arms and legs and apnoea (often *not* accompanied by bradycardia but usually associated with other subtle signs).

Multifocal clonic: Non-ordered migratory clonic convulsions.

Focal clonic: Usually a manifestation of metabolic disturbance.

Tonic: Especially preterm infants, often indicating cerebral damage. Extension and stiffening of the body and upward deviation of the eyes.

Myoclonic: Least common. Synchronized jerking of limbs; distinguish from jitteriness by grasping and gently flexing the limb, which abolishes jitters but has no effect on myoclonic jerks.

Causes of convulsions

Neonatal seizures are usually secondary to underlying brain disturbances in contrast to the primary epilepsies of childhood. Up to 90% may be ascribed to definite or probable aetiologies.

Metabolic

Hypoglycaemia (see Chapter 13, page 192)
Hypoglycaemia (see Chapter 13, page 193)
Hypomagnesaemia (see Chapter 13, page 197)
Hyper- and hyponatraemia (see Chapter 17, page 256)
Inborn errors of metabolism, including:
    Organic acidaemias (Chapter 13, page 208)
    Pyridoxine dependency
    Non-ketotic hyperglycinaemia (Chapter 13, page 206)
    Urea-cycle disorders (Chapter 13, page 208)

Haemorrhagic/ischaemic encephalopathy

Perinatal asphyxia
Subarachnoid haemorrhage
Tentorial tear
Subdural haemorrhage
Periventricular brain lesions in preterm infants
Cerebral contusion

Infections

Meningitis

Severe systemic infection (e.g. septicaemia, urinary tract infection)
Herpes, rubella, toxoplasmosis, cytomegalovirus, Coxsackie B and
   echovirus infections
Other CNS infections

Drugs and toxins

Drug withdrawal (narcotics, barbiturates, amphetamines)
Local anaesthetic (accidentally given into fetal scalp before delivery)
Kernicterus

Others

Idiopathic
Fifth day fits (? zinc deficiency)
Benign familial
Polycythaemia
Cerebral malformation or arteriovenous malformation
Cerebral venous thrombosis
Incontinentia pigmenti

Investigation

Must include: Blood sugar (check BM stix IMMEDIATELY)
                   Serum electrolytes (calculate anion gap – normal
                      <15 mmol/l (see page 407)
                   Serum calcium (total or ionized)
                   Blood gases and pH
                   Sepsis screen including lumbar puncture (see
                      Chapter 14, page 216)
                   Packed cell volume (PCV), white blood cell (WBC)
                      count and platelets
                   Cerebral ultrasound

May include: Magnesium
                   Metabolic screen
                   Clotting screen
                   EEG
                   CT scan

NB   The EEG may be useful in confirming seizure activity in the
presence of subtle neurological signs, for assessing control in children
treated with sedatives or muscle relaxants, and for prognosis.
Seizures may arise from deep neural seizures and some (e.g. tonic)
may not be associated with EEG discharges.

Management

Treatment of a prolonged seizure is urgent as the enormously increased oxygen consumption during a fit may outstrip its delivery.

Correct underlying disorder

For example, hypoglycaemia, hypocalcaemia (Chapter 13, page 192) or meningitis (Chapter 14, page 218).

Anticonvulsant drugs (in order of preference)

Phenobarbitone: Give a loading dose of 20 mg/kg as 10 mg/kg followed by a further 10 mg/kg 30–60 min later if no response. Maintenance treatment may be started after 3–4 days if required: half-life 60–180 hours; therapeutic range: 20–30 microg/ml (45– 110 micromol/l).

Phenytoin: Give a loading dose of 20 mg/kg over 15 min followed by maintenance. Beware of dysrhythmias during i.v. administration: therapeutic range 10–20 microg/ml (40–80 micromol/l).

Paraldehyde: Stat dose of rectal preparation or i.v. infusion of 5% solution at 0.5–2.0 ml/kg/hour (dilute paraldehyde (100%) with 5% dextrose; protect from light; avoid prolonged contact of undiluted paraldehyde with plastics; change infusion sets 12 hourly).

Other anticonvulsants: Clonazepam, sodium valproate and thiopentone may be useful for rapid seizure control. **Avoid** diazepam which has very prolonged elimination characteristics and is particularly depressant to the respiratory system.

Prognosis

Mortality after seizures has recently declined but a consistent 30 –35% children have neurological sequelae, usually neuromotor and developmental impairments, the remainder having no long-term sequelae.

Favourable aetiologies include primary subarachnoid haemorrhage and hypocalcaemia. Children with seizures due to symptomatic hypoglycaemia, hypoxic ischaemic encephalopathy and group B streptococcal meningitis have a better than 50% chance of normal development. Children with structural anomalies of the brain have the least favourable outcome, emphasizing the importance of an accurate aetiological diagnosis.

Prognosis is most clearly related to abnormalities of the background EEG activity but interpretation is difficult and must take account of gestational age.

Haemorrhagic and ischaemic brain lesions

Cerebral ultrasound scanning

Routine transfontanelle cerebral ultrasound scanning using a 5–7.5 MHz sector scanner facilitates the detection and management of perinatal brain pathology. All children <33 weeks' gestation should be scanned on admission to the special care baby unit (SCBU) and at intervals of a few days during the acute illness. Follow up scans should be performed weekly in the presence of abnormalities. Even in the absence of early abnormalities one or two later scans should be performed and will occasionally show previously unsuspected abnormality, especially periventricular leucomalacia. In the term infant haemorrhage, ischaemic lesions and gross cerebral oedema may be observed. Most major brain malformations are also detectable.

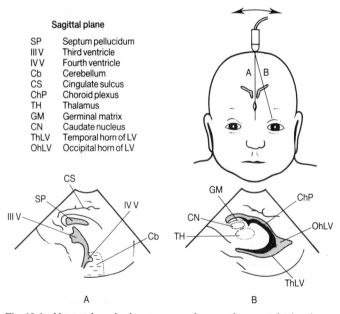

Sagittal plane

SP	Septum pellucidum
III V	Third ventricle
IV V	Fourth ventricle
Cb	Cerebellum
CS	Cingulate sulcus
ChP	Choroid plexus
TH	Thalamus
GM	Germinal matrix
CN	Caudate nucleus
ThLV	Temporal horn of LV
OhLV	Occipital horn of LV

Fig. 10.1 Neonatal cerebral anatomy on ultrasound scan: sagittal and parasagittal planes.

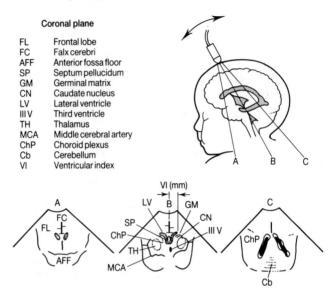

Coronal plane

FL	Frontal lobe
FC	Falx cerebri
AFF	Anterior fossa floor
SP	Septum pellucidum
GM	Germinal matrix
CN	Caudate nucleus
LV	Lateral ventricle
III V	Third ventricle
TH	Thalamus
MCA	Middle cerebral artery
ChP	Choroid plexus
Cb	Cerebellum
VI	Ventricular index

Fig. 10.2 Neonatal cerebral anatomy on ultrasound scan: coronal plane.

Coronal and parasagital scans (Figs 10.1 and 10.2) should be performed and suspected lesions confirmed in two planes of examination. Haemorrhage and oedema appear as bright echogenic areas, clotted blood within the ventricle being particularly easy to identify (Levene, 1985).

Early scans (<7 days) will identify the severity of any haemorrhagic lesion by size, position and distribution. No grading scheme is perfect; it is better to describe exactly what is seen.

Later scans (>7 days) will indicate the extent of any ventriculomegaly (measure ventricular index; Fig. 10.3) and identify the site, nature and extent of cortical echodensities and cysts as they evolve.

Classification of haemorrhagic lesions

Site	*Comment*
Periventricular haemorhage (PVH)	See below
Subdural	Torn bridging veins (trauma)
(a) *Supratentorial*	Rarely directly fatal
(b) *Infratentorial*	Usually fatal

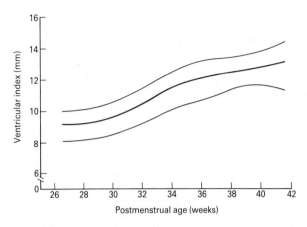

Fig. 10.3 Ventricular index (see B of Fig. 10.2) and postmenstrual age: 3rd, 50th and 97th percentiles. From Levene, M. I. (1981) *Arch. Dis. Childh.* **56**, 900–904.

Subarachnoid	Associated with bleeding tendency and anoxia; may extend from intraventricular haemorrhage; usually venous (contrast with adults)
Intracerebral	Infarction associated with sepsis, asphyxia, embolism and PVH
Cerebellar and brain stem	Rarely detected in life

Diagnosis

Suspect intracranial haemorrhage after traumatic or asphyxial delivery. Symptoms may include cerebral depression, seizures, apnoea, circulatory collapse, poor temperature regulation and rapid fall in haematocrit; although subarachnoid and small periventricular haemorrhages are often asymptomatic. Microscopy of CSF is unreliable.

Investigations

Cerebral ultrasound   First choice for supratentorial lesions.
CT scan   Useful for posterior fossa lesions and if subdural collections are suspected.
Coagulation screen   In children >34 weeks' gestation
Other investigations: for example, subdural taps, largely superceded.

Periventricular haemorrhage

This usually originates in the germinal matrix (26–32 weeks' gestation). It may occur rarely in term infants (usually from the choroid plexus). It is uncommon immediately after birth and appears during the first week. It may be confined to subependymal layers, rupture into ventricles, pass into the subarachnoid space or extend into the periventricular parenchyma. It may be followed by complete resolution, or posthaemorrhagic hydrocephalus (see below) and may be associated with later periventricular leucomalacia.

Risk factors

Infants <33 weeks' gestation (incidence 40–50% in this group but
  may now be less common)
Respiratory distress
Pneumothorax
Hypercapnia and acidosis
Hypotension

Prognosis

Outcome is best evaluated by sequential scanning and relates to the degree of ischaemic changes (see below).

Prevention

Prophylaxis is now substantiated by controlled trials. **Vitamin E** (25 mg/kg i.m. given on admission to SCBU) and **ethamsylate** (12.5 mg/kg qds i.v. for 16 doses) have both been demonstrated in randomized placebo-controlled trials to decrease the frequency of major degrees of PVH.

Avoid acidosis, hypercapnia and pneumothorax.

Pay close attention to the maintenance of peripheral perfusion and blood pressure using colloid and inotropic support if necessary.

Management

Correct bleeding tendency and transfuse if necessary.
Avoid exacerbation by acidosis, hypotension and fluctuations in blood pressure.
Perform serial scans to detect ventriculomegaly.
(Neurosurgical intervention is unnecessary with PVH.)

Classification of ischaemic brain lesions

Persistent ventricular enlargement

Non-progressive dilatation of lateral ventricles (>97th percentile; Fig. 10.3). Probably represents mild cortical atrophy. Significance uncertain.

Cystic periventricular leucomalacia (PVL)

Cystic degeneration in periventricular tissue 10–21 days after ischaemic injury. Cysts are usually small (<1 cm) and multiple. Significance depends upon site: fronto-parietal lesions are usually associated with few sequelae; bilateral occipital changes with neuro-motor impairment.

Subcortical leucomalacia

Cystic changes in more superficial cortical layers, indicating a very severe injury. They are found more frequently in mature infants. Poor neuromotor outcome.

Porencephaly

Large (>1 cm) cysts, usually solitary (occasionally multiple) and unilateral. May represent progression of parenchymal haemorrhage or PVL. High frequency of cerebral palsy.

Aetiology

All are endpoints of ischaemic brain injury of uncertain pathology. May have origins in antenatal period (suspect if cystic changes occur in first week).

Management

See PVH above.
Careful parental counselling.
Close neurodevelopmental follow-up.

Hydrocephalus (See Table 10.2)

Cerebrospinal fluid, produced by the choroid plexuses of the lateral ventricles, passes through the foramina of Monro into the third ventricle, from there through the aqueduct to the fourth ventricle, and then through the central foramen of Magendie and lateral foramina of Luschka to reach the subarachnoid space. In the subarachnoid space it flows over the cerebral hemispheres, to be absorbed by the arachnoid granulations, and also out of the cranial cavity down the spinal cord. Obstruction of this flow may cause hydrocephalus, which is defined as non-communicating (with the subarachnoid space) if at or proximal to the foramina of Magendie and Luschka, and communicating if it involves the arachnoid granulations or flow over the hemispheres and within the posterior fossa.

Table 10.2   Some causes of hydrocephalus

Cause	Level of obstruction
Post-haemorrhagic (following intraventricular haemorrhage	Usually communicating but may progress to obstruction of IVth ventricle foramina
	Occasionally non-communicating, obstruction proximal within ventricular system
Arnold–Chiari malformation of cerebral vermis (commonly associated with meningomyelocele)	IVth ventricle foramina; occasionally cerebral aqueduct
Dandy–Walker malformation – cystic dilatation of IVth ventricle	IVth ventricle foramina; occasionally cerebral aqueduct
Congenital aqueductal stenosis	Cerebral aqueduct
Post-infection (toxoplasma, rubella, CMV, meningitis)	Cerebral aqueduct, IVth ventricle foramina (often also cerebral atrophy)
Cerebral tumours and arterio-venous malformations (rare)	Various
Choroid plexus papilloma (rare)	No obstruction: CSF over-production

Investigations

Ultrasound scan: first-line investigation.

CT scan: may further define posterior fossa lesions.

Intrauterine infection screen: if indicated.

Queckenstedt's test: free rise and fall of lumbar CSF pressure on jugular venous compression confirms communication.

Management

Hydrocephalus is a dynamic condition and should be differentiated from cortical atrophy ('hydrocephalus *ex vacuo*'). Thus, before treatment is started an excessive increase in ventricular size (Fig. 10.3) or head circumference (Figs 19.1 and 19.2) should be documented. CSF production may later fall to match resorption and the hydrocephalus 'arrest'.

After PVH progressive ventricular dilatation may occur. Serial CSF drainage by lumbar puncture or ventricular tap has been advocated, but has little effect on the need for shunting or outcome. Cerebrospinal fluid (CSF) (10–20 ml/kg) may be removed to control symptoms (seizures, apnoea) or rapid head growth until CSF protein level falls below 1 g/l when shunt insertion is possible.

Other medical treatments, e.g. acetazolamide, 100 mg/kg/day, may temporarily reduce CSF production but are of little long-term benefit. Ventriculoperitoneal shunt insertion remains the treatment of choice when hydrocephalus progresses despite more conservative measures.

Perinatal asphyxia and cerebral intensive care

Despite recent improvements in perinatal care, severe asphyxia still occurs in between 3 and 9 per 1000 births and remains an important cause of neurological handicap. Careful postnatal management of the asphyxiated infant may reduce further cerebral injury.

Assessment of perinatal asphyxia

Intrapartum

Cardiotocograph (CTG)
Meconium staining of liquor ⎫ see Chapter 1
Fetal scalp ph <7.20   ⎭ and Chapter 2

Postnatal

Apgar score <5 at 5 min   ⎫
Cord blood pH <7.25 (venous) ⎪
Length of time to establish ⎪
  spontaneous respiration   ⎬ see Chapter 2
  (>10 min = severe asphyxia) ⎪
Neurological examination   ⎭

Neonatal course: Signs of encephalopathy may evolve over the first few hours.

Mild encephalopathy: 'Hyperalert', awake, restless, jittery, poor feeding, resolution by 48 hours to 7 days.

Moderate encephalopathy: 'Lethargic', hypotonic, decreased responsiveness, poor suck, ± seizures (easy to control), some resolution by 7 days.

Severe encephalopathy: 'Stuporose', profound hypotonia, unresponsive, depressed/absent reflexes, seizures common and difficult to control, high mortality, survivors recover over many weeks.

Management of the asphyxiated infant

Fluids

Restrict fluids to 30–50 ml/kg in first 24 hours, as oliguria (from antidiuretic hormone (ADH) secretion and renal ischaemia) is likely.

Fluid overload exacerbates cerebral oedema and may lead to hyponatraemia which increases cerebral irritability and the risk of convulsions.

Assess fluid balance by monitoring:
    urine output and specific gravity (± osmolality)

urine Na, Cl, K, urea
plasma urea, Na, K, Cl, creatinine ($\pm$ osmolality)
weight (daily)
blood pressure
(see Chapter 16 for management of persisting oliguria)

Persistently poor peripheral perfusion (toe temperature >2°C less than core temperature) $\pm$ acidosis with normal PaO_2 suggests hypovolaemia. Treat with i.v. colloid, 10–20 ml/kg, over 1–2 hours.

Respiration

Monitor blood gases 2–4 hourly
Aim to keep PaO_2 >60 mm Hg (7.8 kPa) and $PaCO_2$ <40 mm Hg (5.2 kPa)
Consider intermittent positive-pressure ventilation (IPPV) if $PaCO_2$ >60 mm Hg (7.8 kPa)

Blood glucose

Maintain at 4–7 mmol/l by i.v. infusion of 10–15% dextrose
Check capillary glucose levels 2–4 hourly
Hypoglycaemia may exacerbate CNS damage
Hyperglycaemia may exacerbate acidosis and cerebral oedema

Blood electrolytes

Hyponatraemia (Na < 130 mmol/l) without excessive urinary sodium loss is likely to be due to excess ADH secretion. Manage by further fluid restriction.

Hyperkalaemia may occur during the acidotic phase (as K^+ leaves red cells in exchange for H^+ ions). Do not add potassium to i.v. fluids until good urine flow established.

Hypokalaemia may occur later as renal sodium loss leads to secondary hyperaldosteronism.

(See also Chapter 17 for management of electrolyte disturbances.)

Intracranial pressure (ICP)

Cerebral oedema leads to raised ICP and is associated with a poor outcome. Ultrasound appearances of generalized echogenicity or compressed ventricles reflect only gross changes. Palpation of the anterior fontanelle and transfontanelle measurement of ICP are very inaccurate. Direct monitoring of ICP (indwelling transducer or catheter) should only be attempted in experienced units and is without proven benefit. Doppler ultrasound studies of flow in cerebral arteries indicate that a high velocity, low pulsatility signal carries a poorer prognosis.

Management of raised intracranial pressure

The measures suggested below may help to control raised ICP but none have been clearly shown to improve prognosis.

Raise head of cot 10–15 cm

Frusemide, 1–2 mg/kg, i.v. may be given if the infant is oliguric

Phenobarbitone, 20 mg/kg, i.v. may reduce cerebral irritability and treat convulsions

Hyperventilation IPPV to lower $PaCO_2$ to 28–35 mm Hg may help to control ICP, but lower levels may be associated with a marked reduction in cerebral blood flow

Mannitol, 2 ml/kg, 20% solution over 30 min has been shown to temporarily reduce ICP

Steroids are usually considered unhelpful

Prognosis

Prognosis depends upon the worst grade of encephalopathy recorded and time taken to recover. These are no sequelae for those with mild encephalopathy; 75–100% of those with severe encephalopathy die or have severe impairments. Only half of the infants with seizures will have poor outcome. Areas of attenuation on a CT scan performed in the second week indicate a poorer prognosis.

The floppy infant
Diagnosis

Distinguish between paralytic and non-paralytic conditions. The infant moving limbs against gravity or maintaining posture of a passively elevated limb is not paralysed (see Table 10.3) (Dubowitz, 1976).

Table 10.3 The floppy infant (Dubowitz, 1976, *Clin. Dev. Med.* 76.)

(A) Paralytic conditions with incidental hypotonia
Hereditary infantile spinal muscular atrophy
Werdnig-Hoffman disease
Benign variants

Congenital myopathies

Structural	Central core disease
	Minicore disease
	Nemaline myopathy
	Myotubular myopathy
	Myotubular myopathy with type I fibre hypotrophy
	Myotubular myopathy, X-linked
	Mixed myopathies
	Congenital fibre-type disproportion
	Mitochondrial myopathies
	Other subcellular abnormalities
	'Minimal-change myopathy'
Metabolic	Glycogenosis types II, III, (IV)
	Lipid storage myopathy
	Periodic paralysis

Other neuromuscular disorders
Congenital myotonic dystrophy
Congenital muscular dystrophy
Neonatal myasthenia; congenital myasthenia
Motor neuropathies
Other neuromuscular disorders

(B) Non-paralytic conditions: Hypotonia without significant weakness
Disorders affecting the central nervous system
Non-specific mental deficiency
Hypotonic cerebral palsy
Birth trauma, intracranial haemorrhage, intrapartum asphyxia and hypoxia
Chromosomal disorders; Down's syndrome
Metabolic disorders: aminoacidurias; organic acidurias; sphingolipidoses
    (leucodystrophies)

Connective tissue disorders
Congenital laxity of ligaments
Ehlers–Danlos and Marfan syndromes
Osteogenesis imperfecta
Mucopolysaccharidoses

Prader–Willi syndrome (hypotonia–obesity)

Metabolic, nutritional, endocrine
Renal tubular acidosis, hypercalcaemia, rickets, coeliac disease,
    hypothyroidism

Benign congenital hypotonia (essential hypotonia)

In the paralytic group exclude neonatal and congenital myasthenia (maternal history and edrophonium (Tensilon) test).

Examine the mother for myopathic facies and non-relaxing handshake, which suggests myotonic dystrophy (also commonly a history of polyhydramnios).

Investigations

Muscle biopsy

Usually quadriceps. (This is the definitive investigation.) Electron microscopy, enzyme histochemistry and histology must be performed. Best delayed until 3 months, but infants who may die need earlier investigation.

Nerve condition velocity

Slow in demyelinating peripheral neuropathy and to a lesser degree in axonal neuropathies and spinal muscular atrophy.

Electromyography

Distinguishes myopathies, denervation, myotonia and myasthenia.

Creatine phosphokinase

This is usually unhelpful. It is moderately raised in congenital muscular dystrophy; and very high in Duchenne's dystrophy (asymptomatic at this age).

Management

Establishment of feeding (may need long-term tube-feeding).
Physiotherapy for limb and joint deformities.
Bladder expression may be necessary.
The diagnosis is important for prognosis and genetic counselling.

Spina bifida and meningomyelocele

Definitions

Spina bifida   Failure of mid-line fusion of vertebral bodies.

Spina bifida occulata	Spinal cord intact (but may be damaged by the effects of tethering). Detectable only by X-ray or dissection. Sometimes there is an overlying skin pit, hairy patch or dimple. Very common.
Meningocele	Skin covered lesion usually has a good prognosis.
Meningomyelocele	Cystic herniation of both meninges and cord through the bony defect, commonly a large lumbar or thoracic defect. Frequent major neurological deficit. Most common type diagnosed in the neonatal period.
Myeloschisis or **myelocele**	Failure of closure of the neural tube. The spinal cord forms a flat disc covered by the granulation tissue. Major neurological deficit. Uncommon.

Spina bifida with meningomyelocele is common. Aggressive, non-selective surgical closure of these defects has led to the survival of many children with multiple severe handicaps. Most centres now adopt a selective approach to early surgical closure. While awaiting preoperative assessment, cover the lesion with sterile gauze soaked in saline and pay attention to temperature stability.

Assessment

General   Temperature, colour, respiration and evidence of birth injury.

Head   Circumference, separation of sutures, anterior fontanelle size and pressure. Ultrasound scan (to detect hydrocephalus).

Back   Level and size of lesion, width of bony defect and availability of skin for repair. Intactness of meningeal sac.

Neurological   Especially sensory and motor levels. Beware of interpreting reflex activity in the lower limbs as spontaneous movement.

Sphincter function   Both anal and urinary.

Orthopaedic   Limitation of movement, muscle wasting, and fixed deformities of lower limbs; spinal deformities; dislocated hips.

Radiological   X-ray spine with wire markers around the external lesion.

Factors predictive of severe disability

Gross hydrocephalus at birth (or microcephaly)
Kyphosis or scoliosis
Absence of voluntary movement below L3
Incontinence of urine and faeces
Postural abnormalities of lower limbs
Major associated defects
The final decision on early surgery rests with parents and attending
doctors (see Chapter 30).

Advice for future pregnancies   Multifactorial inheritance (page
320). Preconceptional vitamin supplements may be useful.

Other developmental defects

Encephalocele

A sac of meninges and cortex protruding from the skull, usually with
intact skin cover, and frequently associated with intracerebral anomalies of poor prognosis. When no neurological tissue is contained
within the sac it may be excised with a reasonable prognosis.

Anencephaly

This is due to failure of closure of the anterior neuropore just as
meningomyelocele is due to failure of closure of the posterior
neuropore. Fifty per cent of these pregnancies are associated with
polyhydramnios. Only 25% are liveborn and most die within a week.

Holoprosencephaly

This is due to defective cleavage of the forebrain and is often
associated with mid-line facial abnormalities. Two-thirds are associated with chromosomal anomalies – particularly trisomy 13. Most are
stillborn or die early in the newborn period.

Agenesis of corpus callosum

May be diagnosed by ultrasound scan. It may be associated with
megalencephaly and hypertelorism but generally is clinically silent.

Microcephaly

Commonly due to cerebral damage early in pregnancy due to environmental agents or congenital infection. Many chromosomal anomalies are also associated with microcephaly. There are also autosomal recessive and X-linked forms. Developmental delay is usually evident during infancy.

Porencephalic cysts and hydranencephaly

These are thought to be due to vascular accidents during pregnancy, sometimes associated with congenital infection. Some porencephalic cysts develop postnatally following haemorrhage or infarction. Translumination may be of value.

Bibliography

Dubowitz, V. (1976). The floppy infant. *Clinics in Developmental Medicine*, Number 79. London: Spastics International Medical Publications.

Dubowitz, L. and Dubowitz, V. (1979). The neurological assessment of the preterm and full-term newborn infant. *Clinics in Developmental Medicine*, Number 76. London: Spastics International Medical Publications.

Levene, M. I. (1985). Ultrasound of the infant brain. *Clinics in Developmental Medicine*, Number 92. London: Spastics International Medical Publications.

Levene, M. I., Bennett, M. J. and Punt, J. (Eds) (1988) *Fetal and Neonatal Neurology and Neurosurgery*. Edinburgh: Churchill Livingtone.

Pape, K. E. and Wigglesworth, J. S. (1989). *Perinatal Brain Lesions*. Oxford: Blackwell Scientific.

Volpe, J. J. (1987). *Neurology of the Newborn*, 2nd edn. Philadelphia: W. B. Saunders.

11

Nutrition and gastroenterology

Breast feeding
Artificial feeding
The preterm or sick infant
Food additives
Feeding techniques
Intravenous nutrition
Gastrointestinal problems

Breast feeding

Background

Breast feeding has evolved to provide the newborn human infant with a perfectly balanced and nutritionally complete source of food. Breast milk meets the growing infant's entire needs, provides important defences against infection and diseases of infancy, delivers biochemical triggers which modulate gut function and supplies primed enzymes to aid digestion and nutrient utilization. The natural evolution of breast feeding makes it likely that optimal oro-facial development and optimal ties of affection between mother and infant are promoted.

For the mother breast feeding completes the natural hormonal cycle initiated at conception, allows her to use the reserves of body fat accumulated during gestation and confers a degree of lactational infertility. A well-nourished mother can meet the nutritional demands of her term infant for at least *three or four months*. Additionally breast feeding is the safest form of feeding under unhygienic conditions.

Clinical staff have a duty to highlight these often intangible benefits for mothers whilst not placing them under undue pressure or engendering any sense of guilt in those mothers electing to bottle feed.

Antenatal preparation

There is little evidence that any physical preparation ('nipple toughening') is necessary to prepare for the act of breast feeding, in contrast to the excellent evidence that mental and emotional preparation is highly beneficial. Antenatal education should include the opportunity to observe and discuss issues with a breast feeding mother, simple facts on the physiology of lactation, practical advice on optimal position and fixing, and some awareness of the common problems encountered.

Although the decision on how to feed a baby may be made before pregnancy, it is possible to encourage a large proportion of mothers to breast feed in the immediate neonatal period, irrespective of how feeding is managed long term. Mothers of preterm children often do so when encouraged by clinical staff, to promote early growth and health. Such mothers must be praised for their personal contribution to their baby's course.

Postnatal considerations

Physiology

The *initiation* of breast milk production occurs as a result of the removal of inhibition of high circulating levels of prolactin by placental steroids (mainly oestrogens) following expulsion of the placenta. Milk production and time to achieve it are, however, very variable (2–5 days post-partum: initial output 200–900 ml/24 hours).

Milk production is *sustained* by three factors:

(a) Frequent afferent stimulation of the nipples by sucking
(b) Effective removal of freshly synthesized milk from the breast
(c) The milk ejection reflex, mediated by oxytocin secretion

If milk is not removed, engorgement and milk stasis are followed by involution of mammary tissue – the natural process of events in mothers who elect for artificial feeding. In contrast, adequate milk production may be sustained by the exclusive use of an electric breast pump (e.g. by mothers of preterm infants). As long as there is frequent emptying of the breast, adequate milk output occurs despite the loss of the suckling-induced prolactin response.

Efficient *transfer* of milk from mother to baby is dependent on the milk ejection reflex and active 'sucking' by the baby. Both require that the baby is effectively fixed and positioned during a feed, ensuring an adequate mouthful of breast tissue to optimize reflex milk release and extraction.

Routine breast feeding management

Infants should be put to the breast in the delivery room. Frequent feeds (1–3 hourly) should be encouraged in the first few days, and later demand feeding (usually 5–7 feeds/day by one week). Infants and mothers should be in the same room at night.

There should be *no restriction* in duration or frequency of feeds and babies should *not* be switched between breasts after an arbitrary time. Babies should feed from the first breast until they come off spontaneously. The second breast should then be offered, but whether or not it is taken, and for how long, should be dictated by hunger/satiety on the baby's part. If feeds are excessively long (>30 mins) or over-frequent (<1 hourly), positioning may be incorrect.

It is central to effective pain-free feeding that the baby takes an adequate volume of breast tissue into the mouth (not simply the nipple), thus ensuring that the breast is not traumatized, and reducing the risk of sore nipples. A baby thus receives a balanced feed, in terms of the high volume, low fat *foremilk*, and low volume, high fat *hindmilk*. Adequate emptying of the breast is essential as hindmilk is important in ensuring slower gastric emptying (thereby extending the inter-feed interval), maximizing intake of fat-soluble vitamins, and developing normal appetite control ('conditioned satiety').

Suboptimal positioning is the commonest cause for failed or inadequate lactation, principally by compromising breast emptying. The essential steps for ensuring correct positioning are contained in a Royal College of Midwives' handbook *Successful Breast Feeding*. In the event of *breast feeding problems*, the advice of a skilled midwife should be sought. We also commend the benefits of a recognized local 'expert', with or without the input of local lay support groups (e.g. National Childbirth Trust breast feeding counsellors).

Special considerations

Preterm infants may feed competently from the breast as early as 30 weeks' gestation. Development of feeding skills may be impaired by the presence of, for example, gastric tubes or supplementary fluids given i.v. or enterally. An early trial of breast feeding is thus recommended. Even 'non-nutritive' sucking may improve the infant's progress and the establishment of breast milk supply.

Electric pumps are efficient at establishing breast milk flow, although the suckling-induced surge of prolactin wanes with repeated use. Treatment with *metoclopromide* (10 mg tds orally) will often offset any fall off in milk supply associated with prolonged pump use.

Test weighing is not a routine clinical procedure. When indicated, it should be conducted over a *24 hour period* and preferably in a familiar environment (i.e. home). Simple mechanical scales are too inaccurate and an electronic balance must be used. 'Test weighing' over a single feed is not recommended.

Ultrasound assessment of oral function (using a submental sagittal view in real time or M-mode) may be useful in differentiating temporary problems from intractable neurological dysfunction.

Clinical breast feeding problems

Oral anomalies which impair feeding

Cleft lip and/or palate is one of the more obvious impairments to successful breast feeding, although babies with unilateral cleft lip are often successful. The cleft interferes with the negative pressure achieved normally in the mouth, impairing the teat stripping action of the tongue. The early provision of a palatal prosthesis may allow successful feeding, although the presence of a plate will disturb the tactile stimulation necessary for the smooth translation of the peristaltic wave from the tongue to the pharynx, and may demand greater perseverance by the mother. One advantage is that earlier feeding will be possible after repair of the lesion.

Sub-mucal cleft is a defect in the bony palate, but not involving the soft tissue. It can interfere with feeding. Feeding is often very noisy, with a loud smacking sound generated as air enters the buccal cavity at the point when the soft tissue can no longer resist the high negative intraoral pressure. Surgical repair may be necessary to prevent later speech or feeding problems.

Pierre–Robin syndrome: the poor muscular development and re-trognathia are usually incompatible with early establishment of feeding – breast or artificial. Subsequent forward growth of the jaw may permit graduation from a spoon to the breast, although using new designs of bottle/teat milk may be successfully squeezed into the oral cavity and artificial feeding established.

Laryngomalacia appears to impair the generation of normal negative intraoral pressure, reducing feeding efficiency, milk intake and occasionally contributing to failure to thrive.

'Tongue tie':   a severe tongue tie can prevent the normal forward thrust of the tongue to form a furrow around the nipple. This impairs the onset of the peristaltic stripping movement which forces milk from the lactiferous sinuses into the mouth. In the presence of breast feeding difficulties surgical intervention is indicated.

Nasal obstruction: (mucus, choanal atresia/stenosis, too close approximation of nares to the breast) will impair the normal 1:1 relation of sucking to breathing. In the case of a positioning problem, rotate the baby to a better position, do not press the breast away from the baby's mouth reducing the amount of breast tissue in the mouth.

Oral thrush results in oral discomfort which, if untreated, can lead to an aversion to feeding. If there is itching, pain or discomfort to the mother she should be treated at the same time as the baby (Chapter 14).

Failure of lactation

Retained placental fragments may secrete sufficient oestrogens to continue inhibition of prolactin.

Primary failure of lactation is rare (<2% of mothers), combining normal lactating prolactin levels (800–6000 mIU/l) with milk output below 150 ml/day at one month. Impaired end-organ responsiveness is suspected. Metaclopromide is ineffective despite causing a further rise in prolactin.

Insufficient lactation

Breast milk insufficiency is found in about 5% of mothers. It is defined as milk output between 200 and 450 ml/day at one month. It may reflect the lower end of the normal range of output but more frequently reflects suboptimal management. Careful assessment of technique is important, although supplementation with artificial formulae may be necessary.

Impaired milk release may be due to impairment of the normal 'let down reflex' and may be overcome by providing a relaxing, familiar environment and sensitive, skilled care. Occasionally it is due to reduced sucking efficiency by the baby (see above) and can be encouraged by the use of an electric breast pump.

Apparent lactation insufficiency

(Poor growth of otherwise normal baby despite normal milk output of 500–800 ml/day.)

Incorrect positioning is the commonest cause, the baby taking low fat foremilk resulting in volume or calorie depletion, and is only usually correctable at an early stage before the infant becomes entrenched in a poor feeding habit.

Inappropriate pattern of breast usage: either exclusive single breast feeding or rigid both breast policies may result in inefficient feeding, and may be overcome by the adoption of more flexible policies.

Over-efficient maternal physiology: an over-vigorous ejection reflex, particularly in combination with either of the preceding two problems, may result in symptoms such as 'colic', over-feeding or symptoms of lactose malabsorption – flatus, 'wind', loose frothy acid stools, possibly because of rapid gastric emptying and spillage of lactose into the colon.

Maternal complications of breast feeding

Engorgement is most common in the first week. Vascular engorgement, which resolves spontaneously, should be differentiated from milk engorgement, usually caused by restrictions on baby's access to the breast. If the baby is unable to remove the milk, physical interventions are necessary (showers, manual expression, pump) to draw off milk and reduce areolar oedema.

Mastitis/blocked duct: infective and non-infective inflammation may present similarly. In the latter there is retrograde flow of milk under pressure from the lumen of the breast into the surrounding tissues, with local and general immune responses. Infective mastitis is usually associated with an infected lesion of the nipple and requires antibiotics. Breast feeds should be continued, even in the presence of infection, as cessation will exacerbate local swelling and may predispose to abscess formation, which usually requires surgical drainage. Breast feeding may still continue, unless sucking impinges on the abscess site.

Breast milk contaminants

Drugs (see Chapter 28)

Environmental pollutants: fat soluble contaminants may accumulate during the period of fat deposition during pregnancy and appear in high concentrations in breast milk. No data on acceptable levels of pollutants exist and relative risks can not be estimated.

Viral infections: there are few data to suggest a higher infectivity rate among breast-fed infants of HIV-positive mothers, compared to those artificially fed, suggesting an ante- or perinatal route of infection. Cross-nursing of another child may constitute a risk.

Artificial feeding

The unmodified milk of the cow, goat and ewe are unsuitable for feeding infants in the first months of life because their composition differs from mature human milk (Table 11.1), and may lead to an excessive renal solute load, late hypocalcaemia and to iron, folate or vitamin deficiencies depending upon the milk used. Modern modified cow's milk formulae should be advised when mothers do not wish to, or are unable to, breast feed.

Soya-based formulae may be used as an alternative to modified cow's milk formulae for babies with cows' milk protein intolerance. Evidence that soya formulae reduce the frequency or severity of atopy is inconclusive.

Table 11.1 shows the types and composition of the available modified formulae in the UK. Those with a casein:whey ratio resembling breast milk are most suitable. Of each type, the various brands are so similar that the only basis of preference should be cost. There is no evidence to support the claim that the less modified formulae with a higher casein content are more 'satisfying' for the 'hungry and demanding baby'.
    Offer a feed within 4 hours of birth and then feed on demand. Volumes recommended are given in Table 17.1 (page 255).

Infants at risk of hypoglycaemia (Chapter 13) should be fed early and more frequently, unless contraindicated by gastrointestinal or respiratory disease.

The preterm or sick infant

Wherever possible, preterm or sick infants should be enterally fed, being safer, cheaper and often better nutritionally than i.v. feeding.
    Recommended volumes for feeding preterm infants are given in Table 17.1 (page 255). The preterm infant requires 100–120 kcal/kg/day to grow at the rate achieved *in utero*. This requires 180–200 ml/kg/day of standard infant formula or pooled breast milk. Such high fluid intakes may be poorly tolerated and may predispose to the development of patent ductus arteriosus (PDA) (see Chapter 9) and necrotizing enterocolitis (NEC).

Low birthweight formulae supply extra energy, protein and minerals to achieve intrauterine growth rates at intakes of 150–180 ml/kg/day (Table 11.1) and may be used in infants of <1500 g. Note that certain formulae have a higher sodium content to meet the needs of infants <1500 g (3–6 mmol/kg/day).

If extra fluid is needed (e.g. phototherapy) give water; do not increase the volume of low birthweight formula. Monitor hydration by daily measurements of urine specific gravity (maintain SG <1.015).

Only increase the volume of low birthweight formulae above the volume recommended if facilities are available for full biochemical screening, including plasma amino acid levels.

Low birthweight formulae should only be used in hospital; change to standard formula when the baby reaches 2000 g or a few days before discharge.

Human milk from mothers of preterm infants has a higher sodium and protein concentration than the milk of mothers of full-term infants, and is thus more suitable for preterm infants. However, the composition varies widely and supplementation with calories (e.g. a glucose polymer or medium-chain triglycerides), phosphate and sodium may be necessary.

Special formulae

Special formulae are used in the newborn period for the treatment of gastrointestinal and inherited metabolic disorders (Table 11.2).

Indications for use of special formulae

(a) For specific gastrointestinal disorders after gastroenteritis, necrotizing enterocolitis or neonatal surgery, e.g. cows' milk protein intolerance, disaccharidase deficiencies and fat malabsorption.
(b) Inherited metabolic disorders, e.g. galactosaemia or phenylketonuria (see Chapter 13, page 206).
(c) Conditions with biochemical disturbances, e.g. Di George syndrome, biliary atresia, renal failure.

Food additives
Vitamins

ALL infants should receive vitamin K_1 shortly after delivery. Give preterm infants and those born by abnormal delivery vitamin K_1, 0.5

Table 11.1 Composition of mature breast milk, standard infant formulae, breast milk of mothers of preterm infants, low birthweight formulae, cows' milk, goats' milk, ewes' milk (units/l)

Milk	Energy		Protein (g)	Casein:whey ratio	Carbohydrate (g)	Fat (g)	Na (mmol)	K (mmol)	Ca (mmol)	P (mmol)	Ca/P (molar)	Fe (mg)	Folate (µg)	Vitamin					
	MJ	kcal												A (µg)	B₁₂ (µg)	C (mg)	D (µg)	E (mg)	K (µg)
Mature breast milk	2.93	700	13	32:68	70	42	6.5	15	8.7	4.8	1.8	0.8	52	600	0.1	38	0.1	3.5	17
Standard infant formulae																			
Cows' milk formulae:																			
casein dominant																			
Milumil (M)	2.90	690	19	80:20	84	31	10	22	18	18	1.0	4.3	50	570	2.0	76	10	8.0	40
Ostermilk Two (F)	2.73	650	17	77:23	86	26	11	22	15	16	1.0	6.5	32	970	1.3	64	10	4.6	26
Plus (C&G)	2.75	660	19	77:23	73	34	11	26	21	18	1.2	5.0	100	800	2.0	80	11	11	50
SMA White Cap (Wy)	2.74	650	15	82:18	72	36	8	16	12	12	1.0	6.7	53	790	1.1	58	11	9.5	58
Cows' Milk formulae:																			
Whey dominant																			
Aptamil (M)	2.81	670	15	40:60	73	36	8	22	15	11	1.3	7.0	100	610	1.6	60	10	7.0	40
Ostermilk (F)	2.84	680	15	39:61	70	38	8	15	9	9	0.9	6.5	34	1000	1.4	69	10	4.8	27
Premium (C&G)	2.75	660	15	40:60	73	36	8	17	14	9	1.6	5.0	100	800	2.0	80	11	11	50
SMA Gold Cap (Wy)	2.74	650	15	40:60	72	36	7	14	11	9	1.1	6.7	53	790	1.1	58	11	9.5	58

Breast milk of mothers of preterm infants

1 week age	2.80	670	24	NA	61	38	22	18	6.2	4.6	1.4	NA	NA	NA	NA	NA	NA	NA	NA
4 weeks age	2.93	700	18	NA	70	40	13	16	5.4	4.6	1.2	NA	NA	NA	NA	NA	NA	NA	NA
Low birthweight formulae																			
Cow & Gate LBWF (C&G)	3.36	800	22	41:59	85	44	14	18	27	17	1.6	9.0	480	1000	2.0	280	24	14	90
Osterprem (F)	3.34	800	20	39:61	70	49	20	17	18	11	1.6	0.4	500	1000	2.0	280	80	100	70
Prematil (M)	2.98	700	20	40:60	77	35	13	19	18	11	1.6	1.0	430	630	1.5	150	29	20	28
SMA LBWF (Wy)	3.34	800	20	40:60	82	44	14	19	19	13	1.5	6.7	100	960	2.0	70	13	10	70
Animal milk																			
Cow's milk	2.80	670	34	77:23	46	39	22	39	30	31	1.0	0.5	50	310	3.0	20	0.6	0.9	NA
Goats' milk	3.06	732	37	86:14	49	43	14	47	33	34	1.0	1.0	2	360	1.0	20	0.5	NA	NA
Ewes' Milk	4.64	1110	58	84:16	46	78	14	50	49	50	1.0	1.0	2	600	3.0	30	NA	NA	NA

Note:
Manufacturers' data sheets used except for mature breast milk and cows' milk from DHSS (1980); casein: whey ratio for goats' milk and ewes' milk from Jelliffe and Jelliffe (1980); remaining data for goats' milk and ewes' milk derived from data in Scientific Tables, 7th edition, 1971, Ciba-Geigy Ltd, Basle, Switzerland. Manufacturers: (C&G) Cow & Gate; (F) Farley Health Products; (M) Milupa; (Wy) Wyeth. NA, Not Available. LBWF, Low birthweight formula. Na. sodium; K. potassium; Ca. calcium; P. phosphorus; Fe, iron.

Table 11.2 Composition of special formulae and energy supplements

	Soya protein, vegetable fat, low lactose (per litre)					Special fat and/or special protein (per litre)			Minimal lactose (per litre)		Low phenylalanine (per litre)		Low calcium (per litre)	Energy supplements per 100 g				Energy supplements per 100 ml	
	Formula S (C&G)	Isomil (A)	Ostersoy (F)	Prosobee Powder (M Jo)	Wysoy (F)	Pepti-Junior (C&G)	Pregestimil (M Jo)	Prejomin (M)	Galactomin 17 (C & G)	Galactomin 19 (C&G)	Lofenalac (M Jo)	Minafen (C&G)	Locasol (C&G)	Glucose	Caloreen (R)	Duocal (SHS)	MCT Duocal (SHS)	Calogen (SHS)	Liquid Calogen (SHS)
Energy																			
MJ	2.8	2.7	2.9	2.7	2.8	2.8	2.8	3.1	2.8	2.3	2.9	2.9	2.8	1.7	1.7	2.0	2.0	1.9	1.7
kcal	660	680	700	652	670	660	660	750	660	545	684	690	660	400	400	470	486	450	416
Protein																			
Amount (g)	18	18	20	20	21	20	19	20	19	27.5	23	17	19	–	–	–	–	–	–
Source	Soy	Soy	Soy	Soy	Soy	HW	HC	H Col Soy	CM	CM	HC	HC	CM	–	–	–	–	–	–
Carbohydrate																			
Amount (g)	71	69	70	66	69	76	91	86	74	72.9	91.8	65	73	100	96	73	74	–	–
Source	G, HS	S, HS	G, HS	G, HS	G, HS	G, HS	G, HS	G, HS St	G, HS	F	G, HS	G,HS St	L	G	HS	HS	HS	–	–

Fat																			
Amount (g)	36	37	38	36	36	37	27	36	34	18	27	42	34	—	—	22	23	50	50
Source	V	V	V	V	V An	V MCT	V MCT	V	V	V	V	V	V,An	—	—	V MCT	MCT	V	MCT
Sodium	8	14	11	11	9	9	14	17	11	10	14	19	12	—	<2	1.2	14	11	11
Potassium	17	20	19	15	19	17	19	20	26	15	18	11	25	—	<0.3	0.1	1.3	0.9	1.7
Calcium	14	18	14	14	16	14	16	13	21	23	17	24	<1.8	—	—	0.6	0.1	0.5	0.7
Phosphate	9	16	12	13	14	9	14	8	18	19	16	8	18	—	—	0.1	—	—	—
Special vitamin or minerals needed	No	No	No	No	No	No	No	No	No	No	Yes	Yes	No	No	No	Not applicable			
Similar products	Prosobee Liquid (M Jo)					Protagen (M Jo)										Many alternative preparations available			

Note:

Manufacturers: (A) Abbott Laboratories; (C&G) Cow & Gate; (F) Farley Health Products; (M) Milupa; (M Jo) Mead Johnson; (R) Roussel Laboratories; (SHS) Scientific Hospital Supplies.

An, animal; CM, cow's milk; F, fructose; G, glucose; HC, hydrolysed casein; H Col, hydrolysed collagen; HS, hydrolysed starch; HW, hydrolysed whey; L, lactose; MCT, medium-chain triglyceride; S, sucrose; St, starch; V, vegetable oil; Soy, soya.

Products with medium-chain triglycerides as the predominant fat are useful for infants with biliary atresia. The composition of Pepti-Junior, Pregestimil and Prejomin make them suitable for infants with multiple malabsorption problems following gastroenteritis, necrotizing enterocolitis or bowel surgery.

Lofenalac and Minafen are deficient in phenylalanine. Seek dietetic advice on use.

mg, intramuscularly in the delivery room and others 1 mg orally with the first feed.

The DHSS recommends that all infants should receive 5 drops/day of Children's Vitamin Drops (or a similar preparation) from 1 month to 2 years (or preferably 5 years) or until the mother's professional adviser believes the infant is receiving an adequate vitamin intake from other sources. The compositions of suitable vitamin drops are:

	Vitamin A	*Vitamin C*	*Vitamin D*
Children's Vitamins Drops (5 drops)	214 microg (700 IU)	21 mg	7 microg (280 IU)
Abidec* (Parke Davis) (0.6 ml)	1200 microg (4000 IU)	50 mg	10 microg (400 IU)
Adexoline Liquid (Glaxo) (0.2 ml)	210 microg (700 IU)	21 mg	7 microg (280 IU)

* Also contains B vitamins

An infant breast fed by a well-nourished mother should not need extra vitamins provided an adequate mixed diet is introduced between the fourth and sixth month of life. Formula-fed infants do not need extra vitamins. Proprietary baby foods are fortified with vitamins. Children's Vitamin Drops should be prescribed when the mixed diet is based on an inadequate family diet.

The following infants are particularly at risk of vitamin deficiencies:

(a) Low birthweight infants (see below).
(b) Infants fed unmodified cows', goats' or ewes' milk. These milks should not be recommended for infants less than six months because of their unsuitable composition (Table 11.1), but if used they need vitamin supplements. Give Children's Vitamin Drops *plus* folate (100 microg daily) for those fed goats' milk and ewes' milk. Vitamin B_{12} will be needed if infants fed goats' milk have the milk boiled before use or are weaned onto a diet low in the vitamin. In practice it is easier to give the total vitamin supplement as Ketovite tables and liquid (Paines & Bryne).
(c) Infants in traditional Asian households or other ethnic groups known to be prone to vitamin D deficiency (e.g. Rastafarians). These infants need vitamin supplementation with Children's Vitamin Drops during breast feeding and after the introduction of the family diet. If formula feeding is commenced it should be encouraged until 12 months of age.
(d) Infants of families on non-standard diets who may have nutritional requirements in addition to that provided in Children's Vitamin Drops. Mothers on vegan, vegetarian and macrobiotic

diets should take additional vitamin B_{12}. Expert paediatric dietetic advice should be sought if in doubt.

Fluoride

Fluoride supplementation is recommended where the drinking water contains less than 0.33 ppm in order to reduce the incidence of dental caries. Fluoride drops are available to provide 0.25 mg daily in either two or five drops. A reduced dosage may be given for water supplies containing between 0.33 and 1.00 ppm fluoride. Information on the fluoride content of water in any area may be obtained from the Local Water Authority. Fluoride supplementation should be stopped when fluoride-containing toothpaste is used.

Special requirements of the very preterm infant

Vitamin D, calcium, phosphorus

Very preterm infants are at risk of metabolic bone disease or osteopenia. This probably results from a failure to achieve intra-uterine rates of phosphate and calcium accretion.

Vitamin D supplements are given as Children's Vitamin Drops (5 drops bd) – 560 IU daily. (Note: a double dose of Abidec is not recommended as this will cause a high vitamin A intake.)

Calcium and phosphate are not routinely supplemented for infants receiving artificial formulae, but phosphate supplementation (K_2HPO_4 2 mmol/kg/day) is necessary for very preterm children (<30 weeks) receiving breast milk. Plasma calcium, phosphate and alkaline phosphatase are monitored weekly. If signs of metabolic bone disease ensue – hypocalcaemia, hypophosphataemia or high alkaline phosphatase (>5 times the upper limit of the adult reference range) – we supplement calcium (3–4 mmol/kg/day as chloride) and phosphorus (2 mmol/kg/day as K_2HPO_4). If alkaline phosphatase levels continue to rise we halve the dose of Children's Vitamin Drops (to 5 drops daily) and give 1-alpha-hydroxy vitamin D (0.05 microg/kg/day).

Vitamin E

The well-described vitamin E-deficient haemolytic anaemia is now rarely seen with modern formulae with the recommended vitamin E: polyunsaturated fatty acid ratio. Randomized trials suggest that a single dose of Vitamin E (25 mg/kg *intramuscularly*) may reduce the risk of severe degrees of intraventricular haemorrage in babies below 33 weeks' gestation (see Chapter 10, page 140).

Folic acid

Folic acid, 0.1 mg, daily orally is given from 14 days until 3 months post-term.

Iron

Preterm infants have low iron stores and become deficient after 3 months as blood volume expands during rapid growth. The little iron in breast milk is very well absorbed. Low birthweight and standard formulae contain extra iron, but probably insufficient to meet the needs of the smallest infants. Extra iron may saturate the iron-binding capacity of lactoferrin, which may increase the risk of gastroenteritis as *E. coli* require free iron to multiply. Additionally, little is probably absorbed before 2 months after birth. We supplement very preterm babies with iron (2 mg/kg/day) from 4 weeks until weaned (5–10 drops of Niferex, an iron–polysaccharide complex containing 0.6 mg elemental iron per drop).

All babies fed unmodified milks need iron supplements until weaned.

Feeding techniques

Infants of 34 weeks gestation can usually coordinate sucking and swallowing and should be offered breast or bottle feeds, but if unsuccessful, tube feeding may be necessary.

Gastric feeding

Orogastric tubes are preferable to nasogastric tubes as they cause less airway obstruction. If taped over the mid-point of the lower lip orogastric tubes are well tolerated.

Gastric feeding should be intermittent (1–4 hourly) and the tube position checked (by testing aspirate for acidity) before each feed. Use a 5FG PVC tube, which should be changed every 2–3 days as PVC becomes stiff in use.

Transpyloric (TP) feeding

This may be used in preference to i.v. feeding in infants who cannot tolerate gastric feeding (e.g. those with cardiac or respiratory disease).

The tube (silicon rubber *not* PVC) should be passed orally if tolerated, and may be fixed in place with a grooved dental plate or taped over the lower lip. Mark the tube at a distance from the tip equal to the baby's mouth to ankle length and, with the baby lying on the right side, pass the tube through the mouth (or nose). When the mark is at the level of the umbilicus, the tip is in the stomach (check aspirate for acidity). Slowly inject 1–2 ml sterile water and continue to advance the tube 1–2 cm every 5–10 min until the mark is at the mouth or nose. Slowly inject 1 ml sterile water and gently aspirate on syringe. If there is resistance to aspiration the tip is probably in the duodenum or jejunum. Insert a gastric tube, inject a further 2–3 ml sterile water into the transpyloric tube and aspirate the gastric tube. If nothing is obtained the tube is almost certainly in the duodenum or jejunum, and the position may be checked by X-ray. The ideal position being in the second part of the duodenum. The jejunum is too far. Tape the tube securely to the baby's face. Transpyloric feeds are given by continuous infusion, usually starting at 1–2 ml/hour and slowly increasing as tolerated. Aspirate the gastric tube 6 hourly. If milk is obtained from the stomach or abdominal distension occurs, stop feeds and X-ray the abdomen. The transpyloric tube may have been pulled back into the stomach or there may be bowel obstruction, sepsis, ileus or NEC.

Intravenous nutrition

Intravenous feeding (i.v. nutrition) is an expensive and complex way of providing nutrition and should be reserved for those situations when enteral feeds are not practicable. It should only be undertaken by experienced medical and nursing staff and where adequate biochemical, bacteriological and pharmaceutical services are available.

Indications

(1) After gastrointestinal surgery.
(2) Ileus, due to extreme prematurity or general ill-health (e.g. septicaemia, cardiac failure).
(3) Necrotizing enterocolitis.
(4) Respiratory illness (until enteral feeds established).

Nutritional requirements

These are similar to those of enteral nutrition. Fluid volume calculations are similar (Tables 17.1 and Table 11.3).

Table 11.3 Intravenous feeding regimen

Day of life	Day of i.v. feeding	Volume (ml/kg/day)					Sodium content of Vamin-glucose (mmol/kg/day)
		Total volume intake*	10% glucose + NaCl (30–50 mmol/l)	Intra-lipid mixture	Vamin-glucose mixture	Glucose mixture	
1	–	60 (80)	60 (80)	–	–	–	–
2	–	90 (100–120)	90 (100–120)	–	–	–	–
3	1	110 (130–140)	–	–	20	90 (110–120)	0.9
4	2	130 (150–160)	–	–	30	100 (120–130)	1.4
5	3	150 (160–180)	–	–	40	110 (120–140)	1.8
6	4	150 (160–180)	–	10 ml of 10%	40	100 (110–130)	1.8
7	5	150 (160–180)	–	15 ml of 10%	40	100 (105–125)	1.8
8	6	150 (160–180)	–	10 ml of 20%	40	100 (110–130)	1.8

* **Recommended** intake for infants >1500 g; figures in brackets for infants <1500 g.
Modify total volume intake by altering intake of 'Solution 1'.
Increase volume intake if abnormal losses; routinely increase by 25 ml/kg/day for phototherapy.
Reduce volume intake if evidence of overhydration or patent ductus arteriosus.

Calories

The newborn infant needs about 100–120 kcal/kg/day for normal growth, this being achieved over the first week. Most energy should be from non-protein sources, allow 150–200 non-protein calories for each gram of nitrogen.

Carbohydrate

Glucose is the main source of carbohydrate, although newborn infants may be relatively intolerant, necessitating a gradual increase. Term infants should tolerate 0.5 g/kg/hour glucose, but the preterm or sick infant may tolerate only half of this.

Protein

Protein is given as a synthetic amino acid mixture. There is uncertainty as to the ideal composition of such solutions. Optimal amino acid requirements at term are about 2.5 g/kg/day and between 24 and 36 weeks about 3.0 g/kg/day.

Fat

Give fat as an emulsion. Fat supplies concentrated calories (9 kcal/g compared to 4 kcal/g for glucose and amino acids) and essential fatty acids. Very small infants tolerate fat poorly. Start at 0.5 g/kg/day increasing to 2.0 g/kg/day. Monitor blood triglyceride levels: do not increase if 100–150 mg/l, reduce infusion if >150 mg/l. *We stop fat infusion* during periods of suspected and proven sepsis, thrombocytopaenia (platelets $<50 \times 10^9/l$), acidosis (pH <7.25) and hyperbilirubinaemia (sufficient to warrant phototherapy). Close monitoring is necessary in children with lung and hepatic disease.

Minerals

Fetal accumulation rates of minerals are the basis for the standard recommendations for preterm children:

Sodium	3.8 mmol/kg/day
Potassium	1.2 mmol/kg/day
Chloride	2.0 mmol/kg/day
Calcium	3 to 4 mmol/kg/day
Magnesium	0.25 mmol/kg/day
Phosphorus	2 to 3 mmol/kg/day

Vitamins

A full range of vitamins must be provided as above. Most are supplied by standard i.v. nutrition additives but vitamin B_{12} supplements are needed after about one month.

Solutions used

We use Kabi-Vitrum products thus:

Glucose electrolyte mixture (GEM)
500 ml 10% glucose solution **plus**
2.5 ml Solivito solution (water-soluble vitamins)
2.5 ml K_2HPO_4 solution (2 mmol K^+ plus 1 mmol PO_4^{2-}) extra sodium (as 30% NaCl; usually 1–3 ml)

Vamin glucose mixture (amino acid source)
90 ml Vamin in 10% glucose **plus** 12 ml Ped-El (trace elements)

Intralipid mixture (soyabean oil emulsion)
Prepare 24 hour requirement in syringe
Add 1 ml/kg/day Vitlipid (fat-soluble vitamins) to a maximum of 4
   ml/day

Prescription

A suggested scheme for prescription of i.v. nutrition is shown in
Table 11.3 to achieve optimal caloric intake by day 8. If starting i.v.
nutrition after the first week start at day 6. Clinical assessment of
water requirement may make changes necessary (e.g. cardiac failure,
use of muscle relaxants). Note that *extra sodium* must be added to the
glucose electrolyte mixture to make up the sodium requirements,
taking account of the sodium content of the Vamin mixture (Table
11.3), arterial line infusate and flush, and the measured losses.

Cautions

Potassium: extra care must be exercised during renal impairment
and K_2HPO_4 omitted or reduced if hyperkalaemic.

Hypocalcaemia rarely occurs secondarily to the phosphate in the
GEM and is corrected by reducing the phosphate concentration.

Never add bicarbonate as this will precipitate as $CaCO_3$.

Never add calcium to GEM as this will precipitate out phosphate.

Administration

Intravenous nutrition may be administered via peripheral or central
venous lines. Peripheral lines should be resited as quickly as possible
to avoid hypoglycaemia. If given centrally the caloric intake may be
increased by the use of 15–20% glucose solutions (sclerosant to
peripheral veins). Arterial lines are not suitable routes for i.v.
nutrition.
   Vamin and GEM may be mixed in a single bag if central sterile
preparation of i.v. nutrition is undertaken (e.g. in a pharmacy).
   Vamin and GEM may be infused via a standard infusion pump
after mixing the correct proportions in a two-entry port burette.
There should be a suitable bacterial filter in line before a Y connector. The fat emulsion is pumped into the other arm of this
connector and thus into the baby.

Strict aseptic techniques are necessary during preparation and administration. Drugs may be given into the line before the bacterial filter if chemically compatible and should be flushed through.

Vamin and GEM are infused continuously; intralipid over 20 hours. Fat infusion should be stopped 2–4 hours before blood samples for biochemical and haematological tests are removed. Lipid levels *in contrast* should be determined during, and after at least 8 hours of, fat infusion.

Modification of glucose concentration is necessary if there is hyperglycaemia and glycosuria (>0.25%). Reduce first to 7.5% and then to 5% if necessary. Remember that hyperglycaemia may indicate infection.

Monitoring

Close clinical (and if possible cardiorespiratory) monitoring is necessary.

Routine nursing observations include:

Daily weight

Temperature: skin and incubator: 4 hourly

Urine: specific gravity, pH, blood, protein and glucose: 12 hourly (glycosuria, see above).

Blood glucose: 4 hourly on first day, 8 hourly after (BM stix or Dextrostix)

Record: activity, apnoea, bradycardia

Routine blood tests include:

Daily (first week, alternate days after)
Full blood count and platelets
Plasma Na^+, K^+, Cl^-, glucose, urea, creatinine, bilirubin
Lipid levels during lipid infusion
Urine Na^+ urea creatinine

Twice weekly (then weekly)
Plasma calcium, magnesium, phosphate and bilirubin

Weekly
Alkaline phosphatase and transaminases
Urinary amino acids
(Blood cultures and clotting studies)

Gastrointestinal problems
Gastro-oesophageal reflux

Simple regurgitation of gastric contents is common in infancy. Gastro-oesophageal reflux may cause concern, however, if it causes failure to thrive, aspiration pneumonia, apnoea or oesophagitis. It may also play a role in some cases of BPD. Predisposing factors include hiatus hernia, delayed gastric emptying and following repair of tracheo-oesophageal fistula.

Investigation

If available *prolonged oesophageal pH monitoring* over 12–24 hours is the most accurate and sensitive method for the detection and quantification of reflux. If the pH is less than 4.0 for more than 5% of the study time, this is an abnormal result, and a value over 15% indicates severe reflux. *Radiology* may be necessary to exclude hiatus hernia.

Management

Clinical reflux spontaneously improves with time, causing confusion over indications for treatment and assessment of its efficacy. The practice of sitting the baby at an angle of 60° is now considered worse than leaving the baby supine; the *anti-Trendelenberg position* (prone with head elevated) is the most effective postural treatment. Other interventions include:

Small frequent feeds thickening agents   such as Carobel or cornflour which make the baby more settled but do not improve reflux. Unsuitable for premature babies.

Antacids,   such as Gaviscon.

Domperidon and Cisapride   new therapeutic agents which have been shown to reduce reflux significantly (and may improve respiratory symptoms in babies with reflux and chronic respiratory symptoms).

H₂ antagonists   may be indicated in severe cases with oesophagitis.

Surgical fundoplication   may be necessary in very severe cases where medical treatment has failed.

Necrotizing enterocolitis (NEC)

Although most common in very low birthweight babies, the frequency of NEC varies widely between centres. It is rare among babies who have not been fed. Recognized risk factors include:

(1) Low birthweight
(2) Asphyxia
(3) Artificial feeds
(4) Intrauterine growth retardation
(5) Polycythaemia
(6) Cardiac catheterization
(7) Early feeding in association with 4 and/or 5

Aetiology

The cause is multifactorial (Fig. 11.1). Developmental factors include immature bowel and transport, abnormal motility and

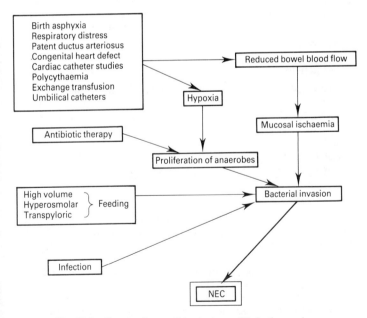

Fig. 11.1 Causes of necrotizing enterocolitis in the newborn.

decreased host resistance. The pathogenesis remains unclear but several important factors have been identified:

(a) Decreased vascular perfusion secondary to hypoxia or hypotension.
(b) Anaerobic bacterial overgrowth, which in association with (a) leads to mucosal damage.
(c) Further exacerbation of mucosal injury by vasoactive agents released by underperfused tissue.
(d) Invasion of damaged mucosa by bacteria such as *Clostridia*, *Klebsiella* or *E. coli*.

The colon and ileum are the sites most frequently affected. Pathological changes include mucosal damage, necrosis, haemorrhage and pneumatosis.

Clinical presentation

Presentation is variable because of difficulty in the early diagnosis of NEC. The classical triad of abdominal distension, bile-stained aspirate and bloody mucousy stools may be accompanied in severe cases with temperature instability, inflammation of the abdominal wall, peritonitis, shock and apnoea. Thirty per cent of suspected cases, however, have no blood in the stools, and most have a much milder illness.

Investigations

Radiological changes are initially non-specific and include reduced bowel gas shadowing, free fluid and thickening of the bowel wall. Later findings include (diagnostic) air in the bowel wall (pneumatosis coli) or even in the portal tract. Free peritoneal gas indicates perforation.

Laboratory findings include thrombocytopaenia, coagulopathy, hyponatraemia, hypoproteinaemia and hyperbilirubinaemia.

Management

Because of the difficulty in diagnosis of early disease and the high mortality, a high index of clinical suspicion is necessary. Medical treatment comprises:

(a) Stop oral feeds (usually for 7–10 days) and continuous low pressure gastric suction.
(b) Full infection screen including stools for virology (usually negative) and begin treatment with antibiotics (we use flucloxacillin, netilmicin and metronidazole).

(c) Correct anaemia, coagulopathy, fluid and electrolyte imbalance. High losses of blood and colloid into the bowel are to be anticipated. Monitor blood pressure and oxygenation.
(d) Isolate the baby (risk of 'cluster' of cases).
(e) Repeat abdominal X-ray 12–24 hourly until pneumatosis is settling (watch for signs of perforation).
(f) Reintroduce feeds slowly after 7–10 days (breast milk or pregestimil preferable to formula as temporary lactose tolerance may occur).

Surgical intervention only indicated if there is intestinal perforation, peritonitis or, rarely, deterioration despite medical treatment.

Complications and prognosis

About 10% will develop stricture and require surgery; short bowel syndrome may follow extensive resections. Mortality is highest in the very preterm. Gut function in most survivors appears normal in later infancy and childhood.

Differential diagnosis of acute diarrhoea

Congenital diarrhoeas – extremely rare
Gastroenteritis – viral and bacterial
Systemic infection – urinary tract infection, septicaemia, meningitis
Necrotizing enterocolitis
Metabolic disorders, e.g. adrenal insufficiency
Surgical conditions – Hirschsprung's disease

Other – Lactose intolerance
       Immunodeficiency
       Prostaglandin therapy
       Opiate withdrawal
       Phototherapy

Gastroenteritis

Acute infectious disease presenting with watery diarrhoea and vomiting which may occur in the newborn. The commonest pathogen is rotavirus, but other viruses, *E. coli*, salmonella, campylobacter, shigella or yersinia may be causative. Less common in breast-fed infants due to presence of IgA, antiviral factors and iron-binding proteins (lactoferrin), which inhibit the growth of *E. coli*.

Management

Stop formula feeds and rehydrate with oral glucose electrolyte solution or i.v. fluids if severe. Some breast feeding can continue. Slowly reintroduce feeds when symptoms settle. Antidiarrhoeal drugs are not indicated.

Lactose intolerance

Secondary

Secondary lactose intolerance may occur after gastroenteritis, NEC or gut surgery. It presents as diarrhoea with acid stools containing reducing substances. To avoid provoking symptoms it is wise to start feeding slowly with breast milk or hydrolysed cows' milk formula (pregestemil). Lactose-containing milk may be reintroduced when the baby is thriving. Very small infants may have a gestation-dependent relative lactose intolerance on formula feeds.

Primary

This is a very rare recessive disorder, presenting in the neonatal period with profuse watery diarrhoea. Sucrose and glucose are well tolerated.

Congenital diarrhoea

This presents as severe diarrhoea at or soon after birth leading to failure to thrive. The baby will need i.v. nutrition until diagnosis is made and appropriate therapy is instituted. It includes defects of intestinal transport (Cl/HCO_3 exchange; chloridorrhoea) and morphology (microvillous atrophy).

Bibliography

American Academy of Pediatrics, Committee of Nutrition (1981). Use of intravenous fat emulsions in pediatric patients. *Pediatrics*, **68**, 738–43.

Anderson, C. M., Burke, V. and Gacey, M. (Eds) (1987) *Paediatric Gastroenterology*. Oxford, Blackwell Scientific Publ.

Bentley, D. and Lawson, M. (1989). *Clinical Nutrition in Paediatric Disorders*. London: Bailliere Tindall.

Bremer, M. J., Brooke, O. G., Oralesi, M. *et al.* (1987). Nutrition and feeding of preterm infants. *Acta. Paed. Scand.* Suppl. 336.

Brooke, O. G. and Lucas, A. (1985). Metabolic bone disease in preterm infants. *Arch. Dis. Child.*, **60**, 682–5.

Bu'Lock, F., Woolridge, M. W. and Baum, J. D. (1990). The development of the co-ordination of sucking, swallowing and breathing; an ultrasonographic study of term and preterm infants. *Devel. Med. Child. Neurol.* **32**, 669–78.

Garza, C., Schanler, R. J., Butte, N. F. and Motil, K. J. (1987). Special properties of human milk. *Clinics in Perinatology*, **14**, 1, 11–32.

Gross, S. J., Geller, J. and Tomarelli, R. M. (1981). Composition of breast milk from mothers of preterm infants. *Pediatrics*, **68**, 490–3.

Jelliffe, D. B. and Jelliffe (1978). *Human Milk in the Modern World*. Oxford: Oxford University Press.

Lindblad, B. L. (1988) *Perinatal Nutrition*. London: Academic Press.

Lucas, A., Morley, R., Cole, T. J. *et al.* (1990). Early diet in preterm babies and developmental status at 18 months. *Lancet*, **i**, 1477–81.

Wooldridge, M. W. and Baum, J. D. (1988). The regulation of human milk flow. In: *Perinatal Nutrition*, (6th Bristol-Myers Nutrition Symposium). Ed. B. S. Lindblad, pp. 243–57. London: Academic Press.

Woolridge, M. W. and Fisher, C. (1988). Colic, 'overfeeding', and symptoms of lactose malabsorption in the breast-fed baby: a possible artifact of feed management? *Lancet*, **ii**, 382–4.

DHSS (1980). *Present Day Practice in Infant Feeding.* Department of Health and Social Security Report on Health and Social Subjects 20. London: HMSO.

World Health Organization (1985) *Energy and Protein Requirements*. WHO Technical Report Series Number 72.4. Geneva: World Health Organization.

12

Neonatal surgical problems

Antenatal diagnosis
Congenital diaphragmatic hernia
Exomphalos (omphalocele)
Gastroschisis
Tracheo-oesophageal fistula (TOF) and oesophageal atresia
Anorectal anomalies
Bowel obstruction
Pyloric stenosis
Inguinal hernia

Antenatal diagnosis (see page 11)

Many surgically treated abnormalities (e.g. diaphragmatic hernia, abdominal wall defects, oesophageal atresia) are suspected from antenatal ultrasound scans. Such infants should, if possible, be delivered in the referral centre with surgical and intensive care facilities rather than transferred after birth. There is no evidence of benefit from elective Caesarean section for infants with abdominal wall defects, diaphragmatic hernia or oesophageal atresia.

Congenital diaphragmatic hernia
Description

Usually, diaphragmatic hernia presenting in the newborn period is posterolateral (foramen of Bochdalek) or complete agenesis of the diaphragm. Herniae are more common on the left.

The incidence is 1 in 2000 live births (Avon County 1981–1983).

Diagnosis

Suspect any baby who fails to respond satisfactorily to intubation or bag-and-mask resuscitation at birth especially in the presence of maternal polyhydramnios. Confirmatory clinical signs such as barrel chest, displaced apex beat and scaphoid abdomen with unequal air entry should then be looked for.

Definite diagnosis is by X-ray of the chest and abdomen combined, showing loops of bowel in the chest and contralateral displacement of the mediastinum.

Management (see also Chapter 7, page 80)

In the labour suite

Bag-and-mask resuscitation may cause gastric distension and worsen respiratory distress. Intubate and insert a nasogastric tube (8F) to decompress the intrathoracic viscera. Nurse head up or flat. Transfer to the Special Care Baby Unit on intermittent positive-pressure ventilation (IPPV) (see Chapter 8, page 86).

In the neonatal intensive care unit (NICU)

Ventilation by IPPV should be maintained. High pressures may be required but these increase the danger of pneumothorax. Positive end-expiratory pressure (PEEP) should not normally exceed 3–4 cm H_2O. High rates of IPPV may also be helpful.

Electively paralyse with pancuronium $\pm$ morphine (for doses see Chapter 28). A preductal right radial and postductal umbilical or posterior tibial arterial line should be inserted (see Chapter 26). If there is a significant oxygen difference between them (>40 mm Hg) indicating shunting through a patent ductus arteriosus (PDA) due to high pulmonary artery pressure, tolazoline or dopamine (for doses see Chapter 23) should be started via a peripheral line. (Dopamine is particularly useful if there is, in addition, a low cardiac output.) As both of these drugs may also cause reduction in systemic blood pressure this must be carefully monitored and plasma given if necessary. (Plasma should be readily at hand when starting treatment.)

Insert a Replogle tube* if available, otherwise use a nasogastric tube (8F) into the stomach and attach to continuous suction (5–10 cm H_2O) to decompress the intrathoracic viscera.

---

*Argyle Replogle Suction Catheter. Catalogue No. 888/256504. Sherwood Medical Industries Ltd., London Road, County Oak, Crawley, Surrey.

Investigations

Check arterial **blood gases** as soon as possible after intubation and IPPV are established. See Chapter 8, page 86 for ventilatory management. If severe metabolic acidosis (pH <7.20) persists despite IPPV, give plasma, 10–20 ml/kg, i.v. over 1 hour.

Perform a combined chest and abdomen X-ray; full blood count and blood culture; then give prophylactic antibiotics immediately prior to operation. Blood group and cross-match mother's and baby's blood: one unit of blood for the operation.

The operation

The optimum time for operation is contentious. Recent evidence suggests that maximum medical support initially, with operative treatment delayed until a stable satisfactory state has been achieved, may improve results. This is not always possible, but operation on a grossly acidotic and hypoxaemic baby is not likely to be successful.

The hernia is repaired through an abdominal or a thoraco-abdominal route, either by a direct suture of the defect or by patching with an abdominal muscle graft or artificial membrane. Intrapleural drains are not generally inserted postoperatively. Air within the pleural cavity will be absorbed slowly. If a tension pneumothorax develops (mediastinal shift to contralateral side) a chest drain should be inserted.

Postoperative care

The *general aim* is to keep the preductal arterial oxygen around 100 mm Hg in term babies (70–90 mm Hg in babies <35 weeks' gestation).

Avoid sudden swings in oxygenation – continue pancuronium ± morphine for 2–3 days.

Moderate fluid restriction for the first 48 hours (60–80 ml/kg/24 hours). Correct assumed plasma losses into chest and peritoneal cavity with 15 ml/kg of fresh frozen plasma daily (or 1 g/kg salt-poor albumin).

Gentle physiotherapy and endotracheal toilet are particularly important in a paralysed baby.

At 3–4 days postoperatively, paralysis is stopped and the patient weaned off the ventilator.

Abdominal splinting with a loosely applied crepe bandage may be useful if abdominal musculature has been used in the repair, and may reduce the work of breathing.

The baby should be nursed head up and preferably prone.

Intravenous alimentation should be started 24–48 hours post-operatively and enteral feeding (via gastric tube) can usually be started by 5–7 days postoperatively.

A persistent patent ductus arteriosus is a common finding; it may lead to significant left-to-right shunting and occasionally requires surgical ligation.

Postoperative investigations

Daily for first 4–5 days postoperatively, then as indicated:

Haemoglobin or packed cell volume
Urea and electrolytes
Calcium and albumin
Chest and abdominal X-ray

Subsequent management

Infants who require minimal ventilatory support have a good outlook and may be out of hospital in 2–3 weeks depending on their gestational age. Those with the more severe defects are difficult to wean from ventilatory support and some develop bronchopulmonary dysplasia with oxygen-dependence which may persist for many weeks or months (see Chapter 8, page 103).

Follow-up

Pulmonary reserve is significantly reduced in the first 1–2 years, and minor respiratory infections commonly lead to severe respiratory symptoms, occasionally requiring ventilatory support. A small proportion of children with the most severe diaphragmatic herniae and secondary bronchopulmonary dysplasia develop cor pulmonale and die in later infancy. The majority of surviving children achieve virtually normal lung function later in childhood.

Exomphalos (omphalocele)
Description

This may be major (large abdominal wall defect covered by a sac of amnion and peritoneum) or minor (hernia of abdominal contents into umbilical cord). Up to 50% are associated with abnormalities of cardiovascular, genitourinary or gastrointestinal systems (e.g. Beckwith's syndrome – exomphalos, visceromegaly, macroglossia and hypoglycaemia).

The incidence is 1 in 10 000 live births.

Management

(see also Chapter 7, page 84)

In the labour suite

Cover the lesion with a plastic bag or cling film (or place the whole body up to the axillae in a plastic bag) to minimize evaporative heat and water loss. Attach a urine bag to measure urine output. Pass a large orogastric tube (8F) and connect to low suction to prevent stomach or bowel distension. This should be continued for several days postoperatively.

Subsequent management

The object is to return the gut to the abdominal cavity in order to reduce the risk of rupture of the sac and or infection. This is a relatively simple procedure in exomphalos minor. In exomphalos major, the abdominal cavity is often very small, and the lungs may be hypoplastic (because of lack of effective diaphragmatic contraction and breathing movements *in utero*). It may be possible to return the sac contents to the abdomen as a primary procedure, but large lesions may require a two or three-stage procedure. If skin cover cannot be achieved at the first operation, a combination of silastic and prolene mesh may be used, and the sac size reduced by progressive application of this covering over a period of several days or weeks, with later closure of the defect.

Raised abdominal pressure after operation may lead to respiratory embarrassment, inferior vena cava obstruction or renal venous thrombosis (see Chapter 16, page 240).

Pre- and postoperatively, sepsis is a major risk and broad-spectrum antibiotics (penicillin and aminoglycoside ± metronidazole) should be started preoperatively (after taking blood cultures) and continued for 5–7 days postoperatively.

Blood pressure, blood gases, blood electrolytes, fluid balance (including frequent urinalysis), and urine microscopy must be carefully monitored.

Intravenous feeding (see Chapter 11, page 167) should be started 24–48 hours postoperatively. Enteral feeding can be started when the infant has passed meconium and gastric aspirate is minimal (usually 5–7 days postoperatively).

Gastroschisis

Description

Coils of intestine herniate through a defect in the anterior abdominal wall, to the right of the umbilical cord. A covering of peritoneal membrane is absent and gangrene or perforation are common in the prolapsed bowel, due to ischaemia. It is not associated with other abnormalities apart from intestinal atresia. Babies are usually small-for-gestational-age and hypoproteinaemic.

The incidence has increased in recent years. It is now approximately 1 in 6000 deliveries. Survival is now >90% (Lafferty *et al*, 1989).

Management

In the labour suite

As for exomphalos.

Subsequent management

General management is similar to that for exomphalos. Surgical management is either primary closure or a two-stage procedure using a silastic silo and reducing the contents gradually over a period of 7–10 days. Bowel resection (for ischaemic damage) is more common with gastroschisis. Extensive protein losses occur into the bowel and peritoneal cavity and regular infusions of plasma or salt-poor albumin are needed to maintain plasma protein levels.

The bowel may take several weeks to work well and i.v. nutrition (usually through a long line) is important during this period.

Extensive bowel resection may lead to a 'short gut' syndrome requiring prolonged hospitalization and i.v. feeding.

Tracheo-oesophageal fistula (TOF) and oesophageal atresia

Description

Five main types exist (see Fig. 12.1). All are due to failure of oesophagus and trachea to differentiate in early embryonic life.

The most common type (87%) is oesophageal atresia with distal tracheo-oesophageal fistula.

The next most common type (8%) is oesophageal atresia without fistula. An X-ray at a few hours of age shows complete absence of

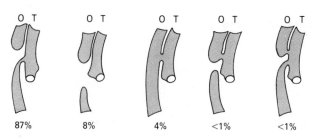

Fig. 12.1 Diagrams of the five most common types of tracheo-oesophageal fistula and oesophageal atresia, in order of frequency. (T = Trachea, O = Oesophagus)

bowel gas shadows. Fifty per cent are associated with other gastro-intestinal abnormalities (duodenal atresia and anorectal anomalies) and cardiovascular malformations. Occasionally there is a family history.

The incidence is 1 in 3000 live births.

Diagnosis

This should be made before feeding, otherwise there is a high risk of aspiration. There is usually a history of maternal polyhydramnios.

All babies born to mothers with polyhydramnios and all 'mucusy' babies should have a gastric tube passed (French 12) as soon as possible after birth. In the delivery suite the distal end of a mucus trap may be used. If oesophageal atresia is present the catheter will usually not pass more than 8–10 cm from the gum margin.

The diagnosis should be confirmed by combined chest and abdominal X-ray with a radio-opaque tube in the oesophagus. This will show the level of the oesophageal pouch and may reveal pulmonary consolidation due to aspiration. In the case of oesophageal atresia without fistula, abdominal X-ray shows a complete absence of bowel gas shadows. Aspiration may occur either from the upper pouch or from the stomach via the distal fistula (the latter is more common and more important).

Management

A Replogle tube should be passed into the oesophageal pouch and kept on low suction. The baby should be nursed head up to avoid aspiration of stomach secretions and to maximize the effect of the

Replogle tube. Surgery is performed as soon as the baby's condition is stable. It may be delayed in order to improve pulmonary function with physiotherapy and antibiotics if aspiration has occurred.

A primary end-to-end anastomosis of the oesophagus and division of the tracho-oesophageal fistula is possible in over 90% of cases, and performed via a right posterolateral extrapleural thoracotomy. A gastrostomy is usually performed and feeding started via a transpyloric tube within 48 hours of operation. An extrapleural drain is usually inserted at operation and removed on day 5 if there is no anastomotic leakage. A barium swallow is performed 5–7 days postoperatively to ensure integrity of the anastomosis before starting oral feeds.

Complications

Pneumonia or anastomotic breakdown may occur.

Coughing during feeds or recurrent chest infections may indicate either recurrence of the TOF or that a second fistula has been missed at operation.

Gastro-oesophageal reflux commonly occurs and requires medical and/or surgical treatment.

A brassy cough is very common and may persist for years. It needs no treatment.

The 'H' type tracheo-oesophageal fistula

This will not be diagnosed by failure to pass a nasogastric tube and usually presents later with episodes of cyanosis after feeds, or recurrent pneumonia.

Diagnosis

Suspected clinically with a positive 'bubble test'. A large nasogastric tube (Jacques No. 12) is passed and then gradually withdrawn up the oesophagus with the proximal end under water. Bubbling should occur when the tip has reached the level of the fistula unless the tube or fistula is full of mucus. The diagnosis should be confirmed at fluoroscopy, when a small amount of Dionesil is trickled down the oesophagus from a fine catheter. The fistula is usually seen at level C_7 or T_1, and usually fills by reflux.

Operation

Division of the fistula is usually possible through a cervical approach.

Anorectal anomalies

Description

For practical purposes lesions of the rectum can be divided into high (supralevator) and low (infralevator).

If the bowel has passed through the 'puborectalis sling', prospects for long-term faecal continence are excellent with relatively minor surgery. If not, then the bowel will have to be brought through the sling without damaging it to obtain continence.

Associated abnormalities include upper urinary tract (15%), cardiovascular (10%), high gut atresias (12%), and also sacral anomalies and oesophageal atresia.

The incidence is 1 in 2000 live births.

Diagnosis

In both boys and girls the low lesion may present with evidence of an anocutaneous fistula, or in girls as an ectopic, anteriorly situated stenotic anus or anovestibular fistula. In boys, the high lesion is frequently associated with a recto-urethral fistula. In girls a high rectovaginal fistula or cloaca may be present.

A lateral X-ray with the infant prone and slightly head down and a smear of barium over the skin dimple at 24 hours of age, may help distinguish the level of obstruction. Earlier X-rays are not usually helpful. Sacral anomalies will be shown on a plain abdominal X-ray.

Management

In low lesions the ectopic stenotic anal opening or covered anus is treated by an anoplasty.

If a high lesion is present a defunctioning high sigmoid colostomy is performed, followed by a 'pull through' operation at 6 months. The colostomy is usually closed 6 weeks after the second operation.

Prognosis in low lesions is excellent, over 90% achieving normal faecal continence, but less good in the high lesions where continence may not be achieved until the teens.

Complications

Urinary tract infections (especially if recto-urethral fistula or upper urinary tract abnormality is present) (see Chapter 16).

Bowel obstruction

Atresia and stenosis of the intestine

Description

Atresia may be of three types:

Type I   lumen completely obstructed by septum or septa
Type II   two ends of gut joined by fibrous cord
Type III ends completely separated with a V-shaped gap in the
          mesentery

Stenotic lesions may be due to localized narrowing of the gut or a perforated septum. They may be single or multiple.

The incidence is rare.

Duodenal atresia is associated with Down's syndrome in a third of cases. It is the commonest site of atresia (1 in 6000 live births). Small bowel atresia may be associated with cystic fibrosis.

Diagnosis

All except duodenal atresia above the ampulla of Vater present with the signs and symptoms of intestinal obstruction, i.e. abdominal distension, bilious vomiting and failure to pass meconium. In general the lower down the small intestine the defect, the later the presentation after birth (usually 24–48 hours). All may be associated with maternal polyhydramnios, fetal growth retardation and prematurity. The amniotic fluid may be green/bile stained due to antenatal vomiting.

An X-ray will show a 'double bubble' appearance in duodenal atresia which is pathognomonic of duodenal obstruction. Otherwise, multiple fluid levels will be seen, sometimes with flecks of calcification, indicating intrauterine perforation. A barium enema should be performed to exclude large bowel obstruction.

Management

Correct any fluid and electrolyte disturbances (see Chapter 17). Duodeno-duodenostomy is the treatment of choice for duodenal atresia. In small bowel lesions, excision of an atretic segment is followed by end-to-end anastomosis if the proximal gut is not too distended. Otherwise a double-barrelled enterostomy is formed to allow decompression of the gut. Anastomosis is usually performed 5–10 days later.

A gastric tube should be passed and connected to low suction preoperatively and for several days postoperatively. Enteral feeding should not be started until meconium has been passed and gastric aspirate is minimal. Intravenous feeding should be commenced 24–48 hours postoperatively and continued until enteral feeding is established (see page 167).

Commence broad-spectrum antibiotics (penicillin and amino-glycoside ± metronidazole) preoperatively (after blood culture) and continue for 5–7 days postoperatively.

Meconium ileus

Description

Fifteen per cent of children with cystic fibrosis present in the neonatal period with bowel obstruction caused by the abnormally tenacious meconium. (NB only 75% of children with meconium ileus have cystic fibrosis.)

Diagnosis

This may be difficult, but the following will suggest the diagnosis:

(1) Family history of cystic fibrosis or neonatal bowel obstruction.
(2) Failure to pass meconium by 48 hours.
(3) Erect abdominal X-ray usually shows no fluid levels but may show:
    (i) characteristic foamy appearance of the gut contents, or
    (ii) if there has been perforation with meconium peritonitis – flecks of calcium.
(4) Blood immunoreactive trypsin level should be assayed. If elevated this is highly suggestive of cystic fibrosis.

Management

A barium enema may reveal a microcolon, and a gastrografin enema may relieve an uncomplicated obstruction by osmotic effect, increasing the water content of the stool.

NB   Loss of water from the circulation may cause hypotension, therefore generous intravenous fluids must be given throughout the procedure.

If this is not successful a laparotomy will need to be performed and a temporary double-barrelled ileostomy fashioned. This is closed after 5–10 days, when the distal loop has been cleared of meconium.

A sweat test can be performed at 4–6 weeks.

Fat globules and low tryptic activity in the stool suggest cystic fibrosis. If weight gain is poor, commence pancreatic supplements (e.g. Pancrex); improved weight gain supports the diagnosis of cystic fibrosis.

Malrotation and volvulus

Description

Failure of complete rotation of the mid-gut around the mesenteric axis.

Uncommon, male:female ratio = 2:1, 75% present in the first month of life.

Diagnosis

Presents with high intestinal obstruction due to volvulus of the small intestine around the mesenteric axis or to duodenal obstruction from tight adhesions (Ladd's bands) to the overlying caecum situated in the right hypochondrium.

The clinical picture is similar to duodenal atresia except that obstruction is usually incomplete so that signs appear more gradually. There may be passage of blood per rectum if strangulation of the bowel occurs. Barium meal will show partial obstruction of the third part of the duodenum and the jejunum in the right upper quadrant of the abdomen.

Management

General management is as for atresia (page 187). *Urgent* surgery is necessary to divide Ladd's bands and undo any volvulus to prevent total gangrene of the whole intestine.

Hirschsprung's disease

Description

Hirschsprung's disease is a congenital absence of ganglion cells in myenteric plexus of Meissner and Auerbach in the rectum and extending proximally for a variable distance.

The incidence is 1 in 5000, male:female ratio = 3:1, increased family incidence.

Diagnosis

The disease generally presents as a large bowel obstruction with vomiting ± distension and failure to pass meconium in the first week. It should be considered in an asymptomatic full-term baby who has not passed meconium by 48 hours, or who passes a meconium plug. Rectal examination may reveal a small conical rectum and be followed by an explosive passage of faeces. A barium enema shows a conical 'transitional zone' where normal dilated colon cones down to the aganglionic segment.

Rectal suction biopsy showing absence of ganglion cells, and hyperplasia of nerve fibres is diagnostic.

Management

General management is as for atresia (page 187).

A defunctioning colostomy in bowel, shown by frozen-section biopsy to have ganglia, should be performed proximal to the obstruction. Excision of the aganglionic segment and a rectosigmoidostomy may be performed at 3–6 months.

Increased sodium losses via the colostomy should be replaced with sodium bicarbonate (a low urinary sodium will indicate the necessity for sodium supplements).

Pyloric stenosis

Description

The muscle of the pylorus is hypertrophic. The cause is unknown. Hereditary factors are involved; siblings of an affected baby are 25 times more likely to be affected than in the normal population.

The incidence is 3 in 1000 live births, male:female ratio = 4:1.

Diagnosis

Presentation is usually around 2–4 weeks with vomiting which becomes projectile but is not bile stained. There is usually constipation and commonly weight loss. The infant looks thin, alert and hungry and may be dehydrated. There is usually a hypochloraemic alkalosis.

A test feed is performed to establish the diagnosis. As well as visible peristalsis (side-lighting is useful to demonstrate this) the hypertrophied pyloric muscle should be felt with the left hand just above and to the right of the umbilicus. Projectile vomiting may occur during or after the feed. An erect plain X-ray of the abdomen usually shows an air-fluid level in the stomach with minimal distal air. Barium swallow is rarely necessary but will show a 'string sign' as the contrast passes through the narrowed pyloric canal.

Treatment

(1) Correct fluid and electrolyte disturbances over 12–24 hours intravenously (see Chapter 17).
(2) *Surgery*: pyloromyotomy.
(3) *Postoperatively*: commonly some vomiting for first 24 hours. Continue i.v. fluids until tolerating oral feeds.

Inguinal hernia

Indirect inguinal hernia is especially common in preterm infants. Eighty per cent occur in boys. In girls the ovary may herniate into the inguinal canal.

Usually a swelling is palpable at the external inguinal ring, but it may extend into the scrotum or labia majora. The swelling may be constant or only noticeable on crying or straining.

There is a high risk of incarceration or strangulation of inguinal herniae in infancy, so surgical repair should be carried out before discharge from hospital.

Older infants noted to have inguinal herniae should have surgical repair carried out within a few days of diagnosis.

Bibliography

Jones, P. G. and Woodward, A. A. (1986). *Clinical Paediatric Surgery*, 3rd edn. Melbourne. Blackwell Scientific Publ.

Kluth, D. (1976). Atlas of esophageal atresia. *J. Pediatr. Surg.*, **11**, 901–19.

Lafferty, P. M., Emmerson A. J., Fleming, P. J. *et al.* (1989). Management of infants with abdominal wall defects. *Arch. Dis. Child.*, **64**, 1029–31.

Nixon, H. H. (1978). *Surgical Conditions in Paediatrics*. Guildford: Butterworth Scientific.

Rickman, P. P., Lister, J. and Irving, I. M. (1978). *Neonatal Surgery*, 2nd edn. Guildford: Butterworth Scientific.

Vidyasagar, D. and Reyes, H. (1989). Neonatal surgery. *Clin. Perinatol.*, **16**, 1.

13

Metabolic and endocrine problems

Disorders presenting as metabolic disturbances
Endocrine problems
Inborn errors of metabolism
Screening for metabolic disease

Disorders presenting as metabolic disturbances

Hypoglycaemia

Definition

Plasma glucose less than 1.7 mmol/l. However, recent evidence suggests that levels below 2.6, particularly if prolonged, may be associated with a poorer outcome. There is no evidence to support the hypothesis that preterm infants can tolerate lower levels than term infants.

Diagnosis

Low capillary glucose (Dextrostix <2.5 or BM stix <2.2 mmol/l). Blood glucose sticks are often inaccurate at low levels, especially if polycythaemic: always confirm with blood glucose measurement.

Causes

Small for gestational age (SGA)
Preterm
Starvation (including delayed resiting of infusions)
Maternal intrapartum treatment with betamimetics or steroids
Decreased adrenal and pituitary function

Inborn errors of metabolism (e.g. galactosaemia, see Table 13.1, page 206).
Congenital heart disease
Cold stress
Hypoxia
Infection
Polycythaemia
Hyperinsulinism   Infant of diabetic mother
                    Beckwith–Wiedemann syndrome
                    Maternal glucose infusion
                    Severe haemolytic disease
                    Nesidioblastosis
                    Islet cell adenoma

Prevention

Avoid risk factors (cold stress etc.)
Check capillary glucose 3–4 hourly for the first 24 hours in at-risk groups (see above).
Early feeding (<4 hours), preferably enteral, if contraindicated (respiratory distress, birth asphyxia, etc.), give 10% glucose, i.v.

Management

Asymptomatic hypoglycaemia: Repeat Dextrostix (check expiry date)
Send blood sugar sample. IF <1.7 mmol/l treat as for symptomatic hypoglycaemia
Correct precipitating cause (e.g. cold stress)
Feed baby (10–15 ml/kg) of breast milk or infant formula
Repeat Dextrostix in 1 hour; if still <2.5 mmol/l (BM stix <2.2 mmol/l) repeat blood sugar and consider need for dextrose infusion
Continue 3–4 hourly Dextrostix until results consistently >2.5 mmol/l (at least 12 hours).

Symptomatic hypoglycaemia: ill-defined symptoms and signs include jitteriness, tremors, apnoea, lethargy, hypotonia, abnormal cry, poor feeding and convulsions.

Immediately

Repeat Dextrostix/BM stix
Send sample for true blood sugar measurement
Stop oral feeds: pass nasogastric tube (to prevent aspiration)
Commence intravenous infusion

(a) Give 2–3 ml/kg 15% glucose solution as bolus *only* if infant is convulsing (beware rebound hypoglycaemia).
(b) Start i.v. infusion of 10% glucose solution at 8–10 ml/kg/hour (15 mg/kg/min) for up to 1 hour – until Dextrostix >2.5 mmol/l (BM stix >2.2 mmol/l).
(c) Slowly reduce infusion rate to 4 ml/kg/hour and continue infusion at this rate until Dextrostix remains stable.

The glucose infusion should be maintained at the rate necessary to maintain blood glucose >2.5 mmol/l. If this results in excessive fluid load, use 15% glucose (see Fig. 13.1).

Glucagon, 0.1 mg/kg, i.m. repeated 6–12 hourly may be used where i.v. glucose is delayed due to poor venous access, but beware of rebound hypoglycaemia. Useful in infants of diabetic mothers who have low glucagon levels at birth.

If the infant requires >12 mg/kg/min of glucose to maintain normoglycaemia then hyperinsulinism is a probable cause. This may be transient (e.g. infant of diabetic mother) or more permanent (e.g. nesidioblastosis).

(a) Take blood for insulin and cortisol measurement.
(b) If the glucose requirement is persistently >12 mg/kg/hour give hydrocortisone 5 mg/kg i.v. or i.m. 12 hourly.
(c) If hydrocortisone is either ineffective or required for >48 hours, start diazoxide 5 mg/kg 8 hourly, with chlothiazide 12.5 mg/kg 12 hourly.
(d) Consider insertion of a central line to enable uninterrupted glucose administration, particularly if high concentrations of glucose are necessary as these are very irritant to peripheral veins.
(e) If nesidioblastosis is present then subtotal pancreatectomy may be ultimately necessary.

Late hypoglycaemia

Hypoglycaemia occurring more than 24 hours after starting feeds, in the absence of an underlying identifiable cause such as sepsis, suggests a metabolic cause (e.g. galactosaemia) and should be fully investigated before recommencing oral feeds (see Table 13.1).

Hyperglycaemia

Definition

Blood glucose >8 mmol/l ± glycosuria.

Causes

Very low birthweight infants tolerate glucose poorly and hyperglycaemia is a common side-effect of total parental nutrition (TPN). A fall in glucose tolerance suggests cold stress or sepsis. Very rarely, transient diabetes mellitus may occur in very small-for-dates infants. Hyperglycaemia may exacerbate acidosis. Glycosuria ($>0.25\%$) may cause osmotic diuresis and electrolyte disturbances.

Management

If acidotic or if glucosuria $>0.25\%$, reduce glucose infusion rate (Fig. 13.1) by decreasing concentration or volume of glucose solution infused. Insulin therapy is dangerous but may be necessary (soluble insulin, 0.05–0.1 units/kg/hour).

Hypocalcaemia

Definition

Serum total calcium* level of less than 1.7 mmol/l or an ionized calcium level of less than 0.7 mmol/l.

Diagnosis

Signs and symptoms are non-specific, e.g. irritability, jitteriness and convulsions.

Aetiology

Early hypocalcaemia   (days 1–3)
Because of low parathormone levels and elevated calcitonin levels, serum calcium normally falls from birth until 48 hours of age, then stabilizes and rises. Any stress (e.g. asphyxia, hypoxia, respiratory distress or infection) may exacerbate this normal pattern.

Risk groups: Preterm infants
Infants of diabetic mothers
During exchange transfusion

Late hypocalcaemia   (days 5–7)
Risk factors: Hypomagnesaemia
Hypoparathyroidism (e.g. Di George syndrome)
Renal failure
Maternal hyperparathyroidism, hypercalcaemia
   or hypovitaminosis D

---

* If available, use calcium level corrected for plasma albumin concentration.

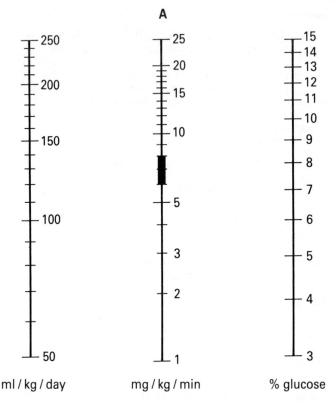

Fig. 13.1   Glucose rate calculator. Use a straight-edge to determine the glucose infusion rate (column A) mg/kg/min. Normal glucose requirement in the newborn infant is 6–8 mg/kg/min. If this is insufficient to maintain adequate blood levels there is evidence of increased utilization e.g. due to cold stress or hyperinsulinism. (From: Klaus M. H. and Fanaroff A. A. Eds. (1979) *Care of the High-Risk Neonate*. London: W. B. Saunders Co.)

Management

Asymptomatic hypocalcaemia: Ensure appropriate milk.
Add calcium supplements to milk (1–2 mmol Ca^{2+}/kg/day).
If already receiving intravenous infusion:
   Check albumin – if low may cause low serum Ca^{2+}, but does not
   need treatment.
   Check phosphate intake – if high may cause reciprocal hypo-
   calcaemia.
   Increase or add calcium to iv fluids .

Symptomatic hypocalcaemia: *For seizures* give 0.2–0.5 ml/kg 10% calcium gluconate diluted 1:4 with water of 10% glucose, under ECG control, *over 15 minutes* or until seizures cease.

For other symptoms, stop i.v. feeding and replace with 10% glucose containing 20–40 mmol/litre NaCl to which has been added sufficient Ca^{2+} as gluconate to ensure 2 mmol Ca^{2+}/kg/day

NB Calcium gluconate 10% contains 0.225 mmol Ca^{2+}/ml. Calcium lactate 10% contains 0.32 mmol Ca^{2+}/ml. Watch *drip sites* carefully during infusion of calcium as extravasation may cause severe tissue injury.

Do not add calcium to solutions containing bicarbonate or phosphate as precipitation may occur.

Resistant hypocalcaemia: Hypocalcaemia resistant to treatment may be associated with hypomagnesaemia.

Hypomagnesaemia

Definition

Serum magnesium less than 0.7 mmol/l.

Diagnosis

Check serum magnesium in unexplained convulsions or persistent hypocalcaemia.

Causes

Idiopathic, often associated with hypocalcaemia
Low skeletal stores due to poor placental transfer
Neonatal hypoparathyroidism (with hypocalcaemia) following exchange transfusion
Gut disorders (poor absorption)

Management

Magnesium sulphate 50%, 0.2 ml/kg, i.m. as a single dose. This is usually sufficient to correct the accompanying hypocalcaemia. Rarely oral maintenance therapy is required (0.2 ml/kg/day). Larger doses may be necessary in malabsorptive states.

NB   Treatment with magnesium may cause neuromuscular block-
ade with transient weakness and hypotonia.

Endocrine problems

Ambiguous genitalia

This includes:
    Bilateral cryptorchidism
    Perineal hypospadias
    Frankly ambiguous genitalia

Assessment

History
Drugs during pregnancy
Family history (ambiguous genitalia; infertile aunts)
Neonatal or infant deaths, congenital adrenal hyperplasia (CAH)

Examination
Any dysmorphic features
Blood pressure
Size of phallus
Position of urethral orifice
Gonads (if both palpable, they are probably testes)
Position of anus

Management

See Fig. 13.2.

NB   Do not rush the choice of gender, and NEVER GUESS.

Explain to parents that it will take time, investigation and discussion
before confirming gender. If the phallus is very small, even a chromo-
somally male child may be better reared as a female. Reassure the
parents that the baby *will* be *either* a boy or girl, *not* 'in-between'.

Congenital adrenal hyperplasia

Presentation

Congenital adrenal hyperplasia may present in the neonatal period as
ambiguous genitalia, sometimes accompanied by pigmentation of
nipples and/or scrotum. These infants may develop a high serum

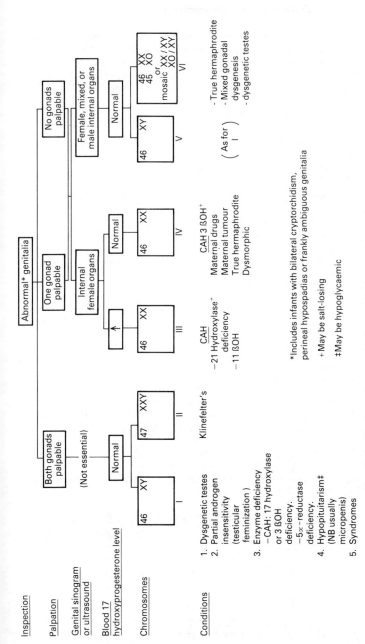

Fig. 13.2 The investigation of infants with abnormal genitalia.

potassium before the classical finding of hyponatraemia with paradoxically high urinary sodium. About half are strong 'salt losers' and
may present with adrenocortical crisis – dehydration and collapse –
during the second or third week of life. A small percentage may be
hypertensive (especially 17-OH or 11-beta-OH deficiency).

Diagnosis

Plasma 17-hydroxyprogesterone level (17-OHP)
Plasma electrolytes (daily)
Blood pressure and weight (daily)

Maintain daily plasma electrolytes, blood pressure and weight.

Normal values   17-OHP <30 nmol/l in blood taken 24 hours after
birth (to exclude placental 17-OHP). In untreated CAH, it is
generally >200 nmol/l.

Immediate management

(a) Infuse 0.9% saline in 5–10% dextrose at 150 ml/kg/day.
(b) hydrocortisone, 25 mg, i.m. 12 hourly (i.v. infusion of 1 mg/hour
    for 24 hours if collapsed).
(c) 9-Alpha-fludrocortisone 100 microg daily orally.

Maintenance

Educate parents in the technique of intramuscular injections which
are essential if the child is vomiting or seriously unwell. Maintenance
hydrocortisone is given intramuscularly for the first few weeks.

Give: Hydrocortisone 25 mg i.m. twice weekly
         9-Alpha-fludrocortisone orally microg daily
         Sodium supplements (2–5 mmol Na/kg/day orally for the first
         few weeks).

When parents can cope well with injections change to hydrocortisone
cypionate 20 mg/m²/day* in 2–3 doses, continue 9-alpha-
fludrocortisone.

* Surface area calculated as $\dfrac{[\text{weight in Kg} \times 4] + 7}{\text{weight in Kg} + 90}$

Illness

Parents should double the steroid dosage and give hydrocortisone 100 mg i.m. if vomiting, diarrhoea or very unwell.

General

Careful maintenance of length essential. Use both longitudinal and velocity data.

Congenital hypothyroidism

Causes

Goitrous cretinism
Maternal goitrogens (antithyroid drugs or iodine)
Dyshormogenesis
Haemangiomata or lymphangiomata of thyroid

Non-goitrous hypothyroidism
Congenital athyreosis
Ectopic thyroid
Thyroid dysgenesis

Presenting features

Commonly *no* clinically apparent features in neonatal period; may have:
   Prolonged gestation
   Normal birthweight
   Temperature instability
   Poor tone
   Large tongue
   Delayed passage of meconium
   Poor feeding
   Lethargy
   Later features include umbilical hernia, prolonged jaundice, large
      fontanelles, hoarse cry, dry skin, constipation etc.

Diagnosis

Thyroid function tests including thyroxine (T_4) and thyroid-stimulating hermone (TSH) assays (X-ray of knee: absent epiphyses in a term infant suggests hypothyroidism).

Normal range: T_4, 90–195 nmol/l (2 weeks–1 year)
                 TSH, <5 mU/l

NB   Small, sick preterm infants may show biochemical evidence of transient hypothroxinaemia.

Treatment

L-thyroxine 8–10 microg/kg/day for preterm infants; 5–8 microg/kg/day for term infants. Increase dose slowly until T_4 and TSH return to normal. Subsequently monitor dosage by maintaining normal TSH level. Dose: 5 microg/kg/day for first 3–4 years of life, subsequently falling to 3–4 microg/kg/day.

Screening

This is now routine in many areas (see page 205).

Neonatal hyperthyroidism

Causes

This may occur in infants born to mothers with active or non-active Graves' disease. It is due to transplacental passage of a thyroid-stimulating IgG immunoglobulin. The infants may be protected initially by maternal antithyroid drugs, but may show signs of thyrotoxicosis at birth. Usually they present at 7–10 days with signs of thyrotoxicosis such as exophthalmos, lid lag, sweatiness and tachycardia – which may progress to heart failure, hyperthermia, weight loss, jitteriness, vomiting and diarrhoea.

Diagnosis

Cord blood for T_4, TSH and thyroid-stimulating immunoglobulin (in mothers with Graves' disease).

Management

Propranolol, 2 mg/kg/24 hours
10% potassium iodide, 8 mg/kg/24 hours
Prophylthiouracil, 5–10 mg/kg/24 hours
(All divided into equal doses 8 hourly)
Digoxin and diuretics may be required

NB   This disorder is self-limiting and therapy is rarely needed beyond two months.

Congenital hypopituitarism

Causes

Mid-line defects
    Septo-optic dysplasia
    Pituitary hypoplasia
    Associated with cleft lip and palate

Presentation

Apnoea, prolonged jaundice, hypoglycaemia, micropenis in males.

Diagnosis

Low plasma cortisol, with poor response to synacthen i.m. $\pm$ low T_4 and TSH.

Treatment

(**a**) Hydrocortisone as for CAH.
(**b**) *L*-thyroxine as for hypothyroidism.
(**c**) If micropenis: testosterone, two doses 1 month apart.
(**d**) Growth hormone replacement may be required when older.

Inborn errors of metabolism

Initial presentation is often non-specific (lethargy, poor feeding, weight loss, hypoglycaemia, tachypnoea). Increased suspicion of an inborn error should occur if there is:
(**1**) Family history of neonatal deaths or unexplained illness
(**2**) Unexplained or persistent symptoms

Initial investigations

Full infection screen
Blood
Full blood count
Glucose
Blood gases
Urea, creatinine, Na, K, Cl
(calculate anion gap: normal <16 mmol/l)
Bilirubin, transaminases

Urine
Reducing substances (clinistix + clinitest)
Ketones

Subsequently illness can usually be classified into one or more of the following four groups:

(1) Acid/base disturbances
(2) Recurrent or persistent hypoglycaemia
(3) Acute liver disease
(4) Neurological deterioration

Further investigations

(1) Acid/base disturbance
    (a) Metabolic acidosis
        Blood: Lactate/3-hydroxy-butyrate
                Ammonia
                Amino acids
        Urine: Amino acids
                Organic acids
    (b) respiratory alkalosis
        Blood: Ammonia
                Amino acids
        Urine: Organic acids
                Amino acids
                Orotic acid

(2) Recurrent or persistent hypoglycaemia
    (collect samples, where possible at time of hypoglycaemia)
    Blood: Insulin
            Cortisol
            lactate
            3-OH-butyrate
            Red blood cell galactose-1-phosphate or galactose-1-P
              uridyl transferase assay
            $Alpha_1$-antitrypsin
    Urine: Organic acids
            Reducing substances

(3) Acute liver disease
    Blood: Amino acids
            Red blood cell galactose-1-phosphate or galactose-1-P
              uridyl transferase assay
            $Alpha_1$-antitrypsin

Urine: Reducing substances
               Amino acids
               Organic acids

(4) Neurological deterioration
    Blood: As for metabolic acidosis
                   Uric acid
    Urine: As for metabolic acidosis
                   Sulphite

NB   Always attempt to discuss with laboratories before samples taken.

Clinical features of specific metabolic disorders (see Table 13.1)

Specimens to be taken if the baby dies

If the baby dies it is still extremely important to try to make a diagnosis, particularly for advice regarding future pregnancies. Specimens must be taken as soon after death as possible.

Blood: 10–20 ml. Separate plasma immediately and freeze at −20°C in 1–2 ml aliquots. Store infranatant at +4°C (up to 2 days) for red and white cells.

Urine: 20 ml in 5 ml aliquots. Freeze at −20°C.

Liver: Needle biopsy. Freeze immediately in liquid nitrogen or dry ice.

Skin: Full thickness skin biopsy. Use aseptic conditions, clean skin with Hibitane in spirit and clean off with alcohol swab. Take at least 1 mm^2 of skin. Place in culture medium, or if not available, in normal saline. Store at +4°C.

Screening for metabolic disease

Two neonatal metabolic screening procedures are routinely performed in the UK at present:

Phenylketonuria (PKU) (incidence 1 in 12 000 births)
Heel prick spot of blood collected onto filter paper >48 hours after baby is on full feeds (age 5–10 days). Amino acid chromatogram on

Table 13.1 Clinical features and management of some inborn errors of metabolism that may present acutely in infancy

Condition	Hypogly-caemia	Acid/base disturbance	Neurological deterioration	Liver failure
Carbohydrate disorders				
Galactosaemia	++	+/−	+/−	+
Gluconeogenic disorders	++	+	−	−
Glycogen storage disease				
Type 1a	++	++	−	−
1b	++	++	−	−
111	+	+/−	−	−
Amino acidaemias				
Tyrosinaemia (type 1)	+/−	−	−	++
MSUD	+/−	++	++	−
Non-ketotic hyperglycinaemia	−	−	++	−

Other features	Diagnosis	Treatment	Prognosis
Cataracts +/− *E. coli* septicaemia	Reducing substances in urine (but may be absent) Red cell enzyme diagnosis	Galactose free diet	Variable, may be satisfactory with early diagnosis and treatment
Lactic acidosis	Liver/skin biopsy	Initial i.v. dextrose No specific therapy Avoid fasting	Variable
Lactic acidosis	No rise in blood sugar with glucagon Liver biopsy	Dextrose, i.v., followed by continuous tube feeds	Good
Lactic acidosis Neutropenia	As type 1a	As type 1a Prophylactic antibiotics	Guarded Recurrent infections
Normal lactate	No rise in blood sugar with glucagon WBC and RBC enzyme assay	As type 1a	Good
Raised plasma tyrosine and methionine	Succinylacetone in urine	Low phenyl-alanine, tyro-sine and methionine diet	Guarded: hepatic failure Liver transplant
Urine smells of maple syrup	Raised plasma and urine leucine, isoleucine and valine	Dextrose, i.v./ bicarbonate +/− exchange transfusion Low leu, isoleu, val diet	Good if early diagnosis and treatment
Early onset of fits Hypergly-cinaemia	Hypergly-cinuria Raised CSF glycine Normal organic acids in urine	None effective	Neonatal onset usually fatal

Table 13.1   *Continued*

Condition	Hypogly-caemia	Acid/base disturbance	Neurological deterioration	Liver failure
Organic acidaemias	+	+ +	+ +	−
Urea cycle disorders	−	+/−	+ +	+
Transient neonatal hyperammonaemia	+/−	+/−	+ +	+/−

AA, amino acid	leu, leucine	val, valine
OCT, otnitrine carboxyl transferase	isoleu, isoleucine	Na, sodium
CPS, carbonyl phosphate synmetase		

spot will detect phenylketonuria and tyrosinaemia (and may detect Maple Syrup Urine disease MSUD).

NB   If bacteriological assay (Guthrie) is used, antibiotics given to the mother or baby may interfere.

Hypothyroidism (incidence 1 in 3500 births)
Heel prick spot of blood collected onto filter paper at age 5–10 days (collected at same time and onto same paper as PKU test). TSH level assayed on blood spot:

TSH level <25 mU/l: normal. (NB   Exact levels vary with laboratory)
>80 mU/l   = Abnormal. Infant recalled urgently for full thyroid function tests.
25–80 mU/l = Equivocal. Repeat on second blood spot on same filter

Other features	Diagnosis	Treatment	Prognosis
Smell of sweaty feet in isovaleric acidaemia +/− hyper-ammonaemia	Characteristic organic acids in urine Neutropenia	Dextrose i.v./ bicarbonate +/− peritoneal dialysis	Variable, may be satisfactory with early diagnosis and treatment
+/− respiratory alkalosis	Hyperam-monaemia Characteristic plasma AA profile Urinary orotic acid (OCT and CPS def) +/− liver biopsy	Dextroxe, i.v. Arginine, i.v. Na phenyl-acetate Na benzoate Exchange transfusion Haemodialysis	Variable, may be satisfactory with early diagnosis and treatment
Early onset (<24 hours) if respir-atory distress			

paper; if still equivocal then infant recalled for repeat sample.

NB   Treatment should start as soon as possible.

Bibliography

Aynsley-Green, A. and Soltesz, G. (Eds) (1985). *Hypoglycaemia in Infancy and Childhood*. Edinburgh. Churchill Livingstone.

Brown, D. and Salsbury, D. (1982). Short term biochemical effects of parental calcium treatment of early onset neonatal hypocalcaemia. *J. Pediatr.*, **100**, 777.

Cornblath, M. and Shwartz, R. (1976). *Disorders of Carbohydrate Metabolism in Infancy*, 2nd edn. London: W. B. Saunders.

DHSS (1981). *Screening for Congenital Hypothyroidism*. Recommendations to Standing Medical Advisory Committee and

Scottish Health Services Planning Council. Appendix to Health Notice H.N. (81) 20. London: HMSO.

Leonard, J. V. (1985). The early detection and management of inborn errors presenting acutely in the neonatal period. *Eur. J. Pediatr.*, **143**, 253–7.

Schaffer, A. J. and Avery, M. E. (Eds) (1977). *Diseases of the Newborn*, 4th edn. London: W. B. Saunders.

Swyer, P. (1975). *The Intensive Care of the Newly Born*. Basel: S. Karger.

Wu, P. Y. K. (Ed.) (1982). Fluid balance in the newborn infant. *Clin. Perinatal.*, **9**, 3.

14

Perinatal infections

Congenital infections
Neonatal infections
Superficial infections
Systemic infections
Investigation of infant suspected of infection
Acute virus infections of the newborn
Fungal infections

The newborn infant is particularly susceptible to infection because of reduced defence mechanisms and is rapidly colonized by whatever organisms are in the environment. Even weak pathogens may cause serious infection. Humoral immunity is mainly by transplacental IgG. The leucocytes have decreased chemotaxis, phagocytosis and bactericidal abilities. Opsonization is defective but can be corrected by infusion of fresh plasma.

Congenital infections
TORCH infections

The commonest non-bacterial organisms causing fetal infection are toxoplasma, rubella, cytomegalovirus and herpes, known as the TORCH infections. Prospective studies suggest that between 1 and 5% of babies may be infected. Although they may present with severe neonatal illness, more than 90% of intrauterine infections are subclinical at birth (for HIV infections see page 5).

Clinical features

(1) Small for gestational age.
(2) Acute neonatal illness characterized by haemolytic anaemia,

jaundice, haemorrhage, thrombocytopenia, hepatitis and hepatosplenomegaly. There may also be a myocarditis, pneumonitis and encephalitis, especially with the disseminated form of herpes.

(3) Subclinical but with specific features as shown:

Toxoplasmosis: Chorioretinitis, microphthalmia, hydrocephalus or microcephaly. Cerebral calcification, high CSF protein.

Rubella: Cataracts. Retinal pigmentation. Congenital heart defect. Microcephaly. Bone lesions (e.g. 'celery stalk' femur).

Cytomegalovirus: Haemolytic anaemia, thrombocytopenia. Microcephaly. Cerebral calcification. Chorioretinitis.

Herpes: Skin vesicles. Chorioretinitis, keratitis. If acquired at the time of birth, herpes may not present for up to 21 days.

Investigations

A firm diagnosis of the disease in the mother is unusual but a history of contact or non-specific illness should be asked for. Blood from mother and baby should be sent for antibody titres against the TORCH organisms, but this is of limited value and more specific tests are necessary:

Blood: for rubella, CMV specific IgM.
Urine: (fresh × 3) for isolation or rubella, CMV virus.
Throat swab: for isolation of rubella, CMV or herpes virus.
Stools: for isolation of toxoplasma, herpes virus.
Skin vesicle fluid: electron microscopy for herpes virus.

Management

Isolate and barrier nurse. Keep pregnant staff away.
General support for acute illness.
Correct thrombocytopenia by platelet transfusion.
Exchange transfusion for unconjugated hyperbilirubinaemia.

Toxoplasmosis May respond to pyrimethamine and sulphadiazine.

Herpes Risk is greatest with primary infection of maternal genital tract, but any case of *active* genital herpes should be delivered by Caesarean section. The need for Caesarean section with non-active infections is controversial. Neonatal herpes usually presents with non-specific signs (lethargy, poor feeding, irritability, vomiting) within one week of birth, but may be delayed until three weeks, and may progress to a fulminating disease as described above. Treatment should be started early and consists of *acyclovir*, 5 mg/kg, by i.v. infusion over 1 hour, repeated 8 hourly, plus full supportive measures (see Chapter 5, page 51).

Other maternal infections during pregnancy

Hepatitis B and HB$_e$Ag carrier

The risk of neonatal hepatitis is greatest if the mother is symptomatic. Give the baby anti-HBs Ig, 2 ml, i.m. (200 IU) as soon as possible after birth and certainly within 48 hours, and hepatitis B vaccine 0.5 ml, i.m. at birth and repeated at 1 and 6 months of age. There are two vaccines available and the recommended doses are HB vaccine 0.5 ml (10 micrograms), Engerix-B 1.0 ml (20 micrograms). (See also Chapter 1.)

Tuberculosis (see Chapter 1)

Mumps

Possible cause of endocardial fibro-elastosis.

Varicella zoster

Maternal rash within 5 days before or after delivery may be associated with severe neonatal illness. Zoster should not affect the baby because of transplacental antibody. Zoster immune globulin may protect the baby from varicella.

Syphilis

Fifty per cent of infants of untreated mothers will be infected. Bloody nasal discharge, septicaemia, anaemia, jaundice, rashes and gummata may be present. Confirm with anti-treponemal IgM. Treat with penicillin.

AIDS (see Chapter 1, page 5)

Neonatal infections

Early onset infections presenting within 48 hours of birth have probably been acquired *in utero* or during birth. An increased risk is associated with:

Prolonged rupture of membranes (>24 hours)
Prolonged labour
Multiple obstetric procedures
Preterm labour
Fetal distress
Maternal pyrexia/infection, especially urinary or enteral
Foul-smelling liquor

The commonest organisms are those in the normal vaginal flora, in particular Group B streptococcus, and less frequently *Escherichia coli, Haemophilus influenzae*, gonococcus, *Listeria*, herpes and *Candida*.

Late onset infections presenting after the age of 48–72 hours have probably been acquired postnatally and may be associated with:

Preterm delivery
Meconium aspiration
Males > females
Malformations, e.g. spina bifida, urogenital anomalies, gastro-intestinal malformations
Intravenous infusions, especially with long lines and parenteral nutrition
Umbilical catheters; peripheral arterial lines
Endotracheal tubes
Cross-infection from staff, parents and other patients
Respiratory Distress Syndrome

The commonest organisms are: *Staphlococcus albus* and *Staph. aureus, E. coli, Pseudomonas*, streptococci, *Candida*, and less commonly *Proteus* and *Klebsiella*.

Management of suspected intrapartum infection

Any infant born after any of the above factors should be regarded as potentially infected.

If **asymptomatic**
Preterm infants: Carry out a full infection screen (page 216) and start penicillin and netilmicin.
Term infants: Observe closely for 24 hours. Consider infection screen and use of antibiotics.

If **symptomatic** (see page 215) carry out full infection screen and start penicillin and netilmicin.

In all cases, if cultures are negative after 48 hours, antibiotics can be stopped. If the mother has been given antibiotics before delivery these may suppress neonatal cultures and baby should be treated for 5 days even if the cultures are negative.

Superficial infections

Ophthalmia neonatorum (see Chapter 23, page 310)

Skin infections

These are usually due to *Staph. aureus*. They may present as scattered pustules or blisters particularly in axillae and groins, paronychia, breast abscess, or rarely as toxic epidermal necrolysis. Routine use of hexachlorophane 0.33% powder will reduce the risk of staphylococcal infection. Isolated spots may be treated with topical Fucidin ointment; more widespread infection needs systemic flucloxacillin.

Umbilicus

The umbilicus should be cleaned daily with alcohol and dusted lightly with hexachlorophene powder (e.g. Ster-Zac). The catheterized umbilicus should be treated daily with povidone-iodine. If the abdominal wall around the umbilicus becomes inflamed, do a blood culture and start systemic antibiotics.

Systemic infections

The clinical signs of sepsis in the newborn are non-specific and overlap with the signs and symptoms of many other disorders, particularly respiratory, cardiac and haematologic. The work-up of any ill infant must include a sepsis screen.

Signs suggestive of infection

Non-specific change in condition: poor colour; lethargy; poor feeding; temperature instability; hypothermia; fever.

Vomiting
Loose stools
Distended abdomen; splenomegaly

Jaundice
Purpura; bleeding
Irritability; convulsions
Cyanotic or apnoeic attacks
Grunting; tachypnoea
Tachycardia
Hypotension
Disordered glucose metabolism } hypoglycaemia
                                    } hyperglycemia and glycosuria

Investigation of infant suspected of infection (sepsis screen)

Sample	Investigation	Abnormal findings
Skin lesions nose, throat umbilical swabs	Gram stain Virology/E.M. Culture	Pus cells and bacteria seen Growth
Stools	Culture and virology	Pathogens isolated
Urine, clean catch or suprapubic aspiration (not bag sample)	Microscopy Culture	Bacteria and white cells seen Growth
Blood	Culture (aerobic and anaerobic)	Growth
	Haemoglobin (HB) Platelets Total WBC Differential WBC	Low $<80\,000$/dl <4000 or $>20\,000$/dl Neutrophils <2000, or $>15\,000$/dl
	Film	Shift to left. Toxic granulation Burr cells
CSF	Microscopy	White cells >30/mm^3 and $>50\%$ polymorphs organisms seen
	Culture/virology Protein Sugar	Growth Raised >1.5 g/l Low compared to blood level ($<0.6 \times$ blood sugar)

Other investigations

Chest X-ray, even in the absence of respiratory symptoms

Abdominal X-ray, if there are any signs suggestive of necrotizing enterocolitis
Blood: Glucose, urea, electrolytes, pH, gases
Urine: Sugar, protein, blood

General management of septic infant

(1) General support as described in Chapter 5.
(2) Respiratory support for apnoea, abnormal blood PaO_2, $PaCO_2$ (see Chapter 8).
(3) Correct hypotension with fresh frozen plasma 10 ml/kg; this may also correct defective opsonization.
(4) Transfuse if anaemic (Hb <12 gm/dl).
(5) Correct fluid, electrolyte, glucose imbalance (see Chapter 13).
(6) In cases of severe toxic shock an exchange transfusion may be beneficial.
(7) Antibiotics must be started at once before bacteriological diagnosis and therefore must be broad spectrum. However, the age at onset of symptoms will help in choosing a suitable antibiotic regimen:

> *Onset within 48 hours of birth:* Use penicillin + aminoglycoside.
> *Onset after 48 hours of birth:* Use flucloxacillin + aminoglycoside.

This regimen should be modified according to the illness being treated (see below) and subsequent isolation of organisms and sensitivities (see Tables 14.1 and 14.2).

Septicaemia

Probable organism depends on route of infection and age of onset (page 213). Treat as above.

Pneumonia

May be congenital due to ascending or intrapartum infection, especially streptococcal. Postnatal infection is related to aspiration syndromes, endotracheal intubation and hypostatic. Treat as above.

Group B streptococcal (GBS) disease

(1) *Early onset* GBS is acquired from vaginal flora, usually in pre-term infants, with prolonged rupture of membranes, but may be normal term delivery. Early respiratory symptoms occur, which mimic respiratory distress syndrome (RDS) and may progress to apnoea and severe shock. Group B streptococcal are found in

Table 14.1 Common organisms causing neonatal infection and recommended antibiotics

Organism	Recommended antibiotics (for parenteral use)
Group B streptococcus	Penicillin Ampicillin
Staph. aureus	Flucloxacillin Cefuroxime. fusidic acid
Staph. epidermidis	Netilmicin Flucloxacillin Cefuroxime Vancomycin
E. coli *Klebsiella* *Proteus*	Netilmicin Cefuroxime Cefotaxime Ceftazidime Chloramphenicol
Pseudomonas	Netilmicin + ceftazidime
Haemophilus	Ampicillin Chloramphenicol Cefuroxime, Cefotaxime
Listeria	Ampicillin Netilmicin
Chlamydia	Erythromycin
Candida (systemic infections only)	Amphotericin + 5-flucytosine

Wherever possible monitor blood levels of antibiotics and adjust dosage accordingly.

gastric aspirate. The baby may have septicaemia and meningitis as well as pneumonia. There is a high mortality rate. Treat with high-dose penicillin and full intensive care support.

(2) *Late onset* (1–2 weeks old). It is probably a nosocomial infection. Typically, meningitis presents in a previously well term infant, often due to type III GBS. The mortality rate is low. Treat with high-dose penicillin.

Neonatal meningitis

There may be no physical signs of meningitis in the neonate and all babies with suspected sepsis, fits or apnoeic attacks must have their

Table 14.2   Neonatal infections and their treatment

Disorder	Recommended antibiotics*
Septicaemia (<48 hours old)	Penicillin + netilmicin
(>48 hours old)	Flucloxacillin + netilmicin
Second-line therapy for failure of above	Cefotaxime (cefuroxime)
Meningitis†	Cefotaxime (chloramphenicol)
Pneumonia	As for septicaemia
Urinary infection	Ampicillin + netilmicin
Necrotizing enterocolitis	Penicillin + netilmicin + metronidazole
Osteomyelitis‡ (*Staph. aureus*)	Flucloxacillin + fusic acid

* All confirmed infections should be treated for 7 days at least.
† Continue treatment for 14 days after the first negative CSF culture.
‡ Continue treatment for 4–6 weeks.

CSF examined. Normal values are given in Table 31.3 (page 416). In cases of a bloody tap the 'normal' ratio of WBC to RBC is taken as 1:1000. The baby will usually have septicaemia as well and general environmental and respiratory support may be needed. The most suitable antibiotics are cefotaxime, or chloramphenicol (or penicillin for streptococcal infection). Aminoglycosides have poor CSF penetration and are not suitable for treatment of meningitis; intrathecal administration by the lumbar route is of no value though intraventricular aminoglycosides may be useful in treating ventriculitis.

Examination of the CSF should be repeated daily for 2–3 days to ensure effective therapy, and antibiotic therapy continued for 2 weeks from the date the CSF becomes sterile. When using aminoglycosides or chloramphenicol it is essential to monitor drug levels in blood and CSF.

Urinary tract infection (UTI)

Usually presentation is insidious with poor feeding, vomiting and jaundice, but may be acute. Always culture the urine of every sick infant (see Chapter 16, for Management of UTI).

Necrotizing enterocolitis

(See Chapter 11)

Gastroenteritis

Uncommon in the newborn in the UK, but epidemics of rotavirus in special care baby units (SCBU) have been reported. Sporadic cases of *Salmonella*, *Shigella*, *Campylobacter* and pathogenic *E. Coli* enteritis do occur; usually acquired from the mother during delivery. Isolate. Stop feeds and give i.v. fluids if dehydrated. Antibiotics not necessary.

Osteomyelitis

Insidious onset, usually not moving a limb, which is inflamed, oedematous and tender to touch. Do blood culture, get orthopaedic advice on aspiration of fluid from infected bone or joint for culture. Commonest organism in neonate is *Staph. aureus*. X-ray changes may not appear for 2–4 weeks. Treat with flucloxacillin and fusidic acid for 6 weeks.

Listeriosis

Infection with *Listeria monocytogenes* acquired transplacentally or intrapartum produces a clinical illness similar to Group B streptococcus. There is commonly a history of maternal pyrexia within a few days before delivery and the amniotic fluid may have a green discolouration. Mothers may acquire the organism from 'cook-chill' foods, paté, soft cheeses, milk etc. *Listeria* will grow at low temperatures (6–10°C) on such foods.

Early onset   Pneumonia: X-ray looks like aspiration pneumonitis but may mimic RDS or miliary pneumonia. Transient salmon-coloured papular rash on trunk. Disseminated disease (granulomatosis) may occur and is commonly fatal unless treatment is started within an hour or two of birth.

Delayed onset   of meningitis at 2–3 weeks old. Peripheral white count usually shows increase in polymorphs and monocytes.

Treatment (early and delayed onset)   Intravenous ampicillin, 200 mg/kg/day (or high dose penicillin) + i.v. netilmicin (or gentamicin).

Chlamydial infections

Infection with *Chlamydia trachomatis* acquired intrapartum from vagina usually presents as ophthalmia at end of first week, unresponsive to usual therapy. May be late onset (1–3 months) of pneumonia and sometimes otitis media. Chest X-ray shows diffuse interstitial infiltration.

Diagnosis   Chlamydial culture of eye swabs and specific IgM.

Treatment   Erythromycin.

Acute virus infections of the newborn

Clinical features are indistinguishable from bacterial sepsis. Investigation and management are similar, and until viral diagnosis is confirmed and bacterial cultures are negative, antibiotics are usually given. Appropriate samples (throat swabs, CSF, urine, stools, blood) should be sent for specific virology.

Viral meningitis

Usually caused by enterovirus. There are clinical signs of infection, but they are not severe.

CSF: normal sugar, raised cell count – polymorphs in first day of illness becoming predominantly lymphocytes. Remember to send separate samples of CSF for bacterial and viral cultures.

No specific treatment. Isolate.

Myocarditis

Usually caused by Coxsackie types B1–5, but may also be caused by TORCH agents, and be one feature of a generalized viral illness (+ meningitis). Presents with pyrexia and signs of cardiac failure, cyanosis and poor cardiac output. Hepatosplenomegaly.

Large heart on X-ray.

The ECG shows low voltage **QRS**, prolonged **QT**, and flat **T** waves. Ventricular ectopics and arrhythmias.

Differential diagnosis of septicaemia, diabetic cardiomyopathy (see Chapter 5), cardiomyopathy, endocardial fibro-elastosis (see Chapter 9).

Give environmental and respiratory support as indicated, digoxin and diuretics. Get cardiological advice. Significant mortality.

ECHO virus infection

A severe illness with collapse, disseminated intravascular coagulation and adrenal, CNS and gastrointestinal haemorrhage. May also cause meningitis, pneumonia, hepatitis and diarrhoea.

Fungal infections
Oral thrush

White spots on tongue and buccal mucosa, may be associated with poor feeding, especially if there is also an oesophagitis.

Treat with oral nystatin or miconazole. Maternal vaginal thrush predisposes.

Perianal thrush

Red rash over napkin area, with scattered satellite lesions, which is commonly associated with oral thrush. Very common.

Keep area as dry as possible; nurse exposed (in warm room); avoid waterproof napkin cover or pants. Treat with oral and topical nystatin or miconazole.

Systemic candidiasis

There is a high risk of candidiasis in association with antibiotic therapy, parenteral nutrition particularly via a central line, and preterm delivery. It usually presents as oral/perianal thrush becoming systemic with candidal septicaemia, meningitis and renal infection. Babies at risk should have regular cultures of blood and supra pubic aspiration urine for candida and should be given prophylactic nystatin.

Presentation and diagnosis

Clinical signs of sepsis failing to respond to antibiotics, and becoming chronic. Recurrent apnoea. Do blood culture (arterial and venous), SPA urine and CSF for candida, taking care to avoid skin contamination of samples.

Treatment

Treat with i.v. amphotericin, 0.1 mg/kg/day, infused over 1 hour, increasing over a period of 1 week to 1.0 mg/kg/day infused over 6 hours. Combine with oral 5-flucytosine 50 mg/kg 6 hourly. Continue therapy for 4–6 weeks. Monitor renal function carefully. Check candidal cultures weekly.

Bibliography

Baker, C. J. (1979). Group B streptococcal infections in neonates. *Pediatric. Rev.*, **1**, 1.

Davies, P. A. and Gothefors L. (1984). *Bacterial Infections in the Fetus and Newborn Infant*. London: W. B. Saunders.

Freij, B. J. and Sever, J. L. (1988). Infectious complications of pregnancy. *Clin. Perinatol.*, **15**, 163–419.

Placzek, M. M. and Whitelaw, A. (1983). Early and late neonatal septicaemia. *Arch. Dis. Child.*, **58**, 728–31.
Remington Klein (1990). *Infectious Diseases of the Fetus and Newborn Infant*, 3rd edn. London: W. B. Saunders.

15

Haematological problems

Normal values
Bleeding and clotting disorders
Anaemia
Polycythaemia

Normal values (see Chapter 31, page 415)
Haemoglobin and haematocrit

Haemoglobin (Hb) and haematocrit (Hct) values are increased by delayed cord clamping and rise after birth (by 2–3 g/dl and 3–6%, respectively) to peak at 3–12 hours of age. Capillary values are consistently higher than venous (or arterial). Therefore the source of the sample should always be stated.

> At 28 weeks' gestation: Mean capillary Hb = 1.2 × venous Hb
> At 40 weeks' gestation: Mean capillary Hb = 1.1 × venous Hb

White cell count

Increase in immature (band) neutrophils suggests infection.

Increase or (more important) decrease in total neutrophil count also suggests infection.

Platelets

A normal platelet count does not change significantly with gestation:

> $275 \pm 60 \times 10^3/mm^3$ at 30 weeks' gestation
> $310 \pm 70 \times 10^3/mm^3$ at 40 weeks' gestation (mean $\pm$ SD)

A platelet count less than $100 \times 10^3/mm^3$ is abnormal at any gestation, and values of $100–150 \times 10^3/mm^3$ warrant further investigation.

Platelet counts commonly fall with neonatal sepsis.

The platelet count rises to $3–400 \times 10^3/mm^3$ by 3–4 weeks in term and preterm infants.

Bleeding and clotting disorders

Assessment of the bleeding infant

History

Family history; maternal illness, e.g. idiopathic thrombocytopenic pupura (ITP), systemic lupus erythematosus (SLE); previously affected siblings; iso-immunization; infections during pregnancy; maternal drugs, e.g. aspirin, indomethacin, phenytoin, phenobarbitone, thiazides; labour and delivery.

Examination

Site of bleeding?
Petechiae?
Hepatosplenomegaly?
Is the infant sick?

Investigations

Platelet count; prothrombin time (PT); activated partial thromboplastin time (PTT); blood film (to look for fragmented red cells) $\pm$ thrombin time (TT); fibrin degradation products (FDP).

Apt's test on vomited blood (to determine whether it is fetal or maternal): to 5 ml water in a test tube add 3 drops vomited blood and 1 ml sodium hydroxide. Adult Hb turns brown in 1–2 min. Fetal Hb stays pink. Always use controls of known Hb F and Hb A.

Differential diagnosis of bleeding in the newborn (see Tables 15.1 and 15.2)

Disseminated intravascular coagulation (DIC)

Disseminated intravascular coagulation results from widespread activation of the clotting mechanism in sick infants, leading to secondary thrombocytopenia and clotting disorder (depletion of factors II, V, VIII and fibrinogen).

Table 15.1 A summary of the results of laboratory screening tests in the differential diagnosis of the bleeding infant*

Platelets	Laboratory Studies PT	PTT	Likely diagnosis
'Sick' infants			
Decreased	Increased	Increased	Disseminated intravascular coagulation
Decreased	Normal	Normal	Platelet consumption (infection, necrotizing enterocolitis, renal vein thrombosis)
Normal	Increased	Increased	Liver disease
Normal	Normal	Normal	Compromised vascular integrity (associated with hypoxia, prematurity, acidosis, hyperosmolality)
'Healthy' infants			
Decreased	Normal	Normal	Immune (auto or iso) thrombocytopenia; occult infection or thrombosis; bone marrow hypoplasia (rare)
Normal	Increased	Increased	Haemorrhagic disease of newborn (vitamin K deficiency)
Normal	Normal	Increased	Hereditary clotting factor deficiencies
Normal	Normal	Normal	Bleeding due to local factors (trauma, anatomic abnormalities); qualitative platelet abnormalities (rare); Factor XIII deficiency (rare)

*From Glader and Buchanan *Pediatrics*, **58**, 548 © 1976.

Causes

Infection (e.g. bacterial, TORCH infections)
Hypothermia
Asphyxia
Acidosis
Hypoxia
Hypotension
Severe Rhesus Disease

Diagnosis

Bleeding from puncture sites ± petechiae ± thromboses (e.g. gangrenous necrosis of skin)
↓ Platelets; ↑ PT and PTT; ↑ TT
↑ FDP in blood and urine
Blood film may show fragmented red cells

Table 15.2 Screening tests of blood coagulation in term and preterm infants

Test	Preterm	Term newborn	>1–2 months
Platelet count ($\times 10^3$/mm^3)	150–400	150–400	150–400
Platelets on peripheral smear*	10–20	10–20	10–20
Prothrombin time (PT) (sec)†	14–22	13–20	12–14
Partial thromboplastin time (PTT) (sec)†	35–55	30–45	25–35
Thrombin time (TT) (sec)†	11–17	10–16	10–12
Fibrinogen (mg/dl)	150–300	150–300	150–300

* Platelets per oil immersion field, including one or two small clumps.
† Normal values may vary from laboratory to laboratory; PT and PTT may remain prolonged in infants <1500 g despite vitamin K_1 having been given.
   Modified from Glader and Buchanan (1976). *Pediatrics*, **58**, 548; and Gross and Stuart (1977). *Clin. Perinatol.*, **4**, 259.

Management

Treat underlying condition (e.g. sepsis, hypoxia).
Replace clotting factors by transfusion with fresh frozen plasma, 10–15 ml/kg.
Give 1 mg vitamin K_1 i.v.
In severely ill infants or those with persisting bleeding/clotting disorder, exchange transfusion (with fresh blood) may be life-saving (see Chapter 26, page 354).

Haemorrhagic disease of the newborn

Vitamin K stores at birth are very small and rapidly depleted. Breast milk contains very little vitamin K and breast-fed infants may develop bleeding from depletion of factors II, VII, IX and X. Phenobarbitone and phenytoin given during pregnancy interfere with vitamin K metabolism and may cause extreme depletion of factors II, VII, IX and X in the fetus with bleeding at birth.

Diagnosis

Bleeding from umbilical cord, melaena, haematemesis, bleeding into the skin or from puncture sites – usually between 24 and 72 hours after birth (occasionally up to 2–3 weeks in breast-fed infants). ↑ PT and PTT; platelets, TT and FDP normal.

Prevention

All infants should be given vitamin K_1 immediately after birth (1 mg orally; or 0.5 mg i.m. to high-risk infants and a further 1 mg i.v. to any infant with actual bleeding).

Management of bleeding infant

(1) **If significant haemorrhage has occurred and infant is shocked** (BP <35 mm Hg; pH <7.25. NB Hb may not fall for 2–3 hours).

Transfuse rapidly over 5–15 min with 10–15 ml/kg uncross-matched O-negative blood. If the infant is still shocked, give a further 10–15 ml/kg over 15–20 min.

Monitor blood pressure and central venous pressure (CVP) closely.

Aim to achieve BP >40 mm Hg (in term infant) and CVP <8 cm H_2O.

If necessary give further transfusion, cross-matched against mother's blood (10–30 ml/kg over 2–3 hours, accompanied by 1–2 mg/kg frusemide i.v.).

(2) **If the infant is not shocked** transfuse with cross-matched packed cells to raise Hb to 10–12 g/dl (over 2–3 hours; with 2 mg/kg frusemide i.v.).

(NB: 10 ml/kg of packed cells will raise Hb by 2–3 g/dl or the Hct by about 10%.)

Hereditary bleeding disorders

These may present with bleeding from puncture sites or incisions (e.g. circumcision).

Haemophilia: X-linked, factor VIII deficiency.

Christmas disease: X-linked, factor IX deficiency.

von Willebrand's disease: Factor VIII deficiency and platelet defect, autosomal dominant.

Diagnosis

Family history; specific factor assay.

Thrombocytopenia

Thrombocytopenia usually presents with petechiae, bruising,

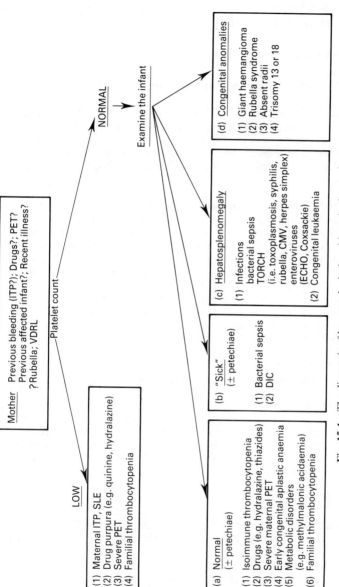

Mother Previous bleeding (ITP?); Drugs?; PET?
Previous affected infant?; Recent illness?
?Rubella; VDRL

Platelet count

LOW

NORMAL

Examine the infant

(a) Normal
(± petechiae)
(1) Isoimmune thrombocytopenia
(2) Drugs (e.g. hydralazine, thiazides)
(3) Severe maternal PET
(4) Early congenital aplastic anaemia
(5) Metabolic disorders
(e.g. methylmalonic acidaemia)
(6) Familial thrombocytopenia

(b) "Sick"
(± petechiae)
(1) Bacterial sepsis
(2) DIC

(c) Hepatosplenomegaly
(1) Infections
bacterial sepsis
TORCH
(i.e. toxoplasmosis, syphilis,
rubella, CMV, herpes simplex)
enteroviruses
(ECHO, Coxsackie)
(2) Congenital leukaemia

(d) Congenital anomalies
(1) Giant haemangioma
(2) Rubella syndrome
(3) Absent radii
(4) Trisomy 13 or 18

LOW box:
(1) Maternal ITP, SLE
(2) Drug purpura (e.g. quinine, hydralazine)
(3) Severe PET
(4) Familial thrombocytopenia

Fig. 15.1 The diagnosis of haematological problems in the newborn.

cephalhaematoma. Rarely major haemorrhage, e.g. intracranial, intrahepatic, may occur as a result of birth injury.

Diagnosis (see Fig. 15.1)

Autoimmune thrombocytopenia (ITP)

Mothers with SLE or ITP may have circulating IgG antiplatelet antibodies which cross to the fetus and cause fetal/neonatal thrombocytopenia in 50% of cases. Neonatal ITP has a variable cause from transient to up to 3 months, and from minor to severe bleeding. Prediction of neonatal ITP before delivery can be assessed by:

(1) Maternal platelet count, 70% risk if her count is <100 000.
(2) Maternal PC^{A1} antigen, 92% risk of levels are elevated.
(3) Maternal splenectomy, high risk. Mother's platelet count may be normal but still have lots of antibodies crossing to the baby.
(4) Fetal scalp blood sample for platelet count in labour. This is not recommended because of the danger of severe fetal bleeding.

There is little evidence that delivery by Caesarean section is of benefit in reducing risk of fetal bleeding, but it is advisable to treat the mother with steroids or immunoglobulin for 5 days before delivery.

Iso-immune thrombocytopenia

Analogous to rhesus disease. The mother produces IgG antibodies to $P1^{A1}$ antigen on infant's platelets, leading to severe neonatal thrombocytopenia. Donor platelets are rapidly destroyed after transfusion (97% population are $P1^{A1}$ positive), so mother's platelets should be used for transfusion. Recurrence rate in subsequent pregnancies is 75%.

Management

Baby's platelet level may be normal at birth and not fall for 2 days, so do platelet count at birth and 12 hourly for 72 hours and thereafter according to level.

Avoid i.m. injections.

If platelet count <10 000, or <50 000 with evidence of continuing bleeding, give platelet transfusion (1 unit; max 20 ml/kg). If platelet count <20 000 treat with either steroids (prednisolone, 2 mg/kg/day) or immunoglobulin (e.g. sandoglobulin, 1 g/kg/day, infused over 12 hours on two consecutive days (see Ballin *et al. J. Pediatr.*, 1988, **112**, 789). Treatment with steroids or repeated courses of immunoglobulin may be needed for several weeks.

Treat significant haemorrhage (see page 228).

Anaemia

Definition

Haemoglobin level <12 g/dl in first week, or <10 g/dl after first week.

Early anaemia

The cause is commonly apparent from the history.

Causes

Haemorrhage

Fetomaternal (NB Kleihauer test)	placenta praevia
	vasa praevia
Twin-to-twin	placental abruption
Placental (during or after delivery)	incision of placenta at caesarean section

Neonatal (e.g. intracranial, intrahepatic, gastrointestinal, pulmonary, sub-aponeurotic, from umbilical cord, from venous or arterial cannula).

Haemolysis
Rhesus iso-immunization
Haemoglobinopathies (e.g. alpha-thalassaemia)
TORCH infections
Bacterial infections

Investigations

Full blood count, film and reticulocyte count
Serum bilirubin (direct and total)
Blood group and Coomb's test
Kleihauer test on mother's blood
Blood culture
(Clotting studies and platelet count)
(TORCH titres)
(Hb electrophoresis)

Management

As for haemorrhagic disease (page 228).

Late anaemia (i.e. >7 days of age)

Causes

Haemorrhage
Small perinatal haemorrhage
Excessive blood sampling
Haemorrhagic disease
Intraventricular haemorrhage
Chronic gastrointestinal blood loss

Haemolysis
Rhesus, ABO incompatibility
Sepsis (± DIC)
Haemoglobinopathies
Red cell defects (e.g. spherocytosis)
Vitamin E deficiency

Decreased red cell production
Anaemia of prematurity (iron deficiency)
Infection (bacterial or viral)
Folic acid deficiency
Drugs
Congenital marrow hypoplasia ⎫
Congenital leukaemia   ⎬ very rare
                                ⎭

Investigations

Full blood count, film and reticulocyte count
Serum bilirubin (direct and total)
Blood group and Coomb's test
Urine microscopy and culture
Check stools for occult blood
Blood culture

Management

Treat underlying cause
Give iron, folate and vitamin E supplements (see Chapter 11)
Transfuse with packed cells (see page 228) if Hb <8 g/dl or if
    symptomatic

Polycythaemia

Definition

Venous Hct (packed cell volume) >65% in a newborn infant (capillary Hct is commonly 3–5% higher). Blood viscosity rises linearly with Hct up to 65%, but exponentially above that, particularly in vessels with low flow velocity (i.e. veins and capillaries).

Causes

(a) Increased intrauterine erythropoiesis

Placental insufficiency (SGA infants)
Post-term infants
Maternal pre-eclamptic toxaemia (PET)
Maternal drugs (e.g. propranolol)
Maternal smoking

Maternal diabetes
Maternal heart disease
Neonatal thyrotoxicosis
Trisomy 13, 18 or 21
Beckwith's syndrome
Congenital adrenal hyperplasia

(b) Secondary to red cell transfusion

Placental transfusion (delayed cord clamping)

Maternofetal transfusion
Twin-to-twin transfusion

(c) Capillary permeability and plasma loss

Cold stress
Hypoxia

Preterm infants
Hypovolaemia

Clinical features

Commonly plethoric but asymptomatic. However, may show:

Lethargy
Irritability
Hypoglycaemia
Vomiting
Hepatomegaly
Thrombocytopenia
Cardiac failure
NEC
Renal venous thrombosis

Hypotonia
Poor feeding
Cyanosis
Acidosis
Jaundice
Respiratory distress
Convulsions
Peripheral gangrene

Investigations

Full blood count, platelet count, venous and capillary Hct
Blood sugar
Serum calcium and bilirubin

If cardiorespiratory symptoms
Chest X-ray (may show cardiomegaly ± prominent vasculature ± pleural fluid)
ECG (see Chapter 9).

Management

Several studies have shown a significant incidence of long-term neurological sequelae, but the precise level of Hct which warrants treatment is controversial.

If symptomatic

(e.g. cardiorespiratory or neurological signs or symptoms). Dilution exchange transfusion with 20–30 ml/kg fresh frozen plasma over 20–30 minutes (see Chapter 26).

If asymptomatic

Repeat venous Hct 6–12 hourly until <65%
Monitor blood sugar carefully
Ensure adequate fluid intake (monitor urine specific gravity)
Dilution exchange as above if venous Hct >75% or infant becomes symptomatic.

Bibliography

Oski, F. A. and Naiman, J. L. (1982). *Haematologic Problems in the Newborn*, 3rd edn London: W. B. Saunders.
Zipursky, A. (Ed.) (1984). Perinatal haematology. *Clinics in Perinatology*, **II**, 249–511.

16

Renal disease in the newborn

Renal physiology
Clinical features of renal disease
Haematuria
Appendix: Peritoneal dialysis
Haemofiltration

Renal physiology

During the last trimester there is rapid structural and functional development of the kidney with functional maturity continuing through into postnatal life.

Renal blood flow and consequently glomerular filtration rate (GFR) is low at birth but increases rapidly during the next three days. Thereafter, GFR increases as a function of postconceptional age (PCA) (i.e. gestational age plus postnatal age) rather than postnatal age, from 0.45 ml/min at 28 weeks' PCA to 5 ml/min at 42 weeks' PCA.

Glomerular filtration rate may be estimated by measuring standard inulin or creatinine clearances, although neither are practical for routine clinical use. Plasma creatinine is the most commonly used marker for GFR. At birth plasma creatinine reflects maternal levels but falls to infant levels by the second week. The level is higher in the preterm infant and is inversely related to gestational age (see Table 16.1). Isolated results should be interpreted with caution as values are highly dependent on the type of assay used and analytical interference is common, e.g. with unconjugated bilirubin, ketones, drugs.

Creatinine excretion is, however, reasonably constant (mean ± sd, 90 ± 17 micromol/kg/day), and urinary creatinine may be used to estimate urine volume and the sodium excretion rate (see Chapter 17). In contrast, urea generation rates may be very variable, and high in preterm infants as a result of catabolism. Urea excretion rates of

Table 16.1 Renal physiology of the newborn – normal values

	Term	Postnatal age (days)	Preterm (<37 weeks gestation)		Postnatal age (days)
Fractional excretion of sodium (FeNa)*	1%	2	>33 weeks 1%	<33 weeks 3–5%	2–14
Maximal attainable urine osmolality (mOsm/kg)	800	<14	500–700		<14
GFR expressed as creatinine clearance (ml/min)‡	Postconceptional age (weeks) 42 40 38 / 5 3.5 2.5	>3	Post-conceptional age (weeks) 36 34 32 30 28 / 1.8 1.3 0.9 0.7 0.45		>3
Plasma creatinine ± 2 SD (micromol/l)	50 ± 36 / 38 ± 20	7 / 14	Gestational age (weeks) 33 – 36 29 – 32 28 / 68 ± 44 83 ± 41 84 ± 32 / 55 ± 36 69 ± 32 72 ± 32		7 / 14

*FeNa = $\dfrac{\text{Urine sodium}}{\text{Urine creatinine}} \times \dfrac{\text{Plasma creatinine}}{\text{Plasma sodium}} \times 100$

‡Postconceptional age = gestational age + postnatal age.

up to 16 mmol/kg/day may be normal (contrast normal values of 1 mmol/kg/day in healthy term infants). A high blood urea in a sick infant does not therefore necessarily indicate dehydration or renal failure.

Renal tubular function is also immature. Urine concentrating ability is limited by a reduced osmotic gradient between the cortex and the medulla, and also a reduced responsiveness to antidiuretic hormone (ADH). There is also a limited ability to excrete a water load. The term infant is able to conserve sodium efficiently; preterm infants, however, have high sodium losses (see Table 16.1).

Drugs

Because of the changes in GFR and functional tubular maturation, dosages of drugs which are eliminated by GFR or tubular secretion must be adapted for use in the newborn (see Chapter 28). In addition the newborn may be unusually susceptible to renal toxicity particularly from those drugs which alter renal blood flow. Commonly used drugs which should be used with caution are:

Aminoglycosides are excreted by glomerular filtration. Their half-life is related to PCA rather than postnatal age and dosage schedules should be adjusted accordingly (see Chapter 28).

Frusemide is excreted by glomerular filtration and secreted by a weak organic acid tubular mechanism. The effects are delayed and prolonged. The magnitude of response varies widely, particularly in sick infants who may have a low GFR.

Indomethicin, a prostaglandin synthetase inhibitor, alters renal haemodynamics and may produce a fall in GFR, fractional excretion of sodium and free water clearance without any change in systemic blood pressure. The effects are usually transient and recover on stopping the drug.

Tolazoline is an alpha-adrenergic blocking agent with a non-adrenergic vascular relaxant effect. It causes an increase in renal vascular resistance and a consequent fall in renal perfusion. The use of tolazoline in the presence of hypoxaemia, if systemic arterial blood pressure is not maintained, may lead to acute renal failure. It is therefore important to maintain adequate blood pressure during its administration (see Chapter 9).

Aminophylline may have a diuretic and naturetic effect when given as a rapid infusion, by temporarily increasing GFR, but maintenance theophylline probably does not have an important effect.

Clinical features of renal disease

Family history

Some renal diseases are inherited in a Mendelian fashion either alone, e.g. polycystic kidney disease (autosomal dominant and recessive), nephrogenic diabetes insipidus (X-linked), congenital nephrotic syndrome (autosomal recessive), or as part of a syndrome, e.g. Alports (X-linked), Townes (autosomal dominant), Meckels (autosomal recessive). Renal abnormalities, particularly tubular defects, are also seen in association with several metabolic disorders inherited in an autosomal recessive pattern, e.g. tyrosinosis, fructose intolerance, galactosaemia and cystinosis. Vesico-ureteric reflux is common and partly genetically determined in a multifactorial way, with a 4% risk of reflux for first degree relatives of index patients, rising to 50% if the index patients have renal scarring.

Perinatal history

Oligohydramnios suggests renal agenesis, dysplasia or hypoplasia, or bilaterally obstructed urinary tract (e.g. posterior urethral valves). It may be associated with deformation of the infant, together with lung hypoplasia, i.e. Potters syndrome (see Chapter 6).

Less than 4% of children with a single umbilical artery have significant associated genitourinary abnormalities.

A placenta weighing more than 25% of the infant's weight is suggestive of congenital nephrotic syndrome. There may be oligohydramnios and the infants are often small for date, preterm and have fetal distress. Prenatally, diagnosis may be suggested by a raised alpha-fetoprotein (see Chapter 1).

Antenatal ultrasound

Congenital abnormalities of the genitourinary tract can be detected as early as 12–15 weeks gestation. Ninety per cent of fetal kidneys can be identified by 17–20 weeks and 95% by 22 weeks. Accuracy, even in the most experienced hands, is limited and misinterpretation common. For example, in the presence of renal agenesis the adrenal is misshapen and may be mistaken for a kidney; the distinction between multicystic kidney and pelviureteric junction obstruction may be difficult, and dilated calyces may mimic renal cysts. In addition, the normal increased echogenicity of the fetal kidney and physiological dilatation of the collecting system, are commonly open to misinterpretation. Therefore, although antenatal ultrasound may

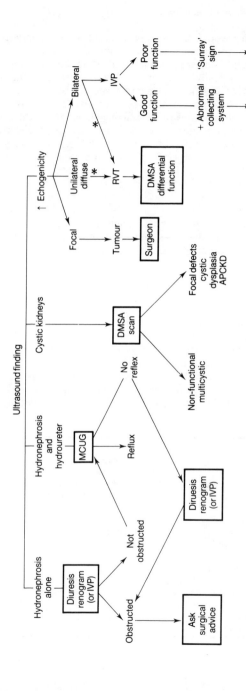

Fig. 16.1 Scheme of investigation of the infant with abnormal renal ultrasound findings.

pick up lesions that would be detectable clinically only in a minority of cases, the technique cannot define the diagnosis accurately.

Therefore, the first stage of postnatal evaluation should be repeat ultrasonography, and only if the abnormality is confirmed is further investigation indicated. The presence of suspected severe bilateral obstruction (e.g. posterior urethral valves or severe pelvi-ureteric junction obstruction) requires prompt management and is the only lesion for which early postnatal investigation is indicated. Elective investigation of other abnormalities, especially where radiology is dependent on renal function (IVP, renal isotope scans) to further define the lesion, is better deferred for a few weeks. It should, however, be remembered that both the presence of vesico-ureteric reflux and obstruction may be associated with urinary tract infections and therefore it may be wiser in the presence of a dilated urinary tract, to commence prophylactic antibiotics (e.g. trimethoprim, 2 mg/kg/day) until the diagnosis and subsequent management is clear. A suggested scheme of investigation is shown in Fig. 16.1.

Abdominal masses

More than two-thirds of abdominal masses detected in the newborn period arise in the genitourinary system. Causes are listed in Table 16.2. Ultrasound will be the first investigation of choice and subsequent examination will be dependent on its appearances and the facilities for investigation available (see Fig. 16.1).

As an enlarged bladder should lead to the suspicion of posterior urethral valves; ultrasound followed by micturating cystourethrogram (MCUG) should be performed. Bladder drainage (urethral or

Table 16.2   Causes of renal enlargement

Unilateral	*Bilateral*
Multicystic kidney	Polycystic kidneys
Solitary cyst	Cystic dysplasia
Hypertrophied single kidney	Acute renal injury (hypoxia, ischaemia)
	Twin-to-twin transfusion (recipient)
Unilateral or bilateral	*Miscellaneous*
Obstructive uropathy:	Horseshoe kidney
Pelvi-ureteric junction	Pelvic kidney
obstruction	
Vesico-ureteric junction	
obstruction	
Bladder outflow obstruction	
Renal vein thrombosis	
Mesoblastic nephroma/Wilm's	
tumour	

suprapubic) should be discussed with the surgeon or specialist centre. Relief of the obstruction may lead to a marked postobstructive diuresis, and natriuresis, which will require careful monitoring and fluid replacement.

Bladder and genital abnormalities

Bladder exstrophy and epispadias requires urgent referral for specialist advice. The bladder mucosa should be protected by applying gauze dressings soaked in saline (see Chapter 20 for details of parent group).

Hypospadias, the site of the meatus, severity of chordee, and any accompanying abnormalities, e.g. meatal stenosis, inguinal hernia, cryptorchidism should be identified. If hypospadias is perineal or is part of an ambiguous genitalia presentation, careful investigation is required (Chapter 13). Infants with coronal and distal shaft hypospadias require surgical review in outpatient clinics. Perineal and penoscrotal hypospadias is an indication for renal investigation which should be done in conjunction with the surgical team. Infants with hypospadias should not be circumcized as the prepuce may be needed for the repair of the defect.

Unilateral **cryptorchidism** is present in 2–3% of term male infants. Follow-up (usually by the family doctor) is required so that if descent has not occurred by the age of one year the child can be referred with a view to orchidopexy being performed before the age of two years. Bilateral cryptorchidism with hypospadias requires urgent investigation (Chapter 13).

Oliguria

To remain in solute balance the minimum rate of urine production depends on the dietary solute load and renal concentrating ability. In infants this is in the range 0.5–1.0 ml/kg/hour. Oliguria may present antenatally as oligohydramnios, or postnatally. It may be due to obstruction, poor renal perfusion, intrinsic renal failure, or increased antidiuretic hormone (see Chapter 17). Obstruction should be excluded by clinical or ultrasonographic examination, and the other conditions differentiated on plasma and urinary biochemistry (see page 245).

Polyuria

Polyuria may be seen in the recovery phase of acute renal failure; following relief of urinary obstruction; with certain drugs, e.g.

diuretics and aminoglycosides; and in nephrogenic diabetes insipidus. A postnatal weight loss of more than 10% in an otherwise healthy infant whose urine is hypo-osmolar, may be the first sign of nephrogenic diabetes insipidus. Rehydrate and ask for advice before embarking on a water deprivation test which may be dangerous.

Haematuria

Gross haematuria is rare although up to 10% of newborns may have microscopic haematuria (>10 RBC/microl). It is important to distinguish between haematuria and pigment discolouration of urine (haemoglobin, urate) and contamination of urine by vaginal blood. Causes include:

Birth trauma
Systemic embolism (e.g. from umbilical artery catheter)
Cortical and medullary necrosis
Acute renal failure
Hydronephrosis
Mesoblastic nephroma/Wilm's tumour
Infection
Following hypoxic, ischaemic or infective episode
Drugs
Alports syndrome
A bleeding disorder may rarely present with haematuria.

Investigation should include microscopy and urine culture, blood count, clotting studies, renal function tests, renal ultrasound and consider referral for specialist advice.

Renal venous thrombosis

Seventy-five per cent of renal venous thromboses occur in the first month of life. Presenting features include macro/microscopic haematuria, oliguria, renal failure and palpably enlarging kidneys. Proteinuria is minimal and nephrotic syndrome is rare. Anaemia and thrombocytopaenia are common.

Haemoconcentration, hyperviscosity and hyperosmolarity predispose to renal venous thrombosis and important risk factors include perinatal asphyxia especially in infants with congenital renal anomalies, infants of diabetic mothers, hypernatraemic dehydration and infusion of hypertonic solutions (e.g. radiological contrast media).

Ultrasound reveals an enlarged kidney with a normal appearance or increased echogenicity. The diagnosis can be made with certainty only by venography which is contraindicated in the sick infant.

Management is conservative. Anticoagulants and fibrinolytics have not been shown to be of value. Radionuclotide scans (DMSA) may be useful to document the function of the unaffected kidney or predict recovery of the affected kidney. Long-term sequelae include renal atrophy and hypertension.

Leukocyturia

Normally there are less than 25 (male) or 50 (female) WBC/μmol. Pyuria is often associated with urinary tract infections but is not pathognomic and an increased white cell excretion rate may be seen in any patient with a fever.

Proteinuria

Protein excretion varies with gestational and postnatal age. Transient proteinuria is common in the first few days of life, and dipsticks frequently give false positive results with alkaline urine. Pathological causes include:

Infection
Renal venous thrombosis
Congenital infection (syphilis, toxoplasmosis, CMV)
Drugs (mercury)
Idiopathic familial congenital nephrotic syndrome

Investigation should include renal function tests, urine protein excretion as protein/creatinine ratio, plasma proteins, congenital infection screen, renal ultrasound and refer for specialist advice.

Oedema

Renal causes include excessive water and salt administration, acute renal failure, obstructive uropathy and congenital nephrotic syndrome. Differentiation from non-renal causes such as anaemia, cardiac failure, tissue injury (anoxia, hypothermia, ischaemia) and hypoproteinaemia (non-renal) is usually evident clinically.

Investigation should include dipstick urinalysis for blood and protein, renal function tests and plasma proteins.

Acidosis

The commonest causes of metabolic acidosis in the newborn will be shock and sepsis, with or without renal failure, and will be associated with an increased anion gap (see Chapter 13). The presence of metabolic acidosis with a normal anion gap suggests a renal tubular acidosis (RTA). During the first few days after birth most infants will have a urine pH around 6 although capacity to alter pH in response to bicarbonate is present. The excretion of an inappropriately alkaline urine in the presence of acidosis may occur in various RTA syndromes and severe respiratory distress syndrome (RDS).

Hyponatraemia and hypernatraemia (see Chapter 17)

Hypertension

The upper limit for systolic and diastolic BP in term infants can be taken as 100 and 75 mm Hg, respectively (see Fig. 31.2). Use a cuff width at least 2/3 of the upper arm length and record BP only when infant is at rest. Blood pressure persistently >110 systolic and/or >80 diastolic requires treatment regardless of the presence of symptoms, although such symptoms (e.g. vomiting, irritability, fits) may occur at lower levels. Of the renal causes of hypertension over 90% will be renovascular, the commonest of which is thrombosis of the renal artery following umbilical artery catheterization.

Treatment of hypertension depends on the cause (see Table 16.3). Hydralazine, 0.5–1 mg/kg, i.v. can be given to control BP acutely. Mild hypertension may respond to diuretics alone but more severe hypertension may require the use of beta-blockers. The latter are

Table 16.3 Causes and management of hypertension

Mechanism	Causes	Management
Renin mediated	Coarctation of aorta Renovascular	See Chapter 9
	Obstructive uropathy Cystic kidneys	Vasodilator and beta-blockade
Salt and water retention	Excess administration Renal failure Adrenal disorders	Fluid restriction diuretic, dialysis (see Chapter 13)
Catecholamine drive	Stress (pain, cold), hypovolaemia, drugs, e.g. dopamine	Correct underlying cause
Raised intracranial pressure	Cerebral oedema; Intraventricular haemorrhage	See Chapter 10

used with caution because of the risk of cardiac failure, and long-term effects of beta-blockade on the endocrine system are unknown. Captopril, 100–300 microg/kg/dose, 8 hourly, may be useful in severe hypertension unresponsive to other agents but renal function should be carefully monitored.

Urinary tract infection

A urinary tract infection should be considered in any infant who is unwell, jaundiced, vomiting, febrile, or failing to thrive.

Diagnosis is confirmed by finding > 100 000 organisms on culture from at least two clean catch specimens; or preferably by obtaining any growth from a suprapubic aspiration sample. No growth from a bag urine will rule out a urinary tract infection, but a bag urine cannot be relied upon to make a positive diagnosis because of the high incidence of contamination.

The baby should be examined for evidence of renal disease and blood culture, lumbar puncture and renal function checked prior to commencing therapy.

Management Before sensitivity results are available an amino-glycoside, e.g. netilimicin i.v. (Chapter 28) plus ampicillin, will almost always prove effective, as the usual organisms are *E. Coli*, *Proteus*, *Pseudomonas*, and *Strep. faecalis*. If there is concurrent meningitis, cefotaxime (Chapter 28) should be added. When sensi-tivities are known, change to the most appropriate, least toxic antibiotic. Sulphonamides should be avoided in jaundiced babies because of the risk of kernicterus.

Many neonatal urinary tract infections are haematogenous in origin with no renal anomaly, but all cases should have radiological investigation of the urinary tract. A renal ultrasound should be performed at the time of diagnosis. All cases should have an MCUG, but this may be performed electively later. However, all babies should be kept on prophylactic antibiotics until vesico-ureteric reflux has been excluded. A DMSA scan several weeks after the infection will identify any scarring.

Acute renal failure

Acute renal failure is characterized by a sudden fall in glomerular filtration rate (GFR) which leads to disturbances in water and electrolyte balance, acid–base homeostasis, and to accumulation of nitrogenous products. Oliguria is usually the first sign of acute renal failure, although a normal urine output does not exclude the diagnosis. In addition, because of the practical difficulties in accurately measuring a baby's urine output, oliguria may escape observation. Diagnosis may be further complicated by the fact that hypercatabolism, common in sick infants, leads to uraemia and hyperkalaemia due to protein breakdown despite a normal GFR. Plasma creatinine is a reliable indicator of GFR. Although a single value is of limited usefulness (see page 235) a rise >20 micromol/24 hours does suggest a fall in GFR.

Acute renal failure may be secondary to circulatory insufficiency without structural damage (prerenal), parenchymal damage (intrinsic renal failure), or due to urinary tract obstruction (postrenal) (Table 16.4).

The symptoms and signs of renal failure may be those of

Predisposing factors e.g. fluid overload (hypertension, oedema, excess weight gain, hepatomegaly, tachypnoea), fluid depletion (poor peripheral perfusion, hypotension), renal abnormality (palpable kidney, bladder).

Table 16.4   Causes of acute renal failure

Prerenal
Hypovolaemic
  Blood loss
  Plasma loss
  Insensible loss (e.g. phototherapy in very low birthweight infants)
  Gastrointestinal loss (diarrhoea, vomiting)
  Polyuria
  Inadequate intake (e.g. fluid restriction after birth asphyxia)
Normovolaemia
  Hypoxia
  Septicaemia
  Hypotensive drugs (e.g. tolazaline)

Intrinsic renal failure
Uncorrected prerenal failure
Acute tubular necrosis
Acute medullary necrosis
Acute cortical necrosis
Renal vessel thrombosis
Nephrotoxins (e.g. gentamicin)
Congenital renal abnormality

Postrenal
Posterior urethral valves
Vesico-ureteric obstruction
Pelvi-ureteric junction obstruction
Neurogenic bladder

Renal failure itself e.g. poor feeding, vomiting, seizures, bleeding, cardiac arrhythmias.

Investigations

Investigations should include weight, blood pressure, infection screen, renal ultrasound and the following:

Urine	Dipstick
	Microscopy (look for casts)
	Urea and electrolytes
	Creatinine
	Osmolality
Blood	Electrolytes
	Urea
	Creatinine
	Acid-base status
	Glucose
	Calcium
	Magnesium
	Albumin
	Full blood count (film and platelets)
	Clotting studies and culture

It is important to differentiate between the three main causes of renal failure as their treatments differ. Obstruction is usually easily confirmed or excluded on renal ultrasound examination; differentiation between prerenal and intrinsic renal failure is often more difficult, and may be further complicated by the fact that the former may lead to the latter.

The indices to differentiate between prerenal and intrinsic renal failure (Table 16.5) are often less helpful than in the older child because a low protein diet and a high urinary sodium excretion affect both osmolality and those indices which rely on urinary sodium. All indices are less reliable in preterm infants, a high fractional excretion

Table 16.5 Indices to differentiate between prerenal and intrinsic renal failure

	Pre-renal	*Renal*
Urine/plasma urea	>10	<10
Urine/plasma osmolarity	>2	<1
FeNa*	<1% term	>3%
	<5% preterm	

* See Table 16.1.

of sodium (FeNa) in particular does not necessarily indicate renal failure.

If doubt exists about the extent of the prerenal component, an intravenous fluid challenge of 10 ml/kg of plasma may differentiate, but should be given with great caution in view of the risk of creating fluid overload.

The management of renal failure

Prerenal   Restore circulating volume with colloid or isotonic saline 10–20 ml/kg i.v. quickly over 30–60 min. With hypotension (see Fig. 31.1) in the absence of fluid depletion give an infusion of an inotrope, e.g. dopamine, 5–10 microg/kg/min.

Postrenal   Relieve obstruction surgically or by suprapubic or urethral catheter as appropriate.

Intrinsic renal failure

Restore circulating volume if indicated. Thereafter replace all fluid losses (urine and gastrointestinal tract) together with insensible losses (see Chapter 17). One-third of insensible loss is respiratory which is negligible if the infant is being ventilated. The volume of infusions of essential supportive drugs may exceed the infant's losses and attempts should be made to use the highest safe concentrations of drugs. In polyuric renal failure (as seen after relief of urinary obstruction) replacement of large urine volumes with glucose solutions may lead to hyperglycaemia and it is important to monitor blood sugar levels especially if glucose infusion rate exceeds the normal utilization rate of 5–8 mg glucose/kg/min.

Electrolyte losses should be calculated and replaced. (Measure urine electrolytes and estimate gastrointestinal losses according to site.)

Severe acidosis (pH <7.2) requires correction (see page 121). Conservative measures to lower plasma potassium (see Chapter 17) should be used only temporarily until the cause of the renal failure is corrected or dialysis instituted.

Caloric needs can rarely be met in an oligo or anuric infant despite infusions of 10–15% glucose and this may be an indication for dialysis. Hypoglycaemia is a common complication and therefore the blood sugar should be monitored regularly.

Regular clinical (input/output charts, weight, blood pressure, peripheral/core temperature gradient) and biochemical assessments are required.

Dialysis

Dialysis is seldom required but urgent indications include:

Severe fluid overload ± pulmonary oedema
Severe metabolic acidosis (pH <7.2 with PCO_2 <40 mm Hg)
Severe hyperkalaemia (K^+ >8.0 despite conservative measures)

If there is immediate prospect for renal recovery dialysis should be commenced prior to the development of fluid and electrolyte imbalance and to allow administration of adequate calories and supportive drugs.

Appendix

Procedure for peritoneal dialysis

This should only be attempted in a non-specialist centre when the infant is too sick to travel or if there are other compelling reasons against transfer. Figure 16.2 shows one type of closed dialysis system which has proved effective.

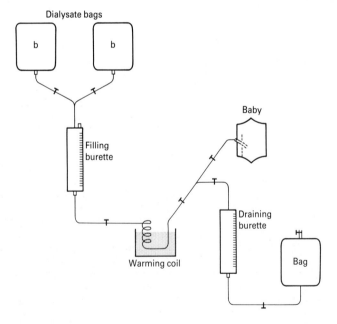

Fig. 16.2 Diagram showing closed system for performing peritoneal dialysis in infants.

Equipment needed Peritoneal cannula (e.g. Wallace paediatric cannula), 1.36 % and 6.36 % glucose dialysis solutions (e.g. Dialaflex 61 and 62), dialysis set (e.g. Avon Medicals type), and water bath set at 37°C.

Procedure Catheterize bladder. Choose a site avoiding enlarged organs – the usual place is the flank, level with umbilicus and lateral to mid-inguinal line (to avoid inferior epigastric artery). Full aseptic technique is required. Cleanse skin and infiltrate site with lignocaine 1 per cent. Introduce 19 g butterfly into peritoneum and run in 20–30 mk/kg of warmed 1.36 per cent dialysate to fill abdomen. Make a small scalpel incision to facilitate insertion of cannula. *Gently* introduce cannula perpendicular to skin and withdraw trocar when all side holes are judged to be within peritoneum. Ensure free flow of fluid in and out of peritoneal cavity. Run fluid into and out of peritoneum rapidly (20–30 ml/kg) until the effluent is clear of blood, then 2 cycles/hr. Use 1.36 per cent solution initially, but if negative balance is not achieved, or if the infant is fluid overloaded, use a mixture of 1.36 per cent and 6.36 per cent solution by adding desired volumes (usually 50/50) to filling burette. Add heparin 500 units/litre to dialysate bags until blood-staining clears, and add 2–4 mmol KCl/litre if plasma K^+ <3.0.

Haemofiltration

Is a simple effective alternative to peritoneal dialysis and may be utilized in infants in whom the abdomen cannot be used for peritoneal dialysis, e.g. postabdominal surgery, or in the present of severe necrotizing enterocolitis. As with peritoneal dialysis it should be performed only in a centre with the necessary local expertise.

Various sites may be used for vascular access and, although the umbilical vein and artery most reliably provide adequate transmembrane pressure gradients, femoral, brachial and jugular access may be used. Cannulae, 18–24 gauge (3.5–5 fg), will provide adequate flow. Total extracorporeal circulating volume using the Amicon minifilter is 12 ml (6 ml filter/6 ml lines). Heparinization is required, and although the standard dose of 40 units/kg followed by 10 units/kg/ hour is appropriate for most patients, this can be reduced to a loading dose of 10 units/kg and maintenance of 5 units/kg/hour, in the presence of increased susceptibility to bleeding. The average ultrafiltration rate achievable is 1–2 ml/min which would be expected to provide, in addition to ultrafiltration, adequate solute clearance for all but the most catabolic in infants.

Bibliography

Donaldson, M. D. C., Spurgeon, P., Haycock, G. B. and Chantier, C. (1983). Peritoneal dialysis in infants. *Br. Med. J.*, **286**, 759–60.

Malcolm, A., Holliday, T., Barratt, M. and Vernier, R. L. (Eds), (1987). *Paediatric Nephrology*, Section 12, The perinatal period. Baltimore: Williams and Wilkins.

Leiberman, K. V. (1987). Continuous arteriovenous haemofiltration in children. *Pediatr. Nephrol.*, **1**, 330–8.

Reuss, A., Wladimiroff, J. W. and Neirmeijer, M. F. (1987). Antenatal diagnosis of renaltract anomalies by ultrasound. *Pediatr. Nephrol.*, **1**, 546–52.

Thomas, D. F. M. and Gordon, A. C. (1989). Management of prenatally diagnosed uropathies. *Arch. Dis. Child.*, **64**, 58–63.

17

Fluid and electrolyte therapy

Water balance
Sodium balance
Hyponatraemia
Hypernatraemia
Potassium balance
Hypokalaemia
Hyperkalaemia

The goal for the management of fluid and electrolyte therapy in newborn infants must be to achieve positive balance without overload. For the well infant this poses little problem and there is a reasonable margin for error. For the sick or very preterm infant the sensible management of fluid balance is crucial to improved outcome.

Water balance

Throughout fetal life water comprises a decreasing proportion of body composition. At 30 weeks water comprises over 90% body volume, 60% in the extracellular compartment. By 40 weeks these proportions have fallen to 80 and 45%, respectively. After preterm delivery there is a reduction in body water to bring the composition closer to that of the term infant (5–10% body weight). In contrast, over the first few days extracellular volume expands resulting in a diuresis that may be delayed if excessive fluids are administered or the child is ill. This may have implications for recovery from respiratory distress syndrome (RDS).

Maturation of renal function is discussed in Chapter 16. Glomerular filtration rate rises rapidly after birth as renal plasma flow increases. Sodium resorption is less efficient in the very preterm compared to the term infant and may lead to high baseline losses.

Water balance is controlled by renal plasma flow and the action of antidiuretic hormone (ADH) on the collecting duct. This posterior pituitary hormone is secreted in response to:

(1) A small rise in plasma osmolality (hypothalamic receptors)
(2) A fall in intravascular volume (left atrial stretch receptors)
(3) A fall in blood pressure (carotid sinus receptors).

In the very preterm infant, ADH action on the collecting duct is partially impaired. In the sick infant, ADH is secreted as a response to stress (oxygenation, intrathoracic pressure, IVH, brain injuries), and this may result in rapid swings in water excretion even with a normal GFR.

Non-renal water loss occurs via the respiratory tract (negligible if the infant is ventilated with humidified air) and, more problematically, via transepidermal evaporative loss. In the very preterm this may result in large losses, even up to 200 ml/kg for infants nursed naked under radiant heaters. For tiny babies, humidification of the environment or the use of barriers such as plastic wrappings or paraffin wax, may reduce this to tolerable levels. These methods also reduce concomitant heat loss (Chapter 5).

Water therapy must be planned with the help of *daily weights*, which are possible in all but the most unstable infants, and electrolytes. For the very preterm, *plasma sodium* may be the most reliable way of assessing loss in the child who is unable to be weighed, water intake being adjusted to maintain plasma sodium in the normal range. The measurement of urine output by collection is often very difficult and inaccurate. Measurement of urine creatinine allows the *estimation* of urine volume from the formula:

$$\text{Urine volume (ml/kg/day)} = 90/\text{Urine creatinine (mmol/l)}$$

where 90 refers to the mean creatinine excretion, which may range from 56 to 124 μmol/kg/day (± 2 sD) (Chapter 16).

Normal water intake in healthy breast-fed infants rises to about 150 ml/kg by the fifth postnatal day, forming the basis for the conventional 60, 90, 120 ml/kg/day steps. This applies only to relatively more mature infants. A suggested scheme for water, sodium and potassium intake is shown in Table 17.1. Any scheme must be tempered by close assessment of the state of hydration for each infant, urine output, insensible and observed losses, and plasma electrolytes. Note that water is an independent variable and the concentration of the various solutes must be altered if the rate of water infusion is altered.

Table 17.1 Suggested water, sodium and potassium intakes (these may need considerable modification from day to day depending on clinical course) for various weight† babies in kilograms

Day	Water				Sodium				Potassium All weights
	<1	−1.5	−2.5	>2.5	<1	−1.5	−2.5	>2.5	
1	100	80	60	60	0	0	0	0	0
2	120	100	90	90	5	4	3	1	0–2
3	150	130	120	110	5*	4	3	1	2–3
4	180	150	150	130	5*	4	3	1	2–3
5	200	180	170	150	5*	4	3	2	2–3
6	200	180	170	150	5*	4	3	2	2–3
7	200	180	170	150	5*	4	3	2	2–3
8–13	200	180	170	150	5*	4	3	2	2–3
14–20	180	160	150	150	4	3	2	1	2–3
21–27	160	160	150	150	3	2	2	1	2–3
>28	160	150	150	150	2	2	2	1	2–3

These figures are for infants nursed in incubators or cots. Infants under radiant warmers may require much higher volumes of water.

* Commonly higher requirements. Check blood sodium daily.

† Use birthweight or most recent weight, whichever is greater.

Remember, when calculating intakes that arterial flush solutions, vamin glucose (Chapter 11) and drugs contain extra sodium and water.

Always use the greater of birthweight or current weight, in calculations.

Management of oliguria and polyuria (see Chapter 16)

Sodium balance

Sodium is normally excreted via the kidney; sweat and bowel losses being negligible. Term breast milk supplies less than 1 mmol/kg/day, implying that the kidney can conserve sodium and achieve positive balance and growth. Control is mediated via the renin–angiotensin –aldosterone system. This is equally active in the preterm, but tubular unresponsiveness leads to sodium wastage which is increased at lower gestation and in sick infants. This usually recovers in 1–3 weeks. Normal requirements are usually 1–2 mmol/kg/day for term and up to 5 mmol/kg/day for very preterm infants.

Monitor urinary electrolytes when there is a disturbance in electrolyte balance. Urinary sodium loss (fractional sodium excretion) may be described using the formula in Table 16.1. Normal is <1% in healthy term infants, sick preterms may have values up to 16%. Sodium excretion may be *estimated* on a spot urine using the formula:

Sodium excretion   = 90 × Urine sodium/Urine creatinine
   (mmol/kg/day)   (mmol/l)

Normative data for electrolyte concentrations are given in Chapter 26.

Hyponatraemia

Definition

Plasma sodium <130 mmol/l.

Causes

Water overload secondary to ADH secretion, commonly occurs with ventilation, pneumothorax or IVH. It may occur in the first 24 hours due to excess administration of intravenous fluids to mother, or later following excess administration to infant.

Acute renal failure in oliguric phase before fluid restriction (dilutional) (see Chapter 16).

Increased losses

Excessive renal loss in preterm infants is commonest, exacerbated during illness and by diuretic or aminophylline therapy.

Inherited tubular disorders mimic poor preterm renal sodium handling. The baby should be given suitable replacements and referred to a specialist unit.

Adrenal insufficiency, associated with hyperkalaemia and dehydration, will require replacement fluids, electrolytes and steroids (Chapter 13).

Excessive gastrointestinal sodium loss during infection (gastroenteritis see chapter 11) or obstruction.

Inadequate intake

Late hyponatraemia may occur during intravenous nutrition (with inadequate sodium concentration) or in preterm infants after 2 weeks of low-solute breast milk or standard formula. Preterm milks

(Chapter 11) contain higher concentrations of sodium avoiding the need for early supplementation, but should probably not be used after 4–6 weeks unless high sodium losses continue.

Calculation of sodium deficit (mmol)

Sodium deficit = (135 − plasma sodium) × 0.6 × body weight (kg)

Try to anticipate high losses, such as in preterm infants or gastrointestinal losses. If hyponatraemic, always slightly underestimate loss and replace *slowly* (e.g. ⅓ deficit over 8 hours followed by ⅓ over 16 hours and last ⅓ over 24 hours). Add as 30% NaCl (5 mmol/ml) to bag or burette. Emergency management of plasma sodium <120 mmol/l with symptoms (irritability, apnoea, convulsions) should be started with a bolus of plasma or normal saline (15–20 ml/kg).

Hypernatraemia
Definition

Plasma sodium >145 mmol/l.

Causes

Net loss of water

Transepidermal water loss in very preterm infants. Requires gentle volume expansion with 0.9% saline or plasma followed by adjustment of water and electrolyte intake (see above). Anticipate higher fluid losses during phototherapy (Chapter 18), due to evaporative loss and stool losses.

High rates of fluid loss occur during episodes of vomiting, diarrhoea or bowel obstruction.

Glycosuria is a common cause for an osmotic diuresis in the sick or very preterm.

It is important to rehydrate *slowly* and to start with isotonic solutions (plasma or 0.9% saline) to reduce the risk of inducing cerebral oedema.

Excess sodium

If fluids are **mismanaged** or excess **bicarbonate** administered. Restrict sodium intake subsequently.

Congenital hyperaldosteronism

Give diuretic (spironolactone) and refer to a specialist unit.

Potassium balance

Healthy term infants ingest about 1 mmol/kg/day and most intravenous nutrition regimens supply about 2 mmol/kg/day, maintaining positive potassium balance after 2–3 days.

Hypokalaemia
Definition

Plasma potassium <3 mmol/l.

Causes

Inadequate intake
Vomiting/diarrhoea
Alkalosis
Diuretics
Hyperaldosteronism

Management

Correct by increasing potassium input by 24 hour infusion or additions to milk. 1–3 mmol/kg/day is usually necessary. Use strong potassium chloride (15%) or dipotassium hydrogen phosphate (17.42%), which contain 2 mmol/ml, diluted in a bag or burette.

Hyperkalaemia
Definition

Plasma potassium >7 mmol/l.
ECG changes are a guide to toxicity – peaked T waves; prolonged PR interval; absent P waves; arrhythmias.

Causes

Artifactual due to sample haemolysis

Severe catabolism in sick infants
Acute renal failure
Hypoxia, shock, acidosis
Congenital adrenal hyperplasia (Chapter 13)

Management

ECG monitoring is needed.

- (a) Calcium gluconate (10%), 0.5–1 ml/kg, i.v. given over 2–4 min, cardioprotective for 30–60 min.
- (b) Correct acidosis (sodium bicarbonate, 1–2 mmol/kg), effective for 1–2 hours.
- (c) Resonium A (sodium polystyrene sulphonate), 1 g/kg/day, orally or rectally.
- (d) Salbutamol, 4 microg/kg, i.v. by bolus injection (as effective as and safer than glucose/insulin infusion).
- (e) Glucose/insulin infusion (*dangerous*): glucose 0.5–1.0 g/kg with 1 unit insulin/4 g glucose (with close blood sugar monitoring) (use in extreme circumstances, until dialysis established).
- (f) Peritoneal dialysis (Chapter 16).

Bibliography

Costarino, A. T., Baumgart, S. (1988). Controversies in fluid and electrolyte therapy for the premature infant. *Clinical Perinatol.*, **15**, 863–878. Philadelphia: W. B. Saunders.

18

Neonatal jaundice

Physiological jaundice
Pathological jaundice

Bilirubin, produced from breakdown of haemoglobin, myoglobin cytochromes and other haem-containing compounds, mainly in the spleen, liver and bone marrow, is fat-soluble and in high concentrations toxic, particularly to the CNS. Conjugated bilirubin (mainly water-soluble diglucuronide) is less toxic. In fetal life unconjugated bilirubin is excreted via the placenta, but from birth it is excreted in the bile, after conjugation in the liver. Unconjugated bilirubin is transported to the liver bound to albumin. An acceptor protein, ligandin, transports bilirubin into the liver cells where conjugation to bilirubin diglucuronide occurs. Water-soluble conjugated bilirubin is then secreted into the bile and excreted via the bowel. Some of the bilirubin reaching the gut is deconjugated by bacterial glucuronidase activity, reabsorbed and returned to the liver (enterohepatic circulation).

Physiological jaundice

The change-over from fetal to neonatal bilirubin metabolism results in a rise in circulating bilirubin levels in normal infants, with a peak on the third or fourth day (mean 120 μmol/l) falling over the next 4–5 days (mean <30 μmol/l at 10 days of age).

Bilirubin levels above 150 μmol/l in the first 48 hours after birth, or above 220 μmol at any time in normal-term infants should not be assumed to be physiological, and warrant investigation (see below). Approximately 6% of term infants develop significant neonatal jaundice (>220 μmol/l).

Pathological jaundice

Pathological processes may affect the metabolism of bilirubin at any stage of the pathway, from production to excretion (Table 18.1).

Table 18.1 Pathophysiology of neonatal jaundice

Unconjugated hyperbilirubinaemia

Acute intravascular haemolysis
  Haemolytic disease (Rhesus, ABO, other)
  Red cell abnormalities (G6PD deficiency, spherocytosis)
  Intrauterine infections (CMV, toxoplasma, herpes, other)
  Bacterial sepsis

High red cell mass (polycythaemia)

Sequestered blood
  Swallowed (fetal or maternal)
  Bruising (cephalhaematoma, breech delivery)
  Intraventricular haemorrhage

Decreased conjugation
  Crigler–Najjar syndrome (glucuronyl transferase deficiency)
  Sepsis

Increased enterohepatic circulation
  Breast milk jaundce
  Delayed passage of meonium (meconium plug, late feeding, hypothyroidism)
  Bowel obstruction (below ampulla of Vater: atresia, stenosis, meconium ileus, Hirschsprung's disease)

Conjugated hyperbilirubinaemia

Impaired hepatocellular function/excretion of conjugated bilirubin
  Intrauterine infections (hepatitic presentation)
  Metabolic disorders (galactosaemia, tyrosinosis, alpha-1-antitrypsin deficiency, other)
  Rare familial conditions (Dubin–Johnson or Rotor syndrome)
  Prolonged intravenous nutrition
  Hepatocellular damage after severe haemolysis

Obstruction to bile flow
  Biliary atresia
  Choledochal cyst
  Common bile duct obstruction by band

Bilirubin toxicity

Albumin binding

Unconjugated bilirubin is carried in plasma bound to albumin. If dissociated from albumin, bilirubin can readily diffuse into cells of the CNS, causing damage by uncoupling oxidative phosphorylation, increasing glycolysis and decreasing protein synthesis. Bilirubin can be displaced from albumin by certain drugs (e.g. sulphonamides, salicylates), by plasma non-esterified fatty acids (NEFA) (which increase with fasting, cold stress and sepsis), or by acidosis.

Bilirubin-binding capacity of albumin varies widely (70–140 mmol bilirubin per gram of albumin), according to clinical circumstances. Numerous techniques (e.g. Sephadex G-25) have been developed to identify 'free' or unbound bilirubin or to quantify the bilirubin-binding capacity of a patient's serum, but the effects of changes in NEFA and pH limit their usefulness.

Bilirubin encephalopathy (kernicterus)

The term kernicterus refers to the yellow staining of the basal ganglia and hippocampus found at autopsy in infants dying with bilirubin toxicity.

The clinical picture of bilirubin encephalopathy may not develop for several hours after toxic levels of bilirubin have occurred. There is a prodromal syndrome of poor feeding, temperature instability, irritability, decreased reflexes, 'cycling' movements of the arms and lethargy. Prompt treatment by exchange transfusion at this stage may prevent further progression. Within a few hours the condition is likely to progress to include generalized stiffening, with extension and tight fisting of the arms, crossed extension of the legs and opisthotonos with rigid arching of the back. The cry becomes high pitched, there may be 'sun setting' of the eyes from paralysis of extra-ocular muscles, and seizures may occur. Gastric or pulmonary haemorrhage may be a terminal event. In survivors the extensor spasms may give way to generalized hypotonia, poor feeding and developmental delay. Long-term consequences vary and may include spastic or choreo-athetoid cerebral palsy, clumsiness, paralysis of upward gaze, mental impairment, dental dysplasia and high-tone hearing loss.

The pattern of bilirubin encephalopathy may be different in very preterm infants, who may only show fisting, increased tone and possibly apnoea in the acute phase.

Bilirubin encephalopathy is rarely seen in term infants without underlying pathology (e.g. glucose 6-phosphate dehydrogenase, G6PD, deficiency) or at bilirubin levels below 380 micromol/l, but in preterm or low birthweight infants, particularly in the presence of acidosis, RDS, sepsis or perinatal asphyxia, it may occur at much lower levels. The risk increases with the bilirubin level, particularly in the presence of factors (e.g. elevated NEFA, acidosis) which decrease albumin binding. These babies also tend to have lower albumin levels.

The jaundiced baby

Jaundice is usually first noticeable in the face and neck; as the level rises it gradually becomes more apparent over the trunk, the limbs and finally on the palms and soles. In black infants jaundice may be difficult to detect, but is usually apparent on the sclera, on the skin of the nose when blanched or, if more severe, on the palms or soles.

History

Important points in the history are mother's (and father's) blood groups; past obstetric history (particularly if any jaundiced infants); ethnic origin of parents; maternal drugs; gestation; mode of delivery; known iso-immune antibody status. Significant jaundice in the first 48 hours of life is usually due to acute haemolysis (see Table 18.1).

Examination

The presence of bruising, cephalohaematomata, or plethora may suggest increased red cell destruction. Hepatosplenomegaly suggests infection or haemolysis and pallor of the mucous membranes supports the latter. Delayed passage of meconium may suggest functional bowel obstruction (e.g. meconium ileus, Hirschsprung's disease) or hypothyroidism.

Investigation (<7 days)

If bilirubin is in or above zone 4 in Fig. 18.1

Check: Blood groups (infant and mother)
Coomb's test (on cord blood or infant's blood)
Haemoglobin, packed cell volume, blood film
Urine for reducing substances (test for galactosaemia; see Chapter 13)

and if baby is unwell: a full infection screen (see Chapter 14)

If bilirubin is close to 'exchange' line in Fig. 18.1

Check: (1) Serum albumin and acid–base status (low pH or albumin increase risk of kernicterus at a given bilirubin level).

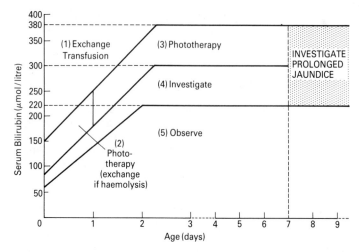

Fig. 18.1 The management of neonatal jaundice in well, term infants (NB. For pre-term and/or sick infants treat as if in the category one (or two) stages higher e.g. if in zone 4, treat as 3 or 2.

(2) Direct (i.e. conjugated) bilirubin (if >10% total bilirubin is conjugated this suggests hepatocellular damage or biliary obstruction – use the *unconjugated* bilirubin level as a guide to the need for exchange transfusion).

Management

Guidelines for management of the term infant with jaundice who is otherwise well are given in Fig. 18.1.

This graph is a *rough guide* only. If the infant is preterm or sick, or particularly if there is hypoproteinaemia or acidosis, then phototherapy and exchange transfusion should be used at considerably lower levels, e.g. for a well infant of 30 weeks' gestation the 'exchange transfusion' line would approximate to the 'phototherapy' line for a term infant (Fig. 18.1). The 'phototherapy' line for such an infant would be correspondingly lower.

If there is evidence of iso-immune haemolytic disease (e.g. positive Coomb's test) then exchange transfusion is likely to be necessary and should be performed if the bilirubin goes into zone 2 in Fig. 18.1, especially if the rate of rise >10 micromol/l/hour.

For preterm or sick infants the early use of phototherapy may reduce the frequency of severe jaundice needing exchange transfusions. However, potential benefits must be weighed against problems with increased insensible water loss and temperature regulation. For term infants there is no evidence that use of phototherapy for lower levels of jaundice than those shown on Fig. 18.1 will decrease the need for exchange transfusion, though it may decrease the duration of jaundice.

Ensure adequate hydration (keep urine specific gravity ≤1012) by giving extra water or feeds if necessary.

Phototherapy

Unconjugated bilirubin when exposed to light is isomerized to a more water-soluble form ('photobilirubin') which can then be excreted in the bile without conjugation. Blue light (wavelength 400–500 nm) is most effective, but is unpleasant for parents and staff, so white lights are commonly used. Efficiency of phototherapy is improved by increasing the area of exposed skin, removing plastic covers, and decreasing the distance from the light to the baby. The intensity of phototherapy may be increased by using two phototherapy units or a high intensity lamp. Stopping phototherapy for up to three hours in six does not significantly decrease effectiveness so it should be stopped for feeding, changing, visiting etc. The main adverse effect of phototherapy is increased fluid loss, particularly in the stools, so extra fluids (about 1 ml/kg/hour extra) are needed. Although there is no good evidence that phototherapy damages the eyes, it is a reasonable precaution to cover the infant's eyes whilst under the light. These covers should be removed when the infant is taken out for feeding etc. Phototherapy reduces skin bilirubin, so the colour of exposed skin is not a good indicator of serum bilirubin and transcutaneous bilirubinometers (e.g. Minolta) are not reliable on such skin. Phototherapy should not be used for infants with high conjugated bilirubin levels as it is unnecessary and may lead to an unpleasant 'bronze baby' appearance of the skin.

Exchange transfusion

Rough guidelines on when exchange transfusion is needed in term infants are given in Fig. 18.1. Practical details are given in Chapter 26, page 354.

If the infant has *severe haemolytic disease* (with hypoproteinaemia, oedema, cardiac failure, severe anaemia or frank hydrops fetalis) exchange transfusion may lead to major, potentially fatal, fluid shifts (see Chapter 2, page 33). For such infants the first exchange transfusion has the aim of correcting anaemia and raising serum albumin, rather than removing bilirubin. This exchange should therefore be of only 30–60 ml/kg. The venous and arterial pressures should be checked frequently, and the infant left with a volume deficit of 10–20 ml/kg (to maintain a central venous pressure of 5–9 cm H_2O).

An exchange transfusion of 160 ml/kg (i.e. twice the infant's blood volume) will remove approximately 80% of the infant's red cells, and reduce the serum bilirubin by about 50%. Check bilirubin level 4–6 hours after the exchange, as there is commonly a rapid 'rebound' rise over the first 4–6 hours, with a much slower rise thereafter.

We do not routinely use prophylactic antibiotics to reduce the risk of NEC following exchange transfusion. Albumin priming (1 g/kg over 30–60 min prior to exchange) may be useful to increase the washout of bilirubin in severe haemolysis or to increase plasma binding capacity if there is a delay in cross-matching.

Prolonged neonatal jaundice

Jaundice persisting beyond the seventh day in a term baby is usually considered pathologically prolonged (Fig. 18.1). The most important investigation is the measurement of **conjugated bilirubin** which dictates further investigation and management.

Unconjugated hyperbilirubinaemia (>90% unconjugated)

Investigations should include:

Thyroid function tests
Urine: Microscopy and culture
         Reducing substances
Full blood count and film

If these investigations are normal and the child breast fed, the jaundice is usually benign ('breast milk jaundice') and probably due to the presence of beta-glucuronidase in the milk. This results in deconjugation of bilirubin in the bowel and an increased enterohepatic circulation. It is of no clinical significance; breast feeding should *not* be interrupted and the mother should be strongly reassured.

Prolonged unconjugated jaundice is common in very preterm infants in whom delayed feeding may lead to both decreased bile flow and gut motility, leading to increased reabsorption of deconjugated bilirubin. It is also common in the presence of polycythaemia.

Conjugated hyperbilirubinaemia

Prolonged jaundice with a high (>20%) conjugated component may occur with damage due to severe haemolytic disease or infection (CMV, toxoplasma, other), metabolic disease or obstruction to bile flow (Table 18.1). Not uncommonly it also occurs after a prolonged period of intravenous nutrition from which most infants make a full recovery.

Investigations Investigations should exclude the common causes as listed in Table 18.1.

Serum for antibodies to CMV, toxoplasma, rubella
Plasma amino acids
Serum for alpha-l-antitrypsin phenotype
Three freshly voided urines for viral culture
Urine: Reducing sugars
           Amino acids
           Organic acids

Further investigation Once the common causes are excluded difficulty may be encountered in distinguishing **biliary obstruction** from '**neonatal hepatitis**'. These probably represent opposite ends of a disease spectrum, arising from damage by an unknown agent to the hepatobiliary system at different stages, from the middle trimester of pregnancy (biliary atresia) to several weeks after birth (neonatal hepatitis). Both conditions are characterized by conjugated hyperbilirubinaemia which may date from the first week or sometimes may not be noticed until 2–4 weeks. Onset after 4 weeks makes biliary atresia unlikely. In both conditions there is commonly enlargement of the liver, disordered coagulation, and elevated transaminase levels. Infants with biliary atresia are often remarkably well despite severe jaundice, and usually have very pale stools. Ninety per cent of infants with biliary atresia have extrahepatic atresia, with absence or hypoplasia of hepatic duct, cystic duct, common bile duct or any combination of these. The importance of distinguishing biliary atresia from neonatal hepatitis is that surgery for the former (Kasai procedure) may be successful if carried out within the first two months of life. Beyond that age irreversible liver damage may occur making surgery unlikely to succeed. Several investigations have been used to try to distinguish between biliary atresia and hepatitis and include: serum alpha-fetoprotein (elevated in hepatitis; usually normal in atresia) and a HIDA excretion scan. Other radionuclides excreted in bile have also been used, but none of these tests is entirely satisfactory. If significant doubt remains, then liver biopsy may show characteristic features of biliary atresia (proliferation of bile ducts and hypertrophy of hepatic artery branches). Giant-cell transformation may occur in either biliary atresia or neonatal hepatitis. If biopsy is equivocal, then a laparotomy with operative cholangiogram may be necessary.

With early diagnosis and biliary drainage through a Roux-en-Y loop of jejunum sutured into the porta hepatitis (Kasai procedure), successful long-term biliary drainage is achieved in about 25% of infants with biliary atresia. Most infants with neonatal hepatitis make a complete recovery, but may have complications from bleeding, sepsis, or malabsorption of vitamins A, D and K.

Infants with prolonged conjugated hyperbilirubinaemia should therefore be given suitable vitamin supplements (see Chapter 11).

Rhesus haemolytic disease

Aetiology

The rhesus antigen system consists of three distinct antigens, Cc, Dd and Ee, where C, D, E are dominant and c, d, e recessive traits. About 85% of Caucasians have 'D' antigen (i.e. are 'rhesus positive').

Leakage of fetal red cells across the placenta into the maternal circulation may lead to the formation by the mother of IgG antibodies directed against fetal antigens which she does not have herself. Most commonly such antibodies are produced by rhesus-negative women (i.e. 'dd' genotype) and directed against rhesus-positive fetal cells (i.e. Dd or DD genotype) but may be produced against 'c' or 'E' antigens. These IgG antibodies cross into the fetus and may cause destruction of circulating red cells.

IgG antibodies are not usually produced on first exposure to an antigen, but require initial sensitization, with an amplified response on second or subsequent exposure. Thus, significant rhesus haemolytic disease is uncommon in first pregnancy, and increases in incidence and severity with increasing parity. Sensitization may occur from mismatched blood transfusion, or from fetomaternal bleeding at abortion. Small fetomaternal leaks may occur spontaneously or after amniocentesis or external cephalic version, and may account for the occasional case of rhesus haemolytic disease in first pregnancies.

Rhesus haemolytic disease is more common if mother and fetus are of the same ABO blood group.

Pathogenesis

The earlier the antibody crosses into the fetus the more severe the disease. Haemolysis starting in the second trimester may cause severe anaemia with hepatosplenomegaly, liver damage, and hypoproteinaemia, cardiac failure and generalized oedema with ascites (hydrops fetalis, see Chapter 2, page 33). In severe cases there is a conjugated hyperbilirubinaemia.

When haemolysis starts nearer to term the infant is born less severely anaemic but develops neonatal jaundice, which may be severe.

Prevention of rhesus haemolytic disease

Since 1969 the incidence of rhesus haemolytic disease has fallen dramatically as a result of the prevention of sensitization of rhesus-negative women. All non-sensitized rhesus-negative women should be given human rhesus hyperimmune gamma globulin (100–200 mg i.m.) within 60 hours after any procedure which might result in sensitization (e.g. birth of a rhesus-positive infant, amniocentesis, termination of pregnancy). The gamma globulin binds to fetal cells and expedites their removal from the maternal cells.

Antenatal management

Routine screening of all rhesus-negative pregnant women for the presence of rhesus antibodies allows the identification of most affected fetuses. The management of an affected pregnancy is controversial. Whereas previously amniocentesis with measurement of the optical density difference and bilirubin concentration was the best estimate of severity, in the second trimester this has been largely replaced in tertiary referral centres by cordocentesis, measurement of haematocrit and blood group, and direct fetal transfusion if necessary. The relative merits and demerits of each technique in the third trimester have not been established and it is still unclear as to whether it is best to proceed to early delivery in the light of excellent neonatal survival from 30 weeks' gestation, or to continue with cordocentesis and transfusion, with their attendant risks, until spontaneous labour ensues.

Management of the infant with rhesus haemolytic disease

The jaundiced baby (page 263); Chapter 2, page 33, hydrops fetalis, and Fig. 18.2.)

Continued low-grade haemolysis in infants who do not need exchange transfusion may rarely lead to late anaemia (after 2–3 weeks) which may necessitate a top-up transfusion. Early supplementation with iron and folic acid may reduce the severity of this anaemia (see Chapter 11).

Jaundice from ABO incompatibility

Infants of blood group A (or more rarely B) born to mothers of blood group O may develop early jaundice from haemolysis caused by transplacental passage of maternal antibodies directed against the A (or B) antigen. The severity of haemolysis does not correlate well with the level of maternal circulating anti-A or anti-B antibody.

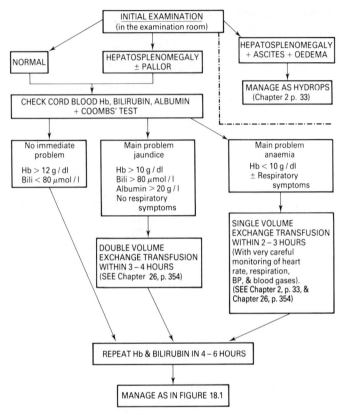

Fig. 18.2 Management of the infant with suspected Rhesus haemolytic disease (e.g. Previous affected sibling or rising Rh. antibody titres during this pregnancy).

Although up to 25% of pregnancies may be potentially affected (mother O, fetus A or B), only 1 in 45 of these infants is affected. The incidence and severity is the same in firstborn or subsequent children.

Most infants with ABO incompatibility show only mild or moderate early jaundice, but in some the bilirubin may rise to levels requiring exchange transfusion. Hepatosplenomegaly is not a feature of ABO incompatibility and late anaemia (see above) is rarely a problem. For management see 'The jaundiced baby', page 263.

Bibliography

Broderson, R. (1980). Bilirubin transport in the newborn infant reviewed with relation to kernicterus. *J. Pediatr.*, **96**, 349.

Cashore, W. J. and Ster, L. (1982). Neonatal hyperbilirubinaemia. *Pediatr. Clin. N. Amer.*, **29**, 1191–1202.

Fraser, I. D. and Tovey, G. H. (1976). Observations on rhesus iso-immunisation past, present and future. *Clinics in Haematology*, **5**, 149–63.

Maisels, M. J. (ed) (1990). Neonatal jaundice. *Clin. Perinatol.*, **17**, 2. Philadelphia: W. B. Saunders.

19

Growth charts and gestational assessment

Growth charts
Gestational assessment

Growth charts

All preterm, low birthweight, high-risk (see Chapters 5 and 1), or sick infants should have weight, length and head circumference measured and plotted on a growth chart at birth, at least weekly until discharge from hospital, and at all follow-up appointments (see Figs 19.1 and 19.2; 29.1 and 29.2).

Gestational assessment

Antenatal

The most reliable assessment of gestational age is obtained from:

(1) First day of mother's last menstrual period if known (add 9 calendar months and 7 days to obtain estimated date of delivery).
(2) Repeated obstetric assessment of gestation before 16 weeks.
(3) Ultrasound assessment of fetal head size (biparietal diameter) before 20 weeks (error ± 7 days between 16 and 18 weeks).

If 1, 2 and 3 are in agreement, then dates are almost certainly correct.
Obstetric assessment of gestational age beyond 28 weeks (including ultrasound scanning) carries a potential error of *at least* ± 2 weeks (see Chapter 1).

Postnatal

The accuracy of postnatal assessment of gestation is at best ± 10

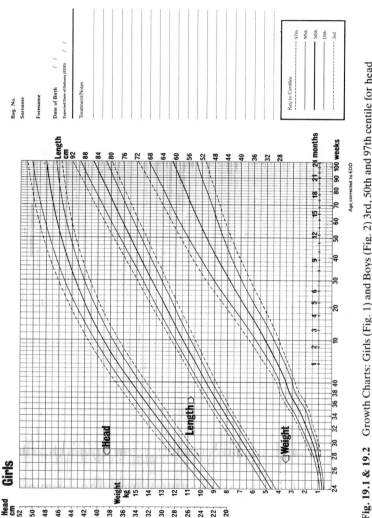

Fig. 19.1 & 19.2 Growth Charts: Girls (Fig. 1) and Boys (Fig. 2) 3rd, 50th and 97th centile for head circumference, length and weight. 24 weeks gestation to 2 years post-term (Reproduced with kind permission from Gairdner, D. and Pearson, J., *Arch. Dis. Childh.* (1971). Published by Castlemead Publications (Reference number GPBA, GPGA).

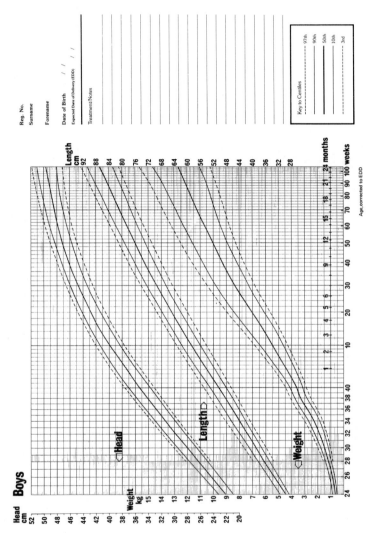

Fig. 19.2

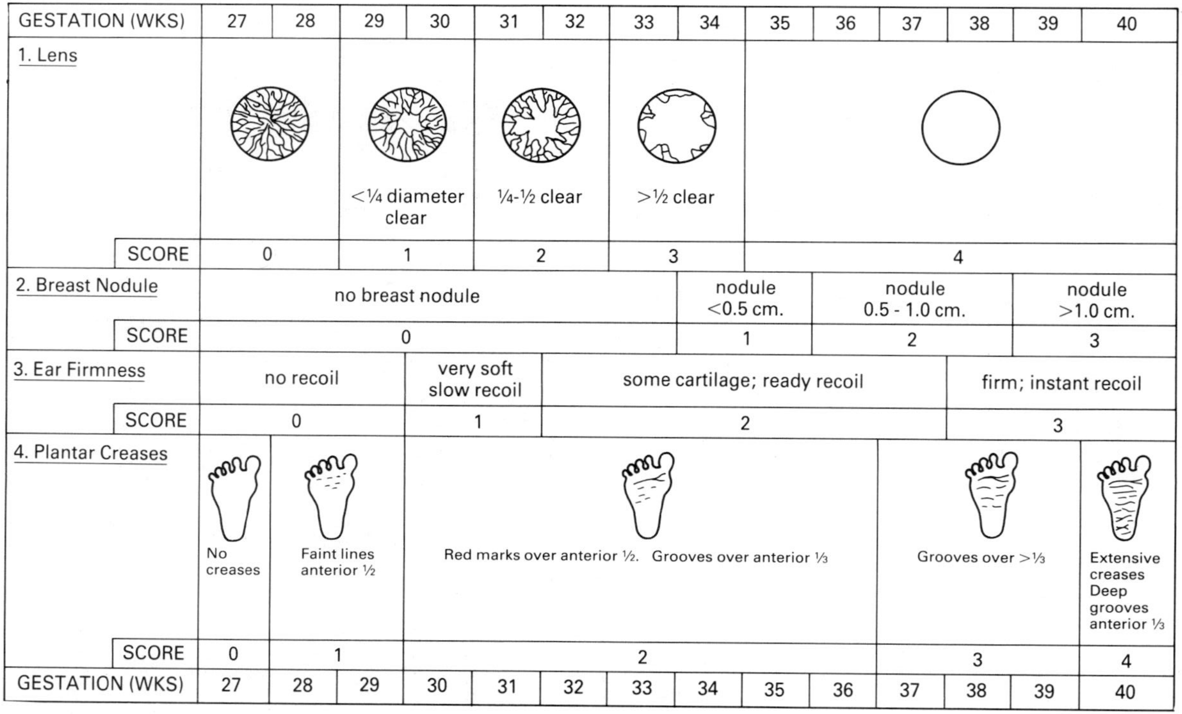

GESTATION (WKS)	27	28	29	30	31	32	33	34	35	36	37	38	39	40
1. Lens														
SCORE	0		<¼ diameter clear 1		¼-½ clear 2		>½ clear 3							
2. Breast Nodule		no breast nodule						nodule <0.5 cm.		nodule 0.5 - 1.0 cm.		nodule >1.0 cm.	
SCORE		0						1		2		3		
3. Ear Firmness		no recoil		very soft slow recoil			some cartilage; ready recoil			firm; instant recoil				
SCORE		0		1			2			3				
4. Plantar Creases	No creases	Faint lines anterior ½		Red marks over anterior ½. Grooves over anterior ⅓						Grooves over >⅓				Extensive creases Deep grooves anterior ⅓
SCORE	0	1		2						3				4
GESTATION (WKS)	27	28	29	30	31	32	33	34	35	36	37	38	39	40

Fig. 19.3 The assessment of getational age (Narayanan *et al.*, *Indian J. Pediatr.*, 1981, **18.** 715–20 reproduced with kind permission)

Table 19.1 Assessment of gestational age.
Relationship between total score and gestational
age (Narayanan *et al.*, 1981) (see Fig. 19.3)

Score	Gestational age (weeks)
0	≤27
1	28
2,3	29
4	30
5	31
6	32
7	33
8	34
9	35
10	36
11	37
12	38
13	39
14	≥40

days. Unless postnatal assessment suggests a 3–4 week discrepancy
with mother's dates, the latter should be accepted. Determination of
gestational age may have serious medicolegal consequences and the
reasons for challenging maternal dates should be clearly stated in the
clinical notes. It is pointless to distress a mother by attempting to
contradict her dates without firm reason.

Many methods have been described. Most rely upon physical
characteristics (e.g. Narayanan *et al.*, 1981; Fig. 19.3; Table 19.1) or
a combination of physical and neurological criteria (e.g. Dubowitz
and Dubowitz, 1970; Figs 19.4 and 19.5).

Neurological assessment is least likely to be accurate in sick or
asphyxiated babies who tolerate handling poorly. Assessment of
gestations below 27 weeks is difficult. If the eyelids are fused the
gestation is probably <26 weeks.

External (superficial) Criteria

EXTERNAL SIGN	SCORE				
	0	1	2	3	4
OEDEMA	Obvious oedema hands and feet. pitting over tibia	No obvious oedema hands and feet. pitting over tibia	No oedema		
SKIN TEXTURE	Very thin. gelatinous	Thin and smooth	Smooth. medium thickness. Rash or superficial peeling	Slight thickening Superficial cracking and peeling esp hands and feet	Thick and parchment-like: superficial or deep cracking
SKIN COLOUR (Infant not crying)	Dark red	Uniformly pink	Pale pink: variable over body	Pale. Only pink over ears, lips, palms or soles	
SKIN OPACITY (trunk)	Numerous veins and venules clearly seen especially over abdomen	Veins and tributaries seen	A few large vessels clearly seen over abdomen	A few large vessels seen indistinctly over abdomen	No blood vessels seen
LANUGO (over back)	No lanugo	Abundant: long and thick over whole back	Hair thinning especially over lower back	Small amount of lanugo and bald areas	At least half of back devoid of lanugo
PLANTAR CREASES	No skin creases	Faint red marks over anterior half of sole	Definite red marks over more than anterior half: indentations over less than anterior third	Indentations over more than anterior third	Definite deep indentations over more than anterior third
NIPPLE FORMATION	Nipple barely visible: no areola	Nipple well defined. areola smooth and flat diameter <0.75 cm	Areola stippled, edge not raised: diameter <0.75 cm	Areola stippled, edge raised diameter >0.75 cm	
BREAST SIZE	No breast tissue palpable	Breast tissue on one or both sides 0.5 cm diameter	Breast tssue both sides: one or both 0.5-1.0 cm	Breast tissue both sides: one or both 1 cm	
EAR FORM	Pinna flat and shapeless. little or no incurving of edge	Incurving of part of edge of pinna	Partial incurving whole of upper pinna	Well-defined incurving whole of upper pinna	
EAR FIRMNESS	Pinna soft. easily folded. no recoil	Pinna soft. easily folded. slow recoil	Cartilage to edge of pinna. but soft in places. ready recoil	Pinna firm. cartilage to edge. instant recoil	
GENITALIA MALE	Neither testis in scrotum	At least one testis high in scrotum	At least one testis right down		
FEMALES (With hips half abducted)	Labia majora widely separated, labia minora protruding	Labia majora almost cover labia minora	Labia majora completely cover labia minora		

TOTAL SCORE	GESTATIONAL AGE IN WEEKS
5	26
9	27
13	28
16	29
20	30
24	31
27	32
31	33
34	34
38	35
42	36
45	37
49	38
53	39
56	40
60	41
63	42
67	43

(Adapted from Farr et al. Develop. Med. Child Neurol. 1966,8,507)

Fig. 19.4 Dubowitz method of assessment of postnatal gestational age.

Neurological Criteria

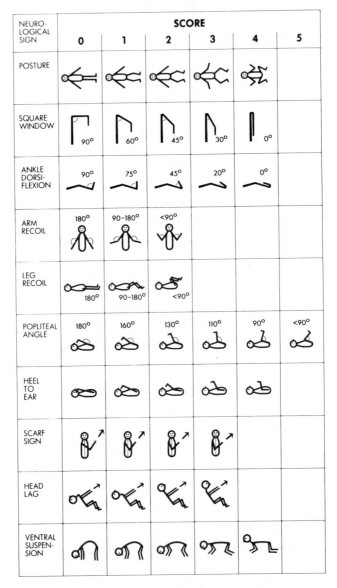

Fig. 19.5 Clinical assessment of gestational age by method of Dubowitz *et al. J. Pediatr.* (1970), **77**, 1. See notes for methods to be used.

Some notes on techniques of Assessment of Neurological Criteria

POSTURE: Observed with infant quiet and in supine position. Score 0: Arms and legs extended; 1: beginning of flexion of hips and knees, arms extended; 2: stronger flexion of legs, arms extended; 3: arms slightly flexed, legs flexed and abducted; 4: full flexion of arms and legs.

SQUARE WINDOW: The hand is flexed on the forearm between the thumb and index finger of the examiner. Enough pressure is applied to get as full a flexion as possible, and the angle between the hypothenar eminence and the ventral aspect of the forearm is measured and graded according to diagram. (Care is taken not to rotate the infant's wrist while doing this manœuvre.)

ANKLE DORSIFLEXION: The foot is dorsiflexed onto the anterior aspect of the leg, with the examiner's thumb on the sole of the foot and other fingers behind the leg. Enough pressure is applied to get as full flexion as possible, and the angle between the dorsum of the foot and the anterior aspect of the leg is measured.

ARM RECOIL: With the infant in the supine position the forearms are first flexed for 5 seconds, then fully extended by pulling on the hands, and then released. The sign is fully positive if the arms return briskly to full flexion (Score 2). If the arms return to incomplete flexion or the response is sluggish it is graded as Score 1. If they remain extended or are only followed by random movements the score is 0.

LEG RECOIL: With the infant supine, the hips and knees are fully flexed for 5 seconds, then extended by traction on the feet, and released. A maximal response is one of full flexion of the hips and knees (Score 2). A partial flexion scores 1, and minimal or no movement scores 0.

POPLITEAL ANGLE: With the infant supine and his pelvis flat on the examining couch, the thigh is held in the knee-chest position by the examiner's left index finger and thumb supporting the knee. The leg is then extended by gentle pressure from the examiner's right index finger behind the ankle and the popliteal angle is measured.

HEEL TO EAR MANŒUVRE: With the baby supine, draw the baby's foot as near to the head as it will go without forcing it. Observe the distance between the foot and the head as well as the degree of extension at the knee. Grade according to diagram. Note that the knee is left free and may draw down alongside the abdomen.

SCARF SIGN: With the baby supine, take the infant's hand and try to put it around the neck and as far posteriorly as possible around the opposite shoulder. Assist this manœuvre by lifting the elbow across the body. See how far the elbow will go across and grade according to illustrations. Score 0: Elbow reaches opposite axillary line; 1: Elbow between midline and opposite axillary line; 2: Elbow reaches midline; 3: Elbow will not reach midline.

HEAD LAG: With the baby lying supine, grasp the hands (or the arms if a very small infant) and pull him slowly towards the sitting position. Observe the position of the head in relation to the trunk and grade accordingly. In a small infant the head may initially be supported by one hand. Score 0: Complete lag; 1: Partial head control; 2: Able to maintain head in line with body; 3: Brings head anterior to body.

VENTRAL SUSPENSION: The infant is suspended in the prone position, with examiner's hand under the infant's chest (one hand in a small infant, two in a large infant). Observe the degree of extension of the back and the amount of flexion of the arms and legs. Also note the relation of the head to the trunk. Grade according to diagrams.

If the score for an individual criterion differs on the two sides of the baby, take the mean.
For further details see Dubowitz et. al., J. Pediat. 1970, 77, 1.

20

Care of the family

During pregnancy
In the delivery room
In the postnatal ward
In the special care baby unit
The death of a baby
Appendix
    Self-help organizations, information and services for young infants
    and their families

During pregnancy

The general practitioner, midwife and obstetrician are usually responsible for answering most of the parents' queries during pregnancy. For some families such as those with a previous perinatal problem (e.g. major malformation or perinatal death) or those for whom problems are anticipated with the present pregnancy (e.g. when preterm delivery is likely, or a major malformation has been detected by antenatal scanning) it is important for the parents to meet and talk to the paediatrician, to see the special care baby unit (SCBU) and meet some of the nursing staff before the birth of the infant. The father should be encouraged to be present at the delivery, particularly if an elective Caesarean section (under epidural anaesthesia) is planned.

In the delivery room

When called to attend a high-risk delivery (see Chapter 2) the paediatrician should arrive with sufficient time to introduce him/herself to the parents and explain what is likely to happen. After resuscitation, the baby should be given to the parents to hold as soon as possible. Skin-to-skin contact between mother and baby is an effective way of keeping the baby warm as well as helping the mother to get to know her baby. The moments soon after childbirth are emotional ones, and the parents should be accorded as much privacy as possible.

The sick or preterm infant

Few if any babies are too sick to be shown to the parents in the delivery room. Parents should be encouraged to touch and stroke their baby (in the incubator or under the overhead heater) before the baby is taken to the neonatal unit. It is important to be positive and encouraging to parents. Negative attitudes may interfere with the process of parent–child 'bonding'.

The child with a congenital abnormality

If there is a major abnormality, the parents should be shown the normal parts of the baby first, the anomaly should then be gently and simply explained to them, and they should then be shown the abnormality. It is a mistake to 'protect' parents from the sight of an abnormality – their imagination of the lesion is very likely to be worse than the real thing.

Parents of sick or abnormal babies need great support. They should be encouraged to touch and hold their baby, to talk to each other and the staff about their feelings, and their natural wish for privacy should not lead to isolation by the staff. Such parents go through a phase of 'mourning' for the perfect baby they wanted but do not have. This may be accompanied by denial and anger, often directed at medical or nursing staff, before the parents can come to terms with the reality of their baby.

If the baby is to be taken to a neonatal unit for care, the parents should be given a polaroid photograph as soon as possible.

In the postnatal ward

'Rooming in'

Babies should routinely be cared for by their mother (with whatever help is needed from nursing staff) and should be kept with their mothers as much as possible. Mothers should be discouraged but not prevented from leaving their babies in the newborn nursery at night, and breast-feeding mothers should routinely be woken to feed their infant (see Chapter 11).

Small infants requiring special care can be safely 'roomed-in' with their mothers provided there is adequate experienced nursing supervision (see Chapter 5).

Visiting

Restrictions on visiting should only be those required for patient care – fathers and siblings should be allowed virtually unlimited visiting.

Help and reassurance

Mothers of newborn infants need help with establishing breast feeding (see Chapter 11), and reassurance about the minor difficulties which most babies experience.

In the special care baby unit

Parents with a baby on a SCBU require careful support – open visiting by parents and siblings; careful, consistent and often repeated explanations by staff (preferably by the same staff); encouraging and optimistic (but honest) attitudes to the baby's outlook. Parents should be encouraged to spend as much time as convenient with their baby and should be involved in his/her care as soon as possible (e.g. tube feeding, nappy changing), but must not be made to feel guilty for wanting to spend some time at home or with other children.

Parents' groups can be of great value. 'Experienced' families who have had their babies on SCBU can give support and encouragement to parents with sick infants. Medical and nursing staff may also benefit from attending, though such meetings are probably best organized by involved medical social workers.

The death of a baby

It is important to involve parents as much as possible in the care of a dying child. Their initial reaction, confronted with a malformed or dying baby, may be to back away. This may be part of a denial, or may simply be because they are frightened to get to love the baby. They may feel that if they do this the loss when the child dies will be even greater. They should be encouraged to spend as much time as possible with the dying child. Many parents say afterwards that the few moments which they had with their dying child were the most precious of their lives. Conversely, parents who have not spent time with their dying baby may feel a deep sense of guilt and regret.

Points to remember in the care of the family of a dying baby

Parents may think that their baby is in pain. Explain to them that if he/she were in pain then adequate analgesia would be given.

Explain to the parents that the baby will be cared for, cleaned and fed as any other baby.

Take one or two polaroid photographs of the baby (with parents holding their child if they wish).

If the decision has been made to withdraw intensive care (see Chapter 30), it may be appropriate for the parents to be present when this is done, or for the baby to be taken to them to hold, free from tubes, electrodes, drips etc. Give them time and privacy with their dying baby.

Parents should be encouraged to see and hold the baby after death, for as long as they wish.

After a baby has died, you may feel inadequate and not know what to say to the parents. An arm round their shoulders may be comforting; and do express your own sorrow at the baby's death.

Table 20.1 gives a check-list to be completed after the death of a baby.

Arrangements for hospital funerals vary from place to place. Find out about the arrangements at your hospital so that you can inform the parents of what will happen if they ask the hospital to handle the funeral. The parents should be able to attend, and according to their wishes there may be a short religious service of their choice; the baby should be buried in a separate, marked and tended grave. If this is not the case in your hospital, then pressure should be applied to the undertakers to meet these basic requirements.

Do talk to your colleagues about your own reaction to the baby's death – to examine your own feelings does not diminish, but increases your professional usefulness.

Many families will benefit from early and continued contact with a medical social worker.

Talk to the parents about the stages of bereavement. Emphasize the importance of talking about their grief to each other and to their friends and relatives. Sudden feelings of intense sadness will come over them at times (often with no warning) for many months or years, but as time passes they may find it easier to think or talk of the dead baby, and to remember the positive aspects of his/her short life.

Acquaintances may have difficulty talking to them about the death of their baby and may actively try to avoid contact with them. This may add to their feelings of alienation.

Older children may develop behavioural disorders, for example, bed wetting, or may themselves become depressed. If they have not been involved in the grieving process and have not seen the baby in

Table 20.1   Neonatal death check-list

(1) Death certificate completed (and parents given instructions on where, when and how to register the death)
(2) Consent for autopsy obtained (and form signed if necessary)
(3) Parents given leaflet explaining the possible types of funeral arrangements
(4) Appointment arranged for parents to see head porter or mortuary attendant (to discuss the funeral arrangements)
(5) Parents given information on the Stillbirth and Neonatal Death Society (see Appendix to this chapter)
(6) Inform obstetric team
(7) GP contacted by telephone and message also left for health visitor
(8) Neonatal discharge form completed
(9) Medical social worker informed
(10) Summary letter written to GP
(11) Follow-up appointment arranged for parents
(12) Community paediatric department notified
(13) ? Whole body X-ray (if not already X-rayed)
(14) ? Check chromosomes
(15) Photograph (of baby, clothed in cot. To be offered to parents at follow-up visit)
(16) Notes sent to pathology with request for autopsy

hospital they may feel alienated and are at a greater risk of developing an abnormal prolonged grief reaction.

Arrange a further appointment in 2–4 weeks' time (when the result of the post-mortem examination should be available). At this appointment explain the post-mortem results, answer any questions they have about their baby's illness or death and explain any genetic implications. It is also important to discuss their feelings about the death, whether they are able to talk freely about him/her to each other, and whether they have developed some insight to their inevitable feelings of guilt and anger surround the baby's death.

Enquire about other children and extended family, particularly the grandparents.

Parents may ask about further children at this stage. They should be warned of the risks of trying to have a 'replacement' baby, and advised to delay a further pregnancy until they feel emotionally and physically ready to cope. There can be no rigid rules, but for most families this involves delaying a further pregnancy for 3–6 months.

References

Redshaw, M. E., Rivers, R. P. A., Roseublatt, D. M. (1985). *Born Too Early: Your Baby in Special Care*. Oxford: Oxford University Press.

Davis, J. A., Rickards, M. P. M., Robertson, N. R. C. (1983). *Parent-Baby Attachment in Premature Infants*. Beckenham: Croom Helm.

Appendix

Self-help organizations, information and services for young infants and their families

Association for the Improvement of the Maternity Services (AIMS)
A pressure group, consisting mainly of parents, but including members of the medical and midwifery professions. AIMS offers information, support and advice to parents about all aspects of maternity care. Produces information leaflets about obstetric and midwifery practices, research and individual experiences.

Contact: S. Warshal, 40 Kingswood Avenue, London, NW6 6LS
(Tel: 081 960 5585)

Association For All Speech Impaired Children (AFASIC)
An association to help children and young people who have disorders of speech and language.

Contact: AFASIC, 347 Central Markets, Smithfield, London, EC1A 9NH
(Tel: 071 236 3632/6487)

Association for Spina Bifida and Hydrocephalus (ASBAH)
The Association provides advisory and welfare services, practical assistance and information to parents, families and individuals; leaflets and publications.

Contact: ASBAH House, 42 Park Road, Peterborough, Cambs, PE1 2UQ
(Tel: 0733 555988)

Bladder Exstrophy Association
Provides practical help and advice to families and professional advisers of children with this condition.

Contact: Mrs Shirley Sparkes, 20 Hill Street, Totterdown, Bristol, BS3 4TW
(Tel: 0272 710067)

British Heart Foundation
Provides information for families of children with heart disorders. Publishes booklets and supports research into heart disease.

Contact: BHF, 14 Fitzharding Street, London, W1H 4DG
(Tel: 071 935 0185)

Cleft Lip and Palate Association (CLAPA)
Provides help and information for families of children with cleft lip and or palate. Useful booklets for parents.

Contact: CLAPA, Mrs Cy Thirlaway, 1 Eastwood Gardens, Kenton, Newcastle upon Tyne, NE3 3DQ
(Tel: 091 285 9396)

The Compassionate Friends
A nationwide self-help organization of parents whose child (of any age, including adult) has died from any cause. Personal and group support, a quarterly Newsletter, a postal library, and range of leaflets. A befriending, not a counselling, service.

Contact: National Secretary, The Compassionate Friends, 6 Denmark Street, Bristol, BS1 5DQ
(Tel: 0272 292778)

Cystic Fibrosis Research Trust
Supports research into CF, provides help and information for families, and produces helpful leaflets on the care of children and adults with CF.

Contact: CFRT, Alexandra House, 5 Blyth Road, Bromley, Kent, BR1 3RS
(Tel: 081 464 7211)

Down's Syndrome Association
Provides help and information for parents and professionals on the care, treatment and training of children with Down's syndrome.

Contact: The Information Officer, 12–13 Clapham Common South
             Side, London, SW4 7AA
             (Tel: 071 720 0008)

The Family Fund
A government fund, administered by the Joseph Rowntree Memorial Trust, to help families with a very severely handicapped child under 16 years of age. Help given includes laundry equipment, family holidays, outings, driving lessons, clothing, etc.

Contact: The Family Fund, PO Box 50, York, YO1 2ZX
             (Tel: 0904 62115)

Foundation for the Study of Infant Deaths
Provides support and information for families bereaved by 'cot deaths'. Useful leaflets for families, nurses, casualty officers, and general practitioners. Also funds research into 'cot deaths'.

Contact: FSID, 4 Grosvenor Place, London, SW1X 7HD
             (Tel: 071 235 1721/0965)

Gingerbread (Association for One-Parent Families)
National network of local self-help groups, providing support, information and advice for one-parent families.

Contact: Gingerbread, 35 Wellington Street, London SE1 1DE
             (Tel: 071 240 0953)

The Haemophilia Society
Provides support, advice and information to families of children with haemophilia. Supports research into haemophilia and similar conditions.

Contact: The Haemophilia Society, 123 Westminster Bridge Road,
             London, SE1 7HR
             (Tel: 071 928 2020)

La Leche League
Provides information and support, primarily through personal help, to women who want to breast feed their babies. Publishes a newsletter, handbook and leaflets aimed at both mothers and health professionals.

Contact: La Leche League, B.M. 3424, London WC1N 3XX
             (Tel: 071 404 5011)

National Association for the Welfare of Children in Hospital (NAWCH)
Provides information and practical support for families, and helps ensure that services are planned with the special needs of children in mind. Also provides an information service for professionals and has published several useful booklets.

Contact: NAWCH, Argyle House, 29/31 Euston Road, London, NW1 2SD
(Tel: 071 833 2041)

National Childbirth Trust
Provides antenatal education and preparation, postnatal support, breast-feeding counselling, and birth education in schools. Publishes leaflets on pregnancy and parenthood and organizes study days for parents and health professionals. Conducts research into maternity care.

Contact: NCT, Alexandra House, Oldham TCE, Acton, London, W3 6NH
(Tel: 081 922 8637)

National Council for One-Parent Families
Helps make the needs of one-parent families known to the public and government, and publishes books and leaflets.

Contact: One-Parent Families, 255 Kentish Town Road, London, NW5 2LX
(Tel: 071 267 1361)

National Deaf Children's Society
Provides advice on welfare and education, a variety of services for deaf children and their families, and information on all aspects of childhood deafness.

Contact: NDCS, 45 Hereford Road, London, W2 5AH
(Tel: 071 229 9272)

Relate: Marriage Guidance
Provides a confidential counselling service for people who have difficulties in their marriage or other personal relationships. Promotes research and publishes literature on topics relating to human relationships.

Contact: Relate: National Marriage Guidance, Herbert Gray
College, Little Church Street, Rugby, CV21 3AP
(Tel: 0788 73241)

or local centres listed in telephone book under 'Marriage
Guidance' or 'Relate'

The Association for Children with Artificial Arms (REACH)
Provides information and support for families of children missing
part of an arm or a hand.

Contact: John Bruce, Secretary, REACH, 13 Park Terrace,
Chard, Somerset, TA20 1LA
(Tel: 0460 61578)

Restricted Growth Association
Provides information and support for families with children affected
by conditions likely to lead to restricted growth. Publishes booklets
for parents and professionals.

Contact: Mrs T. Webb, Administrator, 103 St Thomas Avenue,
Hayling Island, Hants, PO11 0EU
(Tel: 0705 461813)

Royal National Institute for the Blind (RNIB)
The RNIB's Educational and Leisure Division helps visually handicapped children and adults to obtain access to the educational
facilities they need. They provide information, advice and support
for parents, teachers, local authorities and others involved in providing education. The RNIB also provides a range of books and
information pamphlets.

Contact: RNIB, 224 Great Portland Street, London, W1N 6AA
(Tel: 071 388 1266)

Royal National Institute for the Deaf (RNID)
Offers help and advice on all matters concerning deafness, and
produces a wide range of advisory leaflets.

Contact: RNID, 105 Gower Street, London, WC1E 6AH
(Tel: 071 387 8033)

Royal Society for Mentally Handicapped Children and Adults (MENCAP)
MENCAP is concerned with providing support and help for people
with a mental handicap and their families. It runs residential services,

training and employment services, leisure services through the National Education of Gateway Clubs, and holidays. It also offers legal and information services, and mounts conferences and campaigns to improve public awareness of mental handicap and the services for people with a mental handicap.

Contact: Mencap National Centre, 123 Golden Lane, London, EC1Y 0RT
(Tel: 071 454 0454)

SENSE (The National Association for Deaf–Blind and Rubella Handicapped)

Campaigns for and provides advice and support to deaf-blind and rubella handicapped children and young adults, their families and professionals in the field. Services include family advisory service, residential further education centres, long-term residential care, conferences, courses, holidays and respite care, publications and a quarterly magazine.

Contact: SENSE, 311 Gray's Inn Road, London, WC1X 8PT
(Tel: 071 278 1005/1000)

Spastic's Society

Offers a range of services for people with cerebral palsy and their families, including assessment, social work support, education, residential care and independent living schemes, counselling and information services. Campaigns for change in attitudes and greater independence for people with cerebral palsy. Publishes **Disability Now**, a monthly newspaper, and **Developmental Medicine and Child Neurology**, a monthly professional journal as well as many other publications.

Contact: Library and Information Unit, The Spastic's Society, 12 Park Crescent, London, W1N 4EQ
(Tel: 071 636 5020)

Cerebral Palsy Helpline on 0800 62 62 16 (free) from 1.00 pm–10.00 pm Monday–Sunday

STEPS

A support group for families of children with congenital abnormalities of the lower limbs. Publish booklets for parents on talipes and congenital dislocation of the hip.

Contact: Sue Banton, General Secretary, 15 Statham Close, Lymm, Cheshire, WA13 9NN
(Tel: 0925 757525)

Stillbirth and Neonatal Death Association (SANDS)

A support group for families who have suffered bereavement by stillbirth or the death of a baby in the first few weeks after birth.

Contact: 15A Christchurch Hill, London, NW3 1JY
(Tel: 071 794 4601)

Twins And Multiple Births Associations (TAMBA)

Supports families with twins, triplets or more, both individually and through local Twins Clubs, and promotes public and professional awareness of their needs. Specialist sub-groups for parents of Super-twins; Twins with Special Needs; Single Parents; Bereavement Support Group for parents of multiples; small register of parents of Adopted twins. Health and Education Group offers consultancy service for parents, researchers and professionals and produces a range of leaflets, booklets and books.

Contact: TAMBA Secretary, 51 Thicknall Drive, Pedmore, Stourbridge, West Midlands, DY9 0YH (s.a.e. for reply)
(Tel: 0384 373642)

Also
TAMBA Bereavement Support Group
(Tel: 081 363 4743)

Voluntary Council for Handicapped Children (National Children's Bureau)

Offers a comprehensive information and advisory service covering all aspects of childhood disability for statutory and voluntary agencies and for parents. Promotes co-operation between the different voluntary and professional agencies concerned with handicapped children.

Contact: Philippa Russell, VCHC, 8 Wakley Street, London, EC1V 7QE
(Tel: 071 278 9441)

21

Nursing care of newborn infants

Nursing staff levels
Observation and monitoring
Minimal handling
Thermal care
Prevention of infection
Special care baby unit / neonatal intensive care unit nursing procedures

Maximum observation and minimal handling, together with the provision of an *appropriate thermal environment and protection from infection* are the most important aspects of nursing care of the small or sick newborn infant.

Nursing staff levels

See Chapter 5, page 51 and Chapter 29, page 387, for the recommended nursing staff levels for special and intensive care of the newborn.

Observation and monitoring
(see Chapter 4 and 5)

Routine observation of the newborn infant
(see chapter 4)

Should be careful but not obtrusive
Should *not* involve separation of mother and baby
Should aim to identify problems early
Should *decrease not increase* maternal anxiety

Check

Colour and general appearance
Activity (particularly any changes)
Temperature (axillary: on admission to ward and at 12 and 24 hours,
    and then as indicated)
Respiration and heart rate
    Recession?
    Distress?
Feeding difficulties? (avoid test weighing see Chapter 11)
    Vomiting? (bile-stained vomits are *never* normal; see Chapter 12)
Abdominal distension
Stools
    Frequency
    colour
    consistency
Urine
    Frequency
    Urinalysis (preterm, sick or asphyxiated infants)
    Specific gravity
Weight (avoid overemphasis on weight change)
Capillary blood sugar (e.g. Dextrostix, BM glycaemia stix)
    In infants at risk of hypoglycaemia (Chapter 13, page 192)
    After prolonged or difficult labour or delivery
    After cold stress or birth asphyxia
    In infants with feeding difficulties

Frequency of observations

This varies from baby to baby.

e.g. After uncomplicated normal delivery at term: observations
    twice daily for 48 hours, then daily;

    After instrumental or operative delivery at term: observations
    3–4 hourly for 24 hours, then as indicated.

Observation and monitoring of the high-risk infant
(see Chapter 5, page 51)

Skilled nursing observation is not replaced but enhanced by the use
    of electronic monitors.
Observations as for routine care, but *using monitors* to obtain
    information where appropriate.
Remember the importance of minimal handling.
Arrange routine procedures (e.g. washing or changing napkin) to
    allow regular periods without disturbance.

Minimal handling

Sick infants do not like being handled. Minor procedures may cause severe hypoxaemia. Keep disturbances and handling to a minimum. Keep noise levels as low as possible. Careful positioning of the infant is important to avoid pressure sores or obstruction of airway. Use of water pillows will minimize side-to-side flattening of the head.

Thermal care (see Chapter 5, page 52)

Prevention of infection

(a) Staff and visitors

Thorough handwashing is the single most important factor in prevention of cross-infection.

All persons should wash their hands and arms to the elbows before entering any of the nurseries.

Long sleeves should be rolled to the elbows prior to washing.

Watches, bracelets, rings other than simple wedding rings, should be first removed.

Hands should be considered contaminated unless they are washed just before and just after handling an infant or his/her equipment, and after touching contaminated material.

Most useful antiseptics: providone–iodine or chlorhexidine (e.g. Betadine or Hibiscrub).

After initial handwashing, hands may be disinfected before and after handling patients by the use of alcohol-based rub (e.g. Hibisol). If dirty, or contaminated with blood, urine or faeces the hands *must* be thoroughly washed as above.

Whilst handling an infant, care should be taken not to touch one's face, hair, nose, mouth. (A repeat handwash is necessary should this occur.)

Parents and staff with acute respiratory, gastric or wound infections or with herpes simplex infections should not be allowed in the nursery.

Individual gown technique to be observed if the baby is to be held out of cot or incubator.

Use individual stethoscope for each baby.

(b) Equipment

Incubators should be cleaned regularly and changed at least weekly.

Humidifier – water should be changed every 24 hours.

Ventilator or continuous positive airway pressure (CPAP) tubing changed regularly (every 24–48 hours).

Strict and thorough cleaning and *drying* of all equipment.

(c) Babies

Avoid prolonged umbilical catheterization or indwelling lines.

Keep sites of entry clean and dry – spray with povidone–iodine.

Treat cord stump regularly, using alcohol preparation and paying particular attention to base.

Skinfolds (axillae and groins) should be dusted daily with 0.3% hexachlorophane powder.

Isolate infant with known or suspected infection.

Admission swabs from ear, umbilicus, nose, plus gastric aspirate if maternal infection or prolonged rupture of membranes (see Chapter 14).

Weekly swabs from babies on special care baby unit (SCBU), from umbilicus, rectum, nose for culture (to monitor pattern of colonization within the unit).

(d) Infectious infant

Preferably isolate* in a single room.

Keep door closed.

Hang gowns in cubicle, with baby's side outermost.

Wash hands thoroughly on entry.

Don barrier gown – tying tapes.

Only essential equipment, linen etc., to be brought into the cubicle.

Use disposable feeding equipment etc.

Charts to remain inside cubicle.

Notes and X-rays to be left outside.

Wash hands thoroughly after removing gown, and immediately after leaving the cubicle.

Keep a container of alcohol rub (e.g. Hibisol) outside of the cubicle for use on leaving the cubicle.

Wash and disinfect equipment and instruments prior to, and after removing from the cubicle.

The nurse caring for the infant should have as few other assignments as possible.

Special care baby unit / neonatal intensive care unit nursing procedures

(a) Prepare equipment (before arrival of baby)

Incubator – switched on and at appropriate temperature (see Chapter 5, page 52)

---

*NB 'Barrier' nursing is frightening for parents. Ensure the need and nature of cross-infection precautions is carefully (and sympathetically) explained to them.

Air/oxygen/suction apparatus and ⎫ connected up with
   tubing   ⎬ appropriate settings
Humidifier   ⎪ (see Chapter 8)
Ventilator/CPAP circuit/headbox ⎭
Oxygen analyser
Monitors: ECG/respiration, TcPO_2, Temperature, BP
Resuscitation bag and mask
Intravenous/arterial cannulation and infusion equipment
Weighing scales – balanced and ready for use

(b) Admission of infant (transferred in transport incubator; see
   Chapter 7)
Assess general condition and rectify any urgent problems
Note time of admission and perinatal details
Weigh baby (in transit between transport incubator and ward
   incubator)
AVOID COLD STRESS
Connect to monitors ± ventilator or CPAP
Check:
   Head circumference (± length)
   Axillary temperature
   Heart rate
   Respiration rate
Give vitamin K_1, 0.5 mg, i.m. if not already given (i.v. if cannula
   in situ)
Check cord and clamp (leave 3–5 cm long)
Check capillary blood sugar (notify medical staff if <2 mmol/l)
Pass orogastric tube and aspirate stomach contents
Adjust incubator temperature (see Chapter 5, page 52)
Put bonnet and bootees on baby
Cover with heat shield, cling film or bubble plastic if <1500 g or if
   cold (axillary temperature <36° C)
Humidify incubator for infants <1500 g
Assist with cannula placement
Ensure baby is adequately labelled
Take polaroid photograph of baby for parents
WELCOME THE PARENTS – explain treatment, monitors, equip-
   ment, etc. Give them a booklet explaining the SCBU and photo-
   graph of their baby. Ensure parents are seen by medical staff
Complete notes, charts, record books, nursing care plan.

Care of the intubated baby

See Chapter 26, page 350 for the technique of intubation and tube
   fixation.

See Chapter 8, page 96 for ventilator settings and adjustment.
See Chapter 8, page 94 for management of baby on CPAP/IPPV.

Nursing care

Immediately
Ensure endotracheal tube (ETT) is secure
Cut spare ETT to length, attach connector and fixation flange and
    tape to the end of the incubator in packet
Nurse prone whenever possible

Hourly*
Check ETT is secure
Check and record ventilator settings
Check humidifier water level
Check airway temperature
Empty water from tubing
Ensure tubing connections are secure, tubing is not kinked and is not
    dragging on baby

3–4 hourly*
Aspirate gastric tube
Change baby's head position
Endotracheal suction (see below)
Listen to breath sounds on both sides of chest

Technique for endotracheal suctioning

Perform as a sterile technique (gloves and sterile catheter)
Do not leave ETT 'open' (i.e. without CPAP/IPPV) for more than a
    few seconds at a time
Use the smallest catheter that will adequately clear secretions
    (usually 5 or 6 FG)
Use Y suction control valve
Attach a piece of tape measure to the incubator, where it can be
    easily seen, with marks showing the distance from the lower end of
    the ETT to the top of the connector
Procedure (should take <10 sec in total).
Inject up to 0.5 ml 0.9% saline into ETT before suctioning if needed
    to loosen secretions (no more than 4 hourly)

* More frequently if indicated.

Hold suction catheter close to the tape measure showing the length of ETT and connector, add 1 cm

Insert catheter into ETT up to this point. If coughing withdraw 1 cm and suck out ETT by occluding side opening on Y valve using a rotating motion as catheter is withdrawn

If further suctioning is required, rest infant for 1 min, or until recovered, before repeating

Monitor heart rate (and $TcPO_2$) continuously during suction

Clear suction tubing using sterile water and discard catheter

Check breath sounds on both sides of chest after suction

Mouth and pharynx should be suctioned after trachea. Care should be taken not to apply suction to soft tissues or mucous membranes

Send specimens of secretions for culture and sensitivity regularly (2–3 times/week)

Change suction jars and tubing regularly

Tube feeding

See Chapter 11, page 166 for gastric feeding.
See Chapter 11, page 166 for transpyloric feeding.

22

Neonatal skin disorders

Common harmless eruptions
Vesiculobullous eruptions
Pustular disorders
Erythrodermas
Eruptions in the napkin area
Dermatitis

The appearance of the skin at birth is one of the features used to assess gestational age (Chapter 19). The epidermis and dermis of the full-term baby are similar in structure and function to the adult. In the preterm baby the epidermis is more permeable and the dermis is thinner with immature vasculature reflected in the readiness with which generalized hyperaemia, cutis marmorata (marbling) and harlequin colour change occur. Many congenital disorders and acquired diseases are recognized through skin changes.

Table 22.1 Common harmless eruptions

Condition	Clinical Features	Distribution	Pathology
Sebaceous gland hyperplasia	Yellow pinpoint papules	Face, areolae, genitalia	Maternal androgen
Milia	Firm white papules	Face, especially nose	Follicular keratin cysts
Miliaria	Crops of tiny vesicles and/or papules with red background	Head, neck, upper trunk, axillae, groin	Obstruction of sweat ducts Warmth and humidity
Toxic erythaema (erythema neonatorum)	Red macules or papules Occasionally pustules—occurs in first few days	Maximal on trunk Spares palms and soles	Unknown Pustules contain eosinophils

Vesiculobullous eruptions

Blistering occurs more readily in the neonate. Some of these disorders are potentially fatal so early diagnosis is essential. Specialized techniques such as electron microscopy and immunofluorescence may be required and should be discussed with the pathologist.

Condition	Clinical Features	Distribution	Pathology
Sucking blisters	Few blisters	Fingers, lips, forearms	–
Bullous impetigo	Blisters become cloudy	Can be anywhere	Gram stain, culture *Staph. aureus*
Scalded skin syndrome	Fever and malaise Generalized tender erythema with large flaccid bullae, shedding to leave raw area	Anywhere, mucous membranes spared	Gram stain and culture *Staph. aureus*. Histology of blister roof Superficial epidermis only
Epidermolysis bullosa	Depends on clinical/genetic type Blisters at sites of trauma heal with scars in the dystrophic types	Sites of trauma and friction Mucous membranes may be involved	Electron microscopy Immunofluorescence
Toxic epidermal necrolysis	Clinically similar to scalded skin syndrome May have drug aetiology	Anywhere Mucous membranes involved	Histology of blister roof – full thickness epidermis

Neonatal herpes virus infection	Blisters solitary or clustered but can be generalized and mimic epidermolysis bullosa	Anywhere	Electron microscopy Viral culture
Burns, irritants	History of exposure, trauma, use of skin cleansing agents, sticky tape, ECG electrodes etc.	Anywhere	History
Bullous insect bites	Lesions often grouped	Anywhere	Puncture marks evident Exposure feasible (fleas, scabies)
Incontinentia pigmenti	Usually female Linear pattern of blisters, evolve into verrucous lesions grey-brown pigmentation May have eye and CNS anomalies Dominant	Especially trunk and extremities	Eosinophils in vesicles
Epidermolytic hyperkeratosis	Erythroderma with bullae		Histology – vacuolization of upper epidermal cells
Acrodermatitis enteropathica	Blisters evolving into crusts and pustules Glossitis, stomatitis Diarrhoea	Hands, feet, face and genital area	Low serum zinc
Mastocytosis (a) Diffuse	Thickened yellowish skin readily blisters with trauma May have flushing, abdominal and respiratory symptoms	Anywhere	Histology – excess mast cells
(b) Urticaria pigmentosa	Multiple reddish lesions which blister when rubbed	Anywhere	Histology – excess mast cells
(c) Mastcytoma	One or a few nodules which may blister when rubbed	Anywhere	Histology – excess mast cells

Table 22.1 *continued*

Condition	Clinical Features	Distribution	Pathology
Pustular disorders Infection must always be considered. Most of the pustular dermatoses can be diagnosed by Gram and Giemsa stains, and a KOH preparation. Biopsy, bacterial and viral culture of pustule contents are also needed (see Chapter 14).			
Non-infectious disorders			
Pustular toxic	Red macules and papules becoming pustular Onset 24–72 hours old, lasts up to one week	Mainly on trunk	Smear – eosinophils
Pustular miliaria	See miliaria Often high temperature and humidity	Flexures and clothed sites	Histology – pustules in relation to sweat ducts
Acropustulosis of infancy	Itchy pustules Crops may continue for 2–3 years	Hands and feet	Giemsa – neutrophils in pustules
Neonatal pustular melanosis	Transient Mainly black Present at birth Pustules last a few days, followed by melanotic macules which may last for months	Chin, neck, palms, soles	Giemsa – neutrophils in pustules

Mild infections			
Candidiasis			
Congenital	Present at birth Macules, papules, pustules	Widespread	KOH preparation – pseudohyphae. Candida on culture
Neonatal	After first week Pustules at periphery of moist red area	Oral Napkin area	
Staphylococcal impetigo	Vesicles, bullae and pustules on erythematosus base	Anywhere	*Staph. aureus* on culture Gram positive cocci on smear
Scabies	Erythematous papules, vesicles and pustules Scabies in mother or other close contact	Widespread	Mites seen on microscopy of scraping
Severe infections			
Bacterial infections *Staph. aureus.* Group B streptocci, Pseudomonus *Haemophilus influenzae* etc.	Pustules with fever, signs of septicaemia, meningitis etc.	Widespread	Gram stain Positive culture from pustule ± Blood
Congenital syphilis	Vessiculopustular eruption ± Hepatosplenomegaly, chorioretinitis, periostitis Nasal discharge.	Involves palms, soles, face and genitalia	Smear – dark ground micro or direct immunofluorescence to show spirochaetes Serum: Fluorescent treponemal antibody – abs, antitreponemal IgM

Table 22.1 *continued*

Condition	Clinical Features	Distribution	Pathology
Viral infections			
Herpes simplex	Vesicles, often grouped, precede pustules Associated lethargy, irritability etc.	Widespread	Smear – electron microscopy, direct immunofluorescence or Giemsa
Varicella zoster	Chickenpox lesions Severe if acquired less than <5 days before or up to 3 days after delivery	Widespread	As herpes simplex
Cytomegalovirus	Variable rash, usually includes purpura and pustules ± Hepatosplenomegaly, chorioretinitis etc.	Widespread	Urine sediment – intranuclear inclusions Virus isolation from blood, urine, CSF
Candidiasis, disseminated	Like congenital candidiasis plus low birthweight, respiratory distress etc.		*Candida* cultures from blood, urine, CSF
Erythrodermas			
Harlequin fetus	Markedly thickened skin Ectropion Everted lips Hair and nails dysplastic or absent	Generalized	Clinical appearance

Collodion baby	Encased in shiny membrane Ectropion Everted lips Normal hair and nails Membrane shed in 2–12 weeks revealing underlying ichthyoses	Generalized	Clinical appearance
Ichthyoses	Various patterns of scaling with underlying erythema Associated skeletal and neurological disorders in some types	Generalized	Clinical appearance Histology Histochemistry
Seborrhoeic dermatitis	Red scaly patches No itch or impairment of general health	Maximal on scalp, face, intertriginous areas	Clinical appearance
Leiner's disease	Starts off like seborrhoeic dermatitis but becomes generalized with diarrhoea, failure to thrive and Gram negative bacterial and *Candida* infections	Generalized	Complement deficiencies
Psoriasis	Circumscribed red scaly plaques and patches May become pustular	Scalp, trunk, napkin area May become generalized	Histology
Pityriasis rubra pilaris	Follicular papules	Islands of spared skin Marked palmo plantar hyperkeratosis	Clinical appearance
Scalded skin syndrome	Rapidly spreading tender erythema May blister	Anywhere Crusting around mouth, eyes, umbilicus and perineum	*Staph. aureus* in swab from skin site and nose

Table 22.1 *continued*

Condition	Clinical Features	Distribution	Pathology
Drug eruption	Maculopapular erythema	Generalized	Drug exposure
Citrullinaemia	Red scaly skin with moist eroded patches and plaques	Particularly perioral and napkin area	Amino acid analysis in blood and urine
Biotin deficiency	Similar to zinc deficiency (see below)	Generalized	Biochemistry
	Infections, ataxia, hypotonia	Perioral dermatitis	Multiple carboxylase deficiency
			Organic aciduria
Eruptions in the napkin area			
Primary irritant napkin dermatitis	Erythema, erosions in severe cases, maximal on the convexities		Clinical appearance
Perianal dermatitis	Erythema limited to perianal skin		Clinical appearance
Intertrigo	Erythema only, in flexures	Mainly flexures	Clinical appearance
Seborrhoeic dermatitis	Erythema with greasy yellowish scaling	Also scalp, face, axillae	Clinical appearance
Psoriasis	Well-defined red scaly plaques	Often elsewhere, e.g. scalp, trunk	Clinical appearance
			May be family history
Candidiasis	Glazed erythema, raised scaly edge, outlying pustules	Mouth may be involved	*Candida* on culture
Miliaria rubra	Papules and vesicles		Cultures sterile
Bullous impetigo	Thin walled blisters, fluid often cloudy		*Staph. aureus* on culture

Herpes simplex	Clustered umbilicated vesicles, later ulcers	Viral smear and culture
Chronic bullous dermatosis of childhood	Bullae often in annular groups Spread beyond napkin area May occur on scalp, around mouth	Linear IgA on biopsy
Zinc deficiency	Glazed erythema with marginal peeling Perioral dermatitis Failure to thrive, diarrhoea, later alopecia	Low serum zinc
Congenital syphilis	Brownish red macules, papules occasionally bullae (see palms, soles and sometimes elsewhere) ± Hepatosplenomegaly, lymphadenopathy	Syphilis serology
Histiocytosis X	Papules, often purpuric Other sites include scalp, behind ears ± Hepatosplenomegaly	Histology

Dermatitis

Neonatal skin tends to produce an eczematous response to irritants, and such reactions are often short lived. The most common patterns of dermatitis are a seborrhoeic dermatitis, atopic dermatitis which usually begins outside the neonatal period and primary irritant napkin dermatitis. If a bleeding diathesis and evidence of susceptibility to certain infections, especially pneumococci, is present then the Wiskott Aldrich syndrome should be considered. Some other disorders described elsewhere in this chapter in which dermatitis can be a feature include zinc deficiency, Leiner's disease and histiocytotis X.

Bibliography

Maibach H. I. and Boisits E. K. (Eds) (1982). *Neonatal Skin*. New York: Marcel Dekker.
Rook A. J., Wilkinson D. S., Ebling F. J. G., Champion R. H. and Burton J. L. (1986). *Textbook of Dermatology*. Oxford: Blackwell Scientific Publ.

23

Ophthalmic disorders

Examination of the newborn eye
Squint
Conjunctivitis and ophthalmia neonatorum
Retinopathy of prematurity
Disorders of the external eye
Internal eye disorders
Abnormalities of globe size

Examination of the newborn eye

Examination of the eyes of newborn infants forms part of the routine examination (Chapter 4). Unless correctable abnormalities which interfere with the development of vision are detected early, permanent changes develop in the higher visual pathways which preclude good acuity later even if the original condition is successfully treated.

Most neonatal eye conditions are recognizable by simple inspection and testing for a red reflex, with pupillary dilatation and fundal examination with the direct ophthalmoscope if indicated. For detailed examination of the peripheral retina, indirect ophthalmoscopy with an aspheric condensing lens is necessary.

A family history is essential for the detection of inherited eye disorders. Routine examination should include assessment of visual function by observation of fixation and horizontal following of a face, large coloured object, or light. Any definite constant squint is abnormal. The examination should be conducted systematically, starting from the lids and progressing posteriorly to fundus and orbit.

Pupillary dilatation is achieved where necessary with one drop of homatropine (1%), to which one drop of phenylephrine (2.5%) can be added for additional effect. The dose may be repeated after 20 min if necessary.

Indications for direct ophthalmoscopy

Positive family history
Congenital infection
Other external ocular abnormalities

Indications for indirect ophthalmoscopy (usually by an ophthalmologist)

Retinopathy of prematurity suspected
Any fundal abnormality detected
Inability to see the fundus

Parents of children with any significant ocular condition should be counselled by an ophthalmologist and a paediatrician after definition of the lesion.

Squint

An occasional deviation of the visual axis up to the age of 6 months may not be abnormal. A definite diagnosis of squint requires the cover test to be performed accurately.

A constant squint is abnormal at any age and requires investigation by an ophthalmologist. Such a squint causes amblyopia which must be corrected as soon as possible to prevent permanent visual impairment. Fundal examination is mandatory to exclude serious pathology such as retinoblastoma.

Conjunctivitis and ophthalmia neonatorum

The signs of conjunctivitis are purulent discharge, conjunctival injection and lid oedema. The cornea should be bright and clear. If bacterial infection is acquired from the maternal genital tract, the signs are present from the first or second day ('ophthalmia neonatorum') and are usually bilateral. If due to failure of the nasolacrimal duct to open, signs are usually delayed for one week, and though usually bilateral, may be unilateral.

Conjunctivitis may be the result of early bacterial infection (gonococcus, now rare), perinatal infection with *Chlamydia trachomatis* (inclusion conjunctivitis presents after 3 days), later infection with environmental organisms, or occasionally chemical irritation from, for example, meconium. After discussion with the laboratory, conjunctival swabs should be taken for direct microscopy of a smear preparation (gonococcus – first 72 hours), and for a direct immunofluorescent test (*Chlamydia*), in addition to routine bacteriological swabs. *Chlamydia* should be sought even in the presence of gonococcal infection as the two may co-exist.

Suspected gonococcal ophthalmia requires urgent and intensive treatment (before the bacteriological results are available) with penicillin eye drops to avoid possible corneal perforation.

Every 5 min until the discharge ceases, then
Every 15 min for 1 hour, followed by
Every hour for 3 hours, and
Every 4 hours until sensitivities are available

Resistance to penicillin is not infrequent. Other options are tetracycline 1% drops, or a single i.m. injection of cefotaxime. Prophylactic silver nitrate drops are not current UK practice as the frequency of chemical irritation is higher than the frequency of infection.

Chlamydial conjunctivitis is treated with oily 1% tetracycline drops, 4 times a day for 1 month, combined with a full two-week course of oral erythromycin once the infecting agent is confirmed. Ineffective initial treatment of chlamydial conjunctivitis in the newborn may result in chronic subclinical infection with development of corneal neovascularization and scarring in later childhood. A full course of erythromycin is important in the prevention of later pneumonitis.

Infection by other bacteria is usually covered by the administration of 0.5% Neomycin eye ointment/drops, which has the advantage that subsequent cultures for *Chlamydia* are possible, unlike after treatment with chloramphenicol.

Nasolacrimal duct obstruction

This is due to non-pathogenic organisms pooling in the conjunctival sac, and should be treated conservatively with cleaning of the lids, use of antibiotic drops if there is much discharge, and instructions to the parents regarding massage of the lacrimal sac to attempt to open the lower end of the nasolacrimal duct. Only if this has been ineffective by the age of one year should probing of the nasolacrimal ducts be carried out under general anaesthetic.

Retinopathy of prematurity (ROP)

Aetiology

It is probably the result of retinal recovery after the exposure of an immature vascular system to high oxygen tensions. Retinopathy of prematurity particularly affects infants <28 weeks' gestation, and is rare after 32 weeks' gestation. No 'safe' upper limit for PaO_2 has been identified and there is much confusion as to the true aetiology, but traditionally PaO_2 should not be allowed to rise above 100 mm Hg, and perhaps 80 mm Hg for infants below 28 weeks.

Pathophysiology

Retinal vascularization begins at the optic disc from 14 weeks' gestation, progressing outwards to reach the peripheral retina (ora serrata) at term. The growth of retinal vessels is inhibited during this phase. Subsequently, the unvascularized ischaemic peripheral retina may release a vasoproliferative factor (similar to that postulated for proliferative diabetic retinopathy), to stimulate the growth of new vessels from the peripheral edge of the vascularized retina (the demarcation line). These vessels grow forward into the vitreous cavity, stimulate the growth of glial tissue, exert vitreoretinal traction, and thereby cause visual loss from vitreous haemorrhage, retinal distortion and detachment.

Detection

The retinae of all infants born before 32 weeks' gestation should be examined by an ophthalmologist using an indirect ophthalmoscope, starting when the infant reaches the postmenstrual age of 32 weeks (retinopathy does not show up earlier). This is repeated at two-week intervals until 39/40 weeks. No further examination is necessary if no signs have developed by then.

Grading

Stage 1   Flat demarcation line between pink normally vascularized posterior retina and white unvascularized ischaemic peripheral anterior retina.

Stage 2   Demarcation line raised into vitreous cavity.

Stage 3   New vessels elevated into vitreous cavity from raised demarcation line, with or without vitreous haemorrhage

Stage 4   Traction retinal detachment

'*Plus*' is added to each grading if there are dilated retinal vessels in the normal posterior retina and implies progressive disease.

Treatment

Stages 1 and 2 usually resolve spontaneously without sequelae. For Stage 3 ROP, cryotherapy to the ischaemic peripheral retina has been shown to be effective if performed early.

Prevention

Careful monitoring of PaO_2, with the avoidance of high and low levels is recommended. Despite many studies Vitamin E administration has *not* been shown to have a beneficial effect.

Disorders of the external eye

Lids

Coloboma: Gap in lid margin, usually upper and nasal; may lead to exposure keratitis and require surgical repair; associated with Goldenhaar's syndrome.

Cryptophthalmos: Unilateral or bilateral absence of a palpebral fissure and formed globe; no treatment.

Blepharophimosis: Fused lids, partially or completely, normal in very preterm infants (<26 weeks) in whom they open spontaneously; occasionally requires surgery.

Ptosis: Usually unilateral, may be associated with superior rectus muscle weakness, with Horner's syndrome, or may be mechanical due to a lid tumour. Congenital ptosis does not normally require further investigation for a systemic cause. It may require surgery later to avoid amblyopia or for cosmetic reasons.

Tumours

Dermoid cyst: Frequently has orbital component, usually outer part of upper lid; may need excision on cosmetic grounds later.

Capillary haemangioma: Increases in size in first year, spontaneous involution over up to 5 years in most cases. It may cause ptosis and subsequent amblyopia, otherwise best left untreated.

Orbit

Proptosis: Due to traumatic haemorrhage, orbital tumours (haemangioma and lymphangioma are the commonest in the first year), and with shallow orbits, as in craniostenosis, Crouzon's disease (craniofacial dysostosis), and hypertelorism.

Corneal opacities: *In all cases where there is significant corneal opacity, an ophthalmologist should be involved early as corneal grafting may be required to avoid gross amblyopia* (a difficult procedure at this age).

Birth trauma and congenital glaucoma: They may cause splits in Descemet's membrane which allows fluid to enter the cornea causing opacification.

Sclerocornea: A developmental abnormality causing partial or complete opacification. Opacities may be associated with the **anterior chamber cleavage syndrome** where there is incomplete formation of the structures bordering the anterior chamber – cornea, drainage angle, iris and lens.

Dermoid tumours: Tumours of the cornea can occupy a variable extent of the cornea from the limbus – their surface is irregular unlike sclerocornea.

Corneal ulceration: This is a rare cause of opacification. The most likely agent is the gonococcus or pseudomonas. Swabs and ulcer scrapings should be taken for culture and sensitivity as soon as possible. A broad-spectrum antibiotic should be given, before sensitivities are available, topically and by the subconjunctival route (involves a short general anaesthetic).

Metabolic causes: Such causes are very unusual at birth, perhaps because the absent enzyme crosses the placenta from the maternal circulation. Mucolipidosis Type IV does, however, cause opacification at birth.

Internal eye disorders

Iris

Aniridia: This is frequently autosomal dominant with significant later ocular problems. In sporadic cases it is associated with a chromosomal deletion and a high risk of later Wilms' tumour.

Coloboma: This may be autosomal dominant. It is due to failure of closure of the fetal fissure. Always inferior or infero-nasal, it may be associated with a choroidal coloboma, frequently bilateral, the extent of which determines the visual prognosis. No treatment.

Corectopia: An eccentric pupil, may be autosomal dominant, and sometimes associated with subluxation of the lens, otherwise carries a good visual prognosis.

Polycoria: Multiple pupils; is rare, and may sometimes represent partial aniridia; a good visual prognosis provided that there are no associated anterior segment abnormalities.

Anisocoria: Unequal pupils; may be a simple local abnormality with no systemic associations; may be part of congenital Horner's syndrome, or part of a third cranial nerve palsy. In most circumstances, intensive systemic investigation is not required and the visual prognosis is good.

Albinism: Generalized albinism (autosomal recessive) and ocular albinism (X-linked) caused by a lack of melanin pigment in the iris and retinal pigment epithelium, resulting in macula hypoplasia, poor acuity and nystagmus; due to defects in tyrosine metabolism.

Pupil

Leucocoria

An abnormal white reflex from the pupil and a serious prognostic sign. Causes listed are dealt with in the relevant sections:

Causes
Retinoblastoma
Cataract

Coloboma of the choroid
Persistent hyperplastic primary vitreous
Retinopathy of prematurity
Infection – toxoplasma, cytomegalovirus, herpes simplex
Norrie's disease and incontinentia pigmenti (Bloch–Sulzberger
   syndrome)

Lens

Cataract

Causes: Many syndromes include cataract as an occasional feature, reflecting the fact that cataract represents the final common path of many varied insults to the fetal and neonatal lens:

Isolated autosomal dominant and no other abnormality, rarely
   autosomal recessive or X-linked
Intrauterine infection, usually rubella
Metabolic disorders:
   Galactosaemia
   Hypoglycaemia
Chromosomal disorders:
   Trisomy 13, 18, 21
   Turner's syndrome
Associated with other ocular abnormalities:
   Microphthalmos
   Persistent hyperplastic primary vitreous
   Aniridia
   Coloboma of uveal tissue
   Mesodermal dysgenesis of the anterior chamber
Systemic syndromes (see Jones, 1988)

After general examination, investigations include chromosome analysis, intrauterine infection screen (toxoplasma, rubella, cytomegalovirus, herpes simplex), and urine chromatography for aminoaciduria.

Due to the great problems of anisometropic and stimulus deprivation amblyopia, the place of unilateral cataract surgery is still being evaluated. Bilateral congenital cataracts sufficient to obscure the fundus view should be treated at the earliest opportunity.

Vitreous

Persistent hyperplastic primary vitreous: Persistence of the fetal hyaloid vascular system that extends from the optic disc to the posterior lens surface, causing opacity on and behind the posterior lens capsule; immediate referral advised.

Retina

Retinopathy of prematurity (see separate section above)

Retinoblastoma

Pathophysiology: A malignant tumour of embryonic retinal tissue, appearing as a white mass arising from any part of the retina, posterior or peripheral, occasionally present at birth but usually presenting before 5 years. Those that present in the neonatal period are important in that they are often autosomal dominant and may be bilateral or multicentric. The remainder are spontaneous mutations, normally present later and are unilateral (because the mutation is somatic) and not usually inherited.

Presentation: After routine examination in the presence of a relevant family history, or the appearance of a white mass in the pupil (one cause of leukocoria), or squint due to visual loss – an important reason for early fundal examination of any child found to have a constant squint.

Management: Urgent ophthalmological referral is necessary if retinoblastoma is suspected. Children of parents with retinoblastoma must be followed up frequently by an ophthalmological department from birth.

Retinal haemorrhage

Usually due to birth trauma or asphyxia; dome-shaped (under the internal limiting membrane) or flame-shaped (in the nerve fibre layer). They disappear spontaneously, normally without visual sequelae.

Choroid

Albinism (see Iris)

Choroidal coloboma (see Iris)

Congenital toxoplasmosis: Fundal appearance of choroido-retinitis is of a white lesion due to destruction of the pigment epithelium, usually with surrounding pigment proliferation. It is normally inactive at the time of birth, but may cause blindness in the affected eye if the macula region is affected.

Abnormalities of globe size

Megalocornea

Megalocornea is a benign non-progressive condition with a corneal diameter greater than 13 mm. It is consistent with normal sight.

Keratoglobus

This is an X-linked disorder associated with Ehlers–Danlos syndrome with thinning and bulging of the cornea. All must be distinguished from congenital glaucoma causing progressive enlargement of the globe, which must be treated immediately. A small cornea is usually associated with a small globe, microphthalmos, often with multiple other intraocular abnormalities such as cataract and uveal coloboma.

Congenital glaucoma (buphthalmos)

Unilateral or bilateral, usually sporadic, sometimes autosomal recessive. May be associated with *systemic abnormalities* (Jones, 1988).

Signs

Corneal opacity
Watering eye
Enlargement of globe
Photophobia
Eye rubbing

Treatment

Requires urgent referral for glaucoma surgery, usually goniotomy, to prevent permanent visual loss and unsightly enlargement of the globe.

Microphthalmos

Associated with   Other ocular abnormalities
Intrauterine infections
Many syndromes (Jones, 1988)

Bibliography

An International Classification of Retinopathy of Prematurity (1984). The Committee for the Classification of Retinopathy of Prematurity. *Arch. Ophthalmol.*, **102**, 1130–4.

Fielder, A. R., Ng, Y. K. and Levene, M. I. (1986). Retinopathy of prematurity: age at onset. *Arch. Dis. Child.*, **61**, 774–8.

Jones, K. L. (1988). *Smith's Recognisable Patterns of Human Malformation*, 4th edn. Philadelphia: W. B. Saunders.

Lepage, P., Bogaerts, J., Kestelyn, P. and Meheus, A. (1988). Single dose cefotaxime intramuscularly cures gonococcal ophthalmia neonatorum. *Br. J. Ophthalmol.*, **72**, 518–20.

Lucey, J. F. and Dangman, B. (1984). A re-examination of the role of oxygen in retrolental fibroplasia. *Pediatrics*, **73**, 82–96.

Ng, Y. K., Fielder, A. R. and Levene, M. I. (1987). Retinopathy of prematurity in the UK. *Eye*, **1**, 386–90.

24

Clinical genetics in the neonatal period

Diagnosis in the malformed or dysmorphic infant, stillbirth or fetus
Inheritance patterns and recurrence risks
Availability of genetic tests in specific disorders
Prediction of inherited disease in the newborn
Genetic counselling
Other family members at risk
Collection and storage of specimens

Diagnosis in the malformed or dysmorphic infant, stillbirth or fetus

An infant, fetus or stillbirth may appear dysmorphic because of:

(a) **Malformation:** due to a developmental planning problem, often genetic, e.g. polydactyly, craniostenosis, congenital heart disease.

(b) **Deformation:** due to abnormal intrauterine forces on a normal baby, e.g. talipes in oligohydramnios, or due to normal forces on an abnormal baby, e.g. arthrogryposis in congenital spinal muscular atrophy.

(c) **Disruption:** due to interruption or destruction of a normal developmental sequence, e.g. amniotic bands.

Diagnosis is usually made from:

(a) 'Gestalt:' the overall appearance of the infant matched by the observer's past experience.

(b) 'Good handles:' definite dysmorphic features, (e.g. coloboma, mid-line cleft lip, polydactyly, imperforate anus) provide a differential diagnosis.

(c) **Measurements** to recognize if quantitative traits are outside limits of normality, e.g. eye spacing, head circumference.

(d) **Minor congenital anomalies** (e.g. ear lobe creases) can provide confirmatory features. Multiple minor anomalies may be an indicator of a major internal structural anomaly.

(e) **X-rays** are essential for diagnosis of skeletal dysplasia. Also, in dysmorphic infants, the spine and long bone epiphyses and metaphyses often show additional dysmorphic features (e.g. epiphyseal stipping) which can assist in diagnosis.

(f) **Photographs** are invaluable as a record for comparison with literature reports, for consultation with colleagues and for education.

(g) **Chromosomes:** the majority of infants with chromosomal abnormalities (apart from some sex chromosome aneuploidies) are dysmorphic, and often have multiple malformations. Any infant with a definite malformation, and showing other significant dysmorphism, should be karyotyped. Some chromosome abnormalities (e.g. 12p tetrasomy in Pallister–Killian syndrome) are only ever seen as mosaics, demonstration of which may require skin biopsy for fibroblast culture rather than peripheral blood leukocyte cultures.

(h) **Metabolic investigations:** e.g. in suspected peroxisomal disorders.

(i) **Review at a later age:** it may be easier to recognize a particular syndrome diagnosis in a young child than in a newborn infant.

(j) **Comparison with parents and siblings** may give clues to a dominantly inherited condition (e.g. myotonic dystrophy). Some minor dysmorphic features may be normal familial variants.

A specific syndrome diagnosis dictates prognosis, inheritance and management; a diagnostic label should be applied only if it is certain. Diagnosis in dysmorphology is assisted by:

(a) **Reference texts**

(b) **Computerized databases:** these can provide differential diagnoses for combinations of 'good handles', plus syndrome reviews and references.

(c) **Access to relevant past medical literature:** e.g. *American Journal of Medicine, Genetics, Journal of Medical Genetics, Clinical Genetics*.

(d) **Discussion with colleagues:** photographs are essential.

Table 24.1 Inheritance patterns of some conditions with neonatal presentation

Those for which chromosomal regional localization is known and for which closely linked DNA probes can be used for prediction in a family are indicated (*), together with the gene location.

Autosomal dominant
    Achondroplasia
    Crouzon's syndrome
    Marfan's syndrome
    Myotonic dystrophy (*) 19q13
    Neurofibromatosis I (*) 17q11
    Osteogenesis imperfecta I (*) 7q21/17q21
    Retinoblastoma (*) 13q14
    Tuberose sclerosis 9q or 11q

Autosomal recessive
    Cystic fibrosis (*) 7q31
    Congenital adrenal hyperplasia (*) 6p21
    Galactosaemia 9p13
    Infantile polycystic kidney disease
    Jeune's syndrome
    Joubert's syndrome
    Osteogenesis imperfecta IIC
    Osteopetrosis
    Phenylketonuria (*) 12q22
    Roberts' syndrome
    Spinal muscular atrophy I
    Zellweger's syndrome 7q11

Inheritance patterns and recurrence risks

Possible patterns of inheritance are:

(a) Autosomal dominant
(b) Autosomal recessive
(c) X-linked recessive
(d) X-linked dominant
(e) Multifactorial
(f) Chromosomal
(g) Mitochondrial and other extranuclear
(h) Non-genetic

Some common examples of each are given in Table 24.1.

X-linked recessive
Anhydrotic ectodermal dysplasia (*) Xq12
Coffin Lowry syndrome Xp22
Congenital adrenal hypoplasia Xp21
Duchenne muscular dystrophy (*) Xp21
Glucose 6-phosphate dehydrogenase (G6PD) deficiency (*) Xq28
Lesch Nyhan disease (*) Xq26
Lowe's syndrome (*) Xq25
Menke's disease Xq1
Myotubular myopathy (*) Xq27
Norrie disease (*) Xp11

X-linked dominant
Goltz syndrome
Incontinentia pigmenti Xq27
Oral facial digital syndrome I

Multifactorial
Neural tube defects
Congenital heart disease
Hirschsprung's disease
Oesophageal atresia Tracheo-oesophageal fistula (TOF)

Mitochondrial
Kearns Sayre syndrome

Sporadic
VATER association
MURCS association
CHARGE association
Williams syndrome

(a) Autosomal dominant inheritance
Fault in one copy of particular autosomal gene pair
Fifty per cent risk to offspring
Expression may be variable, even within a family
Asymptomatic carriers may occur (non-penetrance)

In an apparently isolated case consider:

New mutation (possibly with raised paternal age)
Parental non-penetrance
Parental germinal mosaicism
Non-paternity
Recurrence risk rarely less than 1%

(b) Autosomal recessive inheritance

Fault in both copies of an autosomal gene pair (one for each parent)

Twenty-five per cent risk to future full siblings

Two-thirds of unaffected siblings are carriers

Consanguinity more likely in rare conditions

Low risk to offspring of affected subject unless partner is related or mutant gene is endemic in population (e.g. sickle cell Hb)

(c) X-linked recessive inheritance

Faulty recessive gene on X-chromosome

Males affected, connected through female line

Two-thirds or more mothers of isolated cases will be carriers (consider also germinal mosaicism)

Fifty per cent risk in sons of carrier females, 50% risk in daughters of being carriers

No risk to sons of affected males, all daughters are obligate carriers

Females can occasionally be affected through:

XO karyotype

Homozygosity for mutant gene

Uneven X-chromosome inactivation in carrier (especially in monozygous twins)

X-autosome translocation with breakpoint through the gene and inactivation of normal X

(d) X-linked dominant inheritance

Rare

Usually considered lethal to affected XY males

Therefore usually only females affected

Fifty per cent risk to daughters of affected female

(e) Multifactorial inheritance

Involves several genes, or genetic susceptibility to environmental triggers

Recurrence risk typically 3–5% in first degree relatives, 1% in second degree relatives

Higher recurrence risk if index case is less commonly affected sex or if the index is more severely affected

(f) Chromosomal inheritance

Autosomal simple trisomies (e.g. t21, t18, t13) not due to translocations, and sex chromosome aneuploidies (i.e. XO, XXY, XXX, YY) are invariably sporadic; parental chromosome analysis is not indicated. For these:

Incidence is related to maternal age (see Table 24.2)

Table 24.2 Birth incidence of chromosomal anomalies by maternal age

Maternal age (years)	t21	t18*	t13*	XO	All chromosome anomalies
20	1/1500				
25	1/1350				
30	1/900				
35	1/380	1/2000	1/5000		
38	1/190	1/700	1/2000		
40	1/110	1/360	1/900		
42	1/65	1/180	1/480		
44	1/40				
All ages	1/650	1/8000	1/14000	1/2500 females	1/150

* Amniocentesis data.

Recurrence risk is usually around 1%, or is double the age-dependent risk if greater

Unbalanced chromosome abnormalities may arise *de novo* or from a balanced rearrangement in one of the parents, which could be familial, necessitating study of the wider family. High-resolution banding may detect small contiguous gene deletions which have now been identified in some cases of previously recognized syndromes (Table 24.3).

(g) Mitochondrial inheritance

Since mitochondria are self-replicating organelles with their own DNA, and are present in the cytoplasm of the oocyte, mitochondrially inherited conditions show matrolineal inheritance with a high proportion of affected offspring from an affected female.

Any of these inheritance patterns could result in an apparently isolated case; clues to increased likelihood of a particular pattern may be:

Multiple congenital abnormality	Chromosomal
Male affected	X-linked recessive
Consanguinity	Autosomal recessive
Recurrent miscarriage	Chromosomal
Raised paternal age	New dominant mutation
Raised maternal age	Chromosomal
'Striped' pigmentation in female	X-linked dominant or chromosome mosaic

Table 24.3   Chromosomal location of some microdeletion syndromes

Location	Syndrome
7p13	Greig's syndrome (Cephalopolysyndactyly)
8q24	Langer Giedion syndrome
11p13	WAGR (Wilms tumour/aniridia/genitourinary/renal) syndrome
13q14	Retinoblastoma/retardation/esterase D deficiency
15q11	Angelman's (happy puppet) syndrome
17p13	Miller Dieker (lissencephaly) syndrome
20p11	Alagille Watson syndrome
22q11	Di George sequence
Xp22	Ichthyosis/chondrodysplasia punctata/Kallmann syndrome
Xp21	Duchenne muscular dystrophy/adrenal hypoplasia etc.
Xq21	Choroideraemia and deafness with stapes fixation

Availability of genetic tests in specific disorders

Following the mapping of the gene for a disorder to a specific chromosomal regional location, molecular genetic (DNA) tests can now be offered in several genetic conditions for predictive tracking of the disease gene through families, including for carrier detection and prenatal diagnosis (Table 24.1). Direct DNA probes which recognize gene deletions or specific mutations can also confirm a diagnosis in syndromes where submicroscopic deletion of continuous genes, or inheritance of both faulty copies of a gene from one parent (uniparental disomy), can be the cause (Table 24.3).

All molecular genetic studies rely on a stored DNA sample from one or more affected members of a family. Consider collecting blood sample (or other tissue) for DNA extraction from all infants, still-births or fetuses which have serious single gene disorders, especially if expectation of survival is low.

Prediction of inherited disease in the newborn

Testing of infants at risk of genetic conditions is important if treatment is available (e.g. phenylketonuria (PKU), hypothyroidism, galactosaemia), and if not, can be helpful if this may relieve parental anxiety through resolution of uncertainty (e.g. by creatine kinase assay in Duchenne muscular dystrophy (DMD).

Genetic counselling

Genetic counselling is the discussion with patients of diagnosis, prognosis, inheritance and recurrence risk; often in relation to the possibility of predictive testing both pre- and postnatally for genetic disorders. Counselling is invariably non-directive; the purpose usually being to enable and help people to take individual, but informed reproductive decisions. The three principal components of genetic counselling are:

(a) **Accuracy of diagnosis**
    This is fundamental to the offer of predictive genetic tests and genetic advice from isolated cases.
(b) **Assessment of inheritance pattern**
    This may assist in making an accurate diagnosis, or may be determined by the diagnosis. For families with single or few cases (e.g. two affected brothers) there may be alternatives for mode of inheritance.
(c) **Individual circumstances and attitudes of the consultant**
    The genetic counsellor should help patients to find decisions which are right for them and should help provide support, whatever decisions are taken. Reproductive decisions may depend on parents' assessment of risk as determined by:

    (i) Chance of recurrence (high, low or negligible)
    (ii) Seriousness of the condition (quality of life, survival, and degree of burden to parents, family or society)

Other family members at risk

Following identification of an index case with a serious genetic disorder, clinicians have a responsibility to identify, inform and counsel other relatives who may be at risk. This is of particular importance in X-linked, autosomal dominant and familial chromosomal disorders, and in families with multiple consanguinity at-risk of recessive disorders.

Collection and storage of samples

Chromosomal analysis

2–5 ml blood in lithium heparin
Remove mixing beads to prevent cell adherence
Send directly to the laboratory (store at 4°C if delayed 24–48 hours)

DNA analysis

5 ml blood in EDTA (10–20 ml from adults)
Samples will keep 24 hours at room temperature or 5 days at 4°C
Extracted DNA will store at −7°C for many years
Fresh (same day) samples may occasionally be required
Amplification of DNA by polymerase chain reaction may allow
   analysis from minute quantities of tissue or blood

Skin biopsy

If blood is not available, if chromosome mosaicism is suspected, or if
certain molecular research or metabolic studies can be anticipated, a
skin biopsy should be considered for establishing fibroblast cultures.
This will also usually grow if taken up to 3 days post-mortem, and
should certainly be taken for chromosome analysis from all stillbirths
or fetuses with multiple malformations.

**The storing of blood or tissue specimens as above should be considered
from all fetuses, stillbirths or infants that may have genetically
based congenital anomalies or other genetic conditions, and whose
expectation of survival is low.**

Bibliography

Harper, P. S. (1989). *Practical Genetic Counselling*, 3rd edn.
   Bristol: John Wright.
Harper, P. S., Frézal, J., Ferguson-Smith, MA *et al.* (1989). Human
   Gene Mapping 10: Report of the committee on clinical disorders
   and chromosomal deletion syndromes. *Cytogenet. Cell Genet.*,
   51, 563–611.
Kingston, H. M. (1989). *ABC of Clinical Genetics*. London: British
   Medical Association.
McKusick V. A. (1988). *Mendelian Inheritance in Man*, 8th edn.
   Baltimore: Johns Hopkins.
Jones, K. L. (1988). *Smith's Recognisable Patterns of Human
   Malformation*, 4th edn. Philadelphia: W. B. Saunders.

Computer databases

Winter, R. and Baraitser, M. (1989). *London Dysmorphology
   Database*. London: Great Ormond Street Hospital.
Bankier, A. (1989). P.O.S.S.U.M. Video disk computerised
   database. Melbourne: Murdoch Institute.

25

Perinatal pathology

The purpose of perinatal post-mortem examination
Consent for post-mortem examination
Requirements for optimal post-mortem examination
Special post-mortems
After the post-mortem examination
Clinicopathological classification of perinatal deaths
Organ weights and footlength charts

The purpose of perinatal post-mortem examination

The perinatal post-mortem seeks to explain why a baby died, and predict risks for future pregnancies. It is both a restrospective and a prospective examination and differs fundamentally from adult necropsy. The objectives of the examination are:

(1) To determine the cause of death
In perinatal medicine there is often no single cause of death, but a sequence of causes starting in pregnancy and compounded by events in parturition and the neonatal period. One quarter to a third of neonatal deaths are due to withdrawal of intensive care. Although necropsy may sometimes reveal a clear 'cause of death' unsuspected in life, expectation of this in every case leads to a falsely low impression of the value of the examination.

(2) To provide information about growth, maturity, mode and time of death
With stillbirths the pathologist will be able to tell whether pregnancy had been proceeding normally until the point of death, or whether intrauterine growth was impaired. It may be possible to determine the mode of death (e.g. sudden and asphyxial or prolonged and

associated with uteroplacental vascular insufficiency) and the approximate time of death (e.g. before the mother entered the hospital, before the onset of labour, during labour). Among neonatals deaths the pathologist's estimate of maturity may give valuable retrospective support to a difficult clinical decision not to offer intensive care to a very immature neonate.

(3) To detect diseases with implications for future pregnancies
This may involve further delineation of conditions recognized in life (e.g. histological demonstration that cystic kidneys were of the autosomal recessive infantile type) or discovery of unsuspected diseases which did not cause the baby's death (e.g. an incidental finding of microscopic evidence of cystic fibrosis).

The post-mortem examination is an opportunity to collect samples for DNA analysis from abnormal babies in case an antenatal diagnostic test becomes available in the future. DNA can be extracted from spleen, or more expensively from fibroblast cultures.

(4) To monitor iatrogenic disease
All medical treatment may have unwanted effects. In the perinatal period these may result from obstetric procedures, obtaining vascular access, maintaining oxygenation and intravenous alimentation.

(5) Teaching, research and epidemiology

(6) Psychosocial
To some parents the post-mortem is helpful in accepting the fact of their child's death. It is an opportunity to provide momentos (photographs, locks of hair, handprints, identity bracelets etc.) Investigation by an uninvolved third party may resolve parental and professional doubts about what might or might not have been done, and restore a doctor–parent relationship strained by the baby's death.

(7) Medicolegal
A properly performed perinatal post-mortem is the best protection against ill-informed litigation.

(8) To provide a basis for counselling parents
This is the single most important purpose of the examination and may draw on any of the above. Parents get much reassurance from the documentation of *normality* which may acquire fresh significance in the light of subsequent abnormal pregnancies.

There is no such thing as a perinatal post-mortem which doesn't show anything. It is unacceptable not to offer a post-mortem because you think you know the causes of death (Table 25.1).

Consent for post-mortem examination

Every parent of a child who has died has the right to be offered a post-mortem examination and it is equally their right in most cases to refuse.

Table 25.1 Agreement between clinical diagnoses and diagnoses after post-mortem examination in a series of 300 perinatal necropsies

Clinical versus pathological diagnosis	Stillbirths (%) (n = 150)	Neonatal deaths (%) (n = 150)
Agree	40	19
Agree, but additional information* from post-mortem	34	66
Clinical diagnosis incorrect	26	15

From Porter and Keeling (1987), *J. Clin. Pathol.*, **40**, 180–4.
* Additional information = information important for counselling parents or care of babies in the future.

Consent for necropsy is required for all liveborn infants regardless of gestational age except in cases referred to the Coroner when he will usually order a post-mortem to be carried out. The rules for referral are the same as for adults (Table 25.2). Consent for a hospital post-mortem is usually recorded on a form provided by the Health Authority; although written consent is not required by law it is a wise precaution. Verbal consent (e.g. by telephone) should be given to two witnesses who must record it in the clinical notes.

Consent is most likely to be obtained if the purpose and benefits of post-mortem examination are sympathetically explained to the parents by the most senior doctor they know well, and who knew their child. They can be reassured that the post-mortem will not delay the funeral, and that although the examination involves incisions the baby will not be disfigured, and can be seen and held by them

Table 25.2 Some circumstances in which deaths must be reported to H. M. Coroner. (The list is not exhaustive, and if in doubt you should discuss a case with the Coroner or his Officer.)

(1) Dead on arrival in hospital or within 24 hours of admission
(2) Unattended stillbirths*
(3) Deaths within 24 hours of an operation, anaesthetic or invasive procedure
(4) Deaths as a result of accident
(5) Unnatural, criminal or suspicious deaths, e.g. neglect, child abuse or poisoning
(6) Deaths as a result of drugs, whether prescribed or not
(7) Deaths as a result of medical or surgical mishap (the doctor should also inform his defence organization)
(8) Deaths in which the doctor is so uncertain of the disease leading to death as to be unable to sign a death certificate.

* The Coroner is not responsible for stillbirths, but in unattended births he must establish that the child was in fact stillborn.

REQUEST FOR POSTMORTEM EXAMINATION

OF ALL FETUSES, STILLBIRTHS AND PERINATAL DEATHS

(All the relevant sections should be completed)

BABY   MOTHER

Name   Name

Registration No.   Registration No.

D.o.b: D.o.b:

Date of Death

Consultant   Consultant

PREVIOUS PREGNANCIES

	Date	Pregnancy	Labour	Puerperium	Sex	Outcome
1						
2						
3						
4						

PRESENT PREGNANCY

LMP   / /   , EDD   / /   , Blood Group ...... Rh ....

Amniocentesis   Yes/No   (Result ....)
Ultrasound Scan   Yes/No   (Result ....)
Threatened Abortion   Yes/No
APH   Yes/No

Hydramnios/Oigohydramnios   Yes/No
Hypertension   Yes/No
PET   Yes/No
Maternal Pyrexia   Yes/No
I.U.G.R.   Yes/No

LABOUR

Spontaneous/Induced (Medical/Surgical)/Accelerated

                    Why ....

Liquor Amount .... Colour ....
Duration of 1st stage .... 2nd stage ....
Fetal distress   Yes/No
Presentation: Vertex/Breech/other

Fig. 25.1

Forceps/Caesarian/other ....
Fetal distress   Yes/No ....
Delivery at .... hr .... min on   / /
Died at   .... hr .... min on   / /

NEONATAL

Birth Weight .... g   Gestation .... wks
Apgar Score .... at 1 min .... at 5 mins.
Resuscitation nil/mucus extraction/O_2 mask/intubation

Neonatal Problems   ### Neonatal Procedures

1 ....   1 ....
2 ....   2 ....
3 ....   3 ....
4 ....   4 ....
5 ....   5 ....

Suspected Causes of Death

1 ....
2 ....
3 ....
4 ....

Any special points of interest to be looked for?

Consent for autopsy examination has been obtained and is supplied with this
request form.
Notes to be suplied if possible

Signature of doctor requesting P.M. ....
Please also print if illegible   ....
Bleep No.   ....

Deliver to Department of Pathology, (Tel ....)

afterwards (exceptions are second trimester fetuses and very macerated stillborn babies).

Some parents may decline a full examination. Key clinical questions can often be answered by a limited post-mortem, e.g. excluding examination of the brain, or limited to the body cavity or organ in question. Even needle biopsies may be helpful. Restrictions must be prominently stated on the consent form.

Views of religious groups should be respected. Sikhs usually have no religious objection to post-mortem examinations, but it is not approved of by strict Hindus or Moslems.

A baby should not be referred to the Coroner as a second line when consent is refused by the parents.

Requirements for optimal post-mortem examinations

The pathologist will require:

(1) A clear history
This is most easily provided in a standard request form (Fig. 25.1) supplemented by the mother's and baby's notes. The junior doctor should remember that he is requesting a consultant opinion.
(2) The placenta
Almost all neonatal deaths follow an abnormal pregnancy or delivery, and every maternity hospital should have a system for collecting all these placentas for the pathologist in case the baby dies.
(3) The baby
Ideally the baby should be sent straight to the mortuary with all tubes still in place. Except in Coroner's cases where this rule is absolute, there is room for compromise between the pathologist's needs and those of the parents, e.g. by tying and cutting off tubes close to the skin.

If there is likely to be a delay before the post-mortem is carried out (or there is no enthusiastic perinatal pathologist!) then the paediatrician should consider doing the following himself if indicated:

Blood culture (from the sagittal sinus)
CSF culture (from the cisterna magna)
Samples for virology (e.g. needle biopsy of liver)
Chromosomes (skin biopsy or tissue from the fetal aspect of the placenta if the baby is at all macerated)
Photographs (any external anomalies)
X-rays (essential in skeletal dystophies. Gas emboli disappear from vessels within 12 hours of death)

In any case the paediatric team should be informed of the time of the examination and attend to give clinical details, ensure that essential questions are answered, and educate and encourage the pathologist.

Special post-mortems

Immediate post-mortem sampling is required when an inborn error of metabolism is suspected. This should be anticipated by obtaining consent before the child's death, warning the pathologist and discussing the samples required with an experienced paediatric chemical pathologist. The tests used are changing rapidly, but if expert advice is not available, then the following samples should suffice:

(1) Unexplained metabolic acidosis or hyperammonaemia etc.: Blood (plasma or serum)

CSF
Urine
Liver
Kidney   } Samples snap frozen at −80°C
Skeletal muscle
Myocardium
Spleen
Culture and save skin fibroblasts

NB   Arrange to save all samples taken in life including blood films)

(2) Suspected storage disorder. In addition to the above:

Liver
Kidney
Skeletal muscle   } In glutaraldehyde
Myocardium   for electronmicroscopy
Spleen

If the storage disorder (or a demyelinating disorder) affects the central nervous system, then a frontal pole of the brain should be frozen and pieces of rectum saved frozen and in glutaraldehyde.

These lists are no substitute for expert advice which will considerably reduce the number of samples required.

A full post-mortem examination with microbiology and histology must then be carried out at leisure, as in many of these cases the metabolic abnormalities are secondary to some other disorder such as infection or congenital heart disease.

Table 25.3   A clinicopathological classification of perinatal deaths (Wigglesworth, 1980). The five categories may be further broken down by birthweight or gestational age

(1) Normally formed macerated stillbirth
(2) Congenital malformation
(3) Conditions associated with immaturity
(4) Asphyxial conditions developing during labour
(5) Specific conditions other than the above

After the post-mortem examination

A provisional report should be available within a few days and a final report within six weeks. The report may be shown to the parents, but the pathologist's consent should be obtained before they are given a copy. Coroner's reports are confidential to him and should not be disclosed to a third party without his consent. However, parents are entitled to a copy from the Coroner, and in practice he usually allows the pathologist discretion to give a copy to the paediatrician concerned.

The post-mortem report must be available for the monthly perinatal mortality meeting held in all good units, and is essential for accurate clinicopathological classification of the death. The classification of Wigglesworth (1980) is widely used because it draws attention to particular aspects of patient care (Table 25.3).

Bibliography

Becker, M. J. and Becker, A. E. (1989). *Pathology of Late Fetal Stillbirth*. Edinburgh: Churchill Livingstone.

Grunewald, P. and Minh, H. N. (1960). Evaluation of body and organ weights in perinatal pathology 1. Normal standards derived from autopsies. *Amer. J. Clin. Pathol.*, **34**, 247–53.

Keeling, J. W. (1987). *Fetal and Neonatal Pathology*. London: Springer-Verlag.

Keeling, J. W., MacGillivray, I., Golding, J. *et al.* (1989). Classification of perinatal death. *Arch. Dis. Child.*, **64**, 1345–51.

Macpherson, T. A., Valdes-Dapena, M. and Kanbour, A. (1986). Perinatal mortality and morbidity; The role of the anatomical pathologist. *Sem. Perinatol.*, **10**, 179–86.

Porter, H. J. and Keeling, J. W. (1987). Value of perinatal necropsy examination. *J. Clin. Pathol.*, **40**, 180–4.

Streeter, G. L. (1921). Weight, sitting height, head size, foot length and menstrual age of the human embryo. *Contributions to Embryology*, Carnegie Institute, **55**, 143–70.

Wigglesworth, J. S. (1980). Monitoring perinatal mortality: a pathophysiological approach. *Lancet*, **ii**, 684–6.

Wigglesworth, J. S. (1984). Perinatal pathology. *Major Problems in Pathology*, Number 15. Philadelphia: W. B. Saunders.

Winter, R. W., Knowles, S.A.S., Bieber, F. R. and Baraitser, M. (1988). *The Malformed Fetus and Stillbirth. A Diagnostic Approach*. Chichester: John Wiley.

Table 25.4   Footlength of the fetus (modified from Streeter 1921)

End of week	Mean footlength (mm)	Minimum footlength (mm)	Maximum footlength (mm)
14	14.0	12.5	15.5
15	16.8	15.2	18.5
16	19.9	18.2	21.6
17	23.0	21.0	25.0
18	26.8	24.8	28.8
19	30.7	28.5	33.0
20	33.3	31.0	35.7
21	35.2	32.5	38.0
22	39.5	36.0	43.0
23	42.2	39.0	45.5
24	45.2	42.0	48.5
25	47.7	44.5	51.0
26	50.2	47.0	53.5
27	52.7	49.0	56.5
28	55.2	51.5	59.0
29	57.0	53.0	61.0
30	59.2	55.5	63.0
31	61.2	57.5	65.0
32	63.0	59.0	67.0
33	65.0	61.0	69.0
34	68.2	64.0	72.5
35	70.5	66.0	75.0
36	73.5	69.0	78.0
37	76.5	72.0	81.0
38	78.5	74.0	83.0
39	81.0	76.0	86.0
40	82.5	77.5	87.5

Table 25.5 Organ weights of newborn infants by body weight

Body weight (g)	Number of cases	Body length (cm)	Heart (g)	Lungs combined (g)	Spleen (g)	Liver (g)	Adrenal glands, combined (g)	Kidneys, combined (g)	Thymus (g)	Brain (g)	Gestational age Weeks	Gestational age Days
500	317	29.4	5.0	12	1.3	26	2.6	5.4	2.2	70	23	5
		±2.5	±1.6	±5	±0.8	±10	±1.7	±2.1	±0.8	±18	±2	3
750	311	32.9	6.3	19	2.0	39	3.2	7.8	2.8	107	26	0
		±3.0	±1.8	±6	±1.2	±12	±1.5	±2.6	±1.3	±27	±2	6
1000	295	35.6	7.7	24	2.6	47	3.5	10.4	3.7	143	27	5
		±3.1	±2.0	±8	±1.5	±12	±1.6	±3.4	±2.0	±34	±3	1
1250	217	38.4	9.6	30	3.4	56	4.0	12.9	4.9	174	29	0
		±3.0	±3.3	±9	±1.8	±21	±1.7	±3.9	±2.1	±38	±3	0
1500	167	41.0	11.5	34	4.3	65	4.5	14.9	6.1	219	31	3
		±2.7	±3.3	±11	±2.0	±18	±1.8	±4.2	±2.7	±52	±2	3
1750	148	42.6	12.8	40	5.0	74	5.3	17.4	6.8	247	32	4
		±3.1	±3.2	±13	±2.5	±20	±2.0	±4.7	±3.0	±51	±2	6
2000	140	44.9	14.9	44	6.0	82	5.3	18.8	7.9	281	34	6
		±2.8	±4.2	±13	±2.7	±23	±2.0	±5.0	±3.4	±56	±3	2
2250	124	46.3	16.0	48	7.0	88	6.0	20.2	8.2	308	36	4
		±2.9	±4.3	±15	±3.3	±24	±2.3	±4.9	±3.4	±49	±3	0
2500	120	47.3	17.7	48	8.5	105	7.1	22.6	8.3	339	38	0
		±2.3	±4.2	±14	±3.5	±21	±2.8	±5.5	±4.4	±50	±3	2
2750	138	48.7	19.1	51	9.1	117	7.5	24.0	9.6	362	39	2
		±2.9	±3.8	±15	±3.6	±26	±2.7	±5.4	±3.8	±48	±2	2
3000	144	50.0	20.7	53	10.1	127	8.3	24.7	10.2	380	40	0
		±2.9	±5.3	±13	±3.3	±30	±2.9	±5.3	±4.3	±55	±2	1
3250	133	50.7	21.5	59	11.0	145	9.2	27.3	11.6	395	40	4
		±2.6	±4.3	±18	±4.0	±33	±3.4	±6.6	±4.4	±53	±4	6
3500	106	51.8	22.8	63	11.3	153	9.8	28.0	12.8	411	40	4
		±3.0	±5.9	±17	±3.6	±33	±3.5	±6.5	±5.1	±55	±1	5
3750	57	52.1	23.8	65	12.5	159	10.2	29.5	13.0	413	40	6
		±2.3	±5.1	±15	±4.1	±40	±3.3	±6.8	±4.8	±55	±1	3
4000	31	52.4	25.8	67	14.1	180	10.8	30.2	11.4	420	41	4
		±2.7	±5.3	±20	±4.0	±39	±3.4	±6.2	±3.2	±62	±2	3
4250	15	53.2	26.5	68	13.0	197	12.0	30.7	11.7	415	41	2
		±2.5	±5.3	±16	±2.5	±42	±3.7	±5.8	±3.7	±38	±2	1

From Gruenwald and Minh (1960). Amer. J. Clin. Pathol., 34, 247–53.

Table 25.6 Organ weights of newborn infants by gestational age

Gestational age*	Number of cases	Body length (m)	Body weight (g)	Heart (g)	Lungs, combined (g)	Spleen (g)	Liver (g)	Adrenal glands, combined (g)	Kidneys, combined (g)	Thymus (g)	Brain (g)
24	108	31.3 ±3.7	638 ±240	4.9 ±1.6	17 ±6	1.7 ±1.1	32 ±15	2.9 ±1.4	6.4 ±2.6	2.7 ±1.4	92 ±31
26	143	33.3 ±3.6	845 ±246	6.4 ±2.0	18 ±6	2.2 ±1.5	39 ±15	3.4 ±1.5	7.9 ±2.9	3.0 ±2.3	111 ±39
28	139	36.0 ±4.2	1020 ±340	7.6 ±2.3	23 ±7	2.6 ±1.4	46 ±16	3.7 ±1.7	10.4 ±3.6	3.8 ±2.1	139 ±48
30	148	37.8 ±3.7	1230 ±340	9.3 ±3.3	28 ±11	3.4 ±2.0	53 ±19	4.2 ±2.2	12.3 ±3.9	4.6 ±2.3	166 ±55
32	150	40.5 ±4.5	1488 ±335	11.0 ±3.7	34 ±11	4.1 ±2.1	65 ±22	4.3 ±2.3	14.5 ±4.8	5.5 ±2.3	209 ±44
34	104	42.8 ±4.5	1838 ±530	13.4 ±3.9	40 ±13	5.2 ±2.1	74 ±27	5.5 ±2.3	17.7 ±5.3	7.5 ±3.8	246 ±58
36	87	45.0 ±4.6	2165 ±600	15.1 ±4.8	46 ±16	6.7 ±3.0	87 ±33	6.4 ±3.0	21.6 ±6.7	8.1 ±4.2	288 ±62
38	102	47.2 ±4.6	2678 ±758	18.5 ±5.5	53 ±15	8.8 ±4.2	111 ±40	8.4 ±3.5	23.8 ±7.0	9.7 ±4.8	349 ±56
40	220	49.8 ±3.9	3163 ±595	20.4 ±5.3	56 ±15	10.0 ±3.9	130 ±45	8.6 ±3.4	25.6 ±6.5	9.5 ±4.4	362 ±55
42	112	50.3 ±3.6	3263 ±573	21.9 ±6.2	56 ±18	10.2 ±4.3	139 ±45	9.1 ±4.0	25.8 ±7.5	10.4 ±4.4	405 ±54
44	42	52.8 ±2.8	3690 ±800	25.8 ±4.5	60 ±17	11.2 ±4.1	149 ±35	9.3 ±4.4	28.4 ±7.5	10.3 ±4.7	417 ±55

From Gruenwald and Minh (1960). *Amer. J. Clin. Pathol.*, **34**, 247–53.
* Gestational age is expressed in weeks from the last menstrual period.

26

Practical procedures

Blood sampling
Insertion of intravenous lines
Insertion of arterial lines
Lumbar puncture
Ventricular tap
Subdural tap
Suprapubic bladder tap
Intubation
Thoracentesis
Exchange transfusion
Pericardial aspiration
Intracardiac injection
Cardiac massage
Abdominal paracentesis
Percutaneous 'long-line' insertion
Bone marrow aspiration

Before performing any practical procedure

(1) Ensure all equipment is prepared.
(2) Ensure any assistants are familiar with the procedure.
(3) Maintain thermal care – use a supplementary overhead heater if the incubator is to be open for any length of time.

Do not persist after three failed attempts – seek a colleague's help or take a break and try again later.

Remember: The procedure is in the *infant's* interest – do not cause avoidable disturbance or trauma.

Blood sampling

Routine precautions for protection against hepatitis B and HIV must be observed. Take particular caution with disposal of needles and sharps.

(a) Capillary samples

See Fig. 26.1 for site of sampling.

Warm or rub the area for 1–2 min to increase perfusion.

Clean the skin surface.

Puncture the skin with a stilette (to depth of 2–3 mm only): Preferably use an Autolet device. This has been shown to reduce the stress caused to the baby by heel-prick sampling.

Gently massage the heel to encourage blood flow.

Avoid adhesive dressings to the area – they keep it moist and increase the risk of infection.

(b) Venous samples

The safest sites are the *antecubital fossa* or the *back of the hand*.

Practical procedures

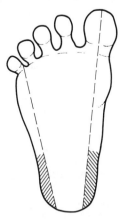

Fig. 26.1 Sites for heel-prick capillary blood sampling. Puncture heel (shaded area) on plantar surface, beyond the lateral and medial limits of calcaneus, to avoid damage to the bone. (Blumenfeld *et al.*, 1979)

Use a large needle (21 or 23 G) for ease of sampling. Blood will drip freely from the needle into the specimen container (but should not be used for blood culture).

For blood cultures clean the skin with an iodine-containing solution and use a new sterile needle to inject the blood into each blood culture bottle. (NB   Beware the anaerobic bottle! It may take *all* the blood sample before you can prevent it!)

Other sites for venepuncture

External jugular vein   This should not be used in infants with respiratory distress. Great care is needed to minimize trauma. The infant is wrapped and held with the head slightly lower than the trunk, and neck flexed away from the side of the venepuncture. The vein is clearly seen, and the sample should be taken through a 21 or 23 G needle with a syringe attached (to minimize the risk of air embolism). After removing the needle, apply firm pressure and sit the infant up.

Femoral vein   This site should be *avoided if at all possible*, as the needle may enter the hip joint and cause septic arthritis. The femoral artery is palpable at the mid-inguinal point, and the vein is medial to this. Clean the skin very carefully and insert the needle vertically, applying gentle suction. Stop advancing the needle as soon as blood is obtained.

(c) Arterial samples

Suitable sites for arterial sampling are the radial, posterior tibial and dorsalis pedis. Brachial and temporal arteries are best avoided for routine sampling (see below). Femoral arterial puncture carries a risk of septic arthritis of the hip and is not recommended.

Radial artery

Check that there is an ulnar artery (it is absent in 1–2% of the population) either by transillumination or by squeezing the hand whilst occluding the sites of the radial and ulnar arteries. If the hand rapidly goes pink when the ulnar artery site is released the ulnar artery is patent.

Hold the wrist in neutral position, or at most slightly extended, with palm of hand upwards.

Locate the radial artery by palpation or transillumination.

Enter the artery just proximal to the wrist crease, at an angle of 25°–30°; use either a heparinized 23 or 25 G scalp-vein needle or a 23 G needle on a heparinized 2 ml syringe.

Posterior tibial

Hold the foot in neutral position or slightly dorsiflexed.

Locate the artery by palpation or transillumination (behind the medial malleolus).

Sampling technique as for radial artery.

Dorsalis pedis

Partially plantar flex the foot.

Locate artery by palpation or transillumination (between first and second metatarsals).

Sampling technique as for radial artery.

Brachial

(NB   The brachial is an end artery and should not be used as a routine site.)

Hold the arm with elbow extended.

Palpate the artery just proximal and medial to the antecubital fossa.

Sampling technique as for radial artery.

Temporal

(NB   Do not insert a cannula into the temporal artery because of the risk of reflex spasm or embolization of other branches of the external carotid (especially the middle meningeal artery).

Branches of the temporal artery can be palpated and samples taken through a 25 G scalp-vein needle.

Intramuscular injections

The preferred injection site is the lateral aspect of the thigh. Avoid the buttocks. Do not give repeated i.m. injections as these may cause fibrosis of the muscles.

Insertion of intravenous lines

(a) Peripheral veins

Site

Veins on the dorsum of the hands and feet, antecubital fossa, long saphenous vein and scalp veins are most often used.

Technique

Clean the skin with antiseptic solution.

Puncture the skin overlying the vein with a needle.

Cannulate the vein with a 24 G or 22 G cannula. Infusion of normal saline through the cannula will help to establish whether or not the cannula is in the vein.

Tape the cannula on securely. Do not cover the skin overlying the cannula tip. This area must be visible at all times in order to observe any extravasation of i.v. fluid.

Immobilize the i.v. site with a splint.

Scalp veins

These should be avoided if possible, as the sight of an intravenous line in an infant's head is particularly distressing to the parents. Hair which is shaved off may take months to regrow.

(b) Umbilical vein

This is used in an emergency situation, e.g. for administering plasma etc., during resuscitation in the delivery room, and occasionally for exchange transfusions.

Technique

Use a full aseptic technique (gloves and gown), carefully clean the cord and surrounding skin, and drape the abdomen with sterile towel.

A tie is placed loosely around the base of the cord to control bleeding.

Cut the cord to 1.0–1.5 cm.

Fill the catheter (size 5.FG) with heparinized saline, attach a syringe, and pass the catheter into the vein.

As the catheter is passed exert gentle traction on the cord.

The catheter tip should be placed between the diaphragm and right atrium. This distance is estimated from the shoulder to the umbilicus length (see Fig. 26.2).

The position of the catheter tip should be checked by X-ray.

Ensure that the infant is not lying in a puddle of alcohol/iodine solution used to clean the skin, as this can cause severe burns to the skin.

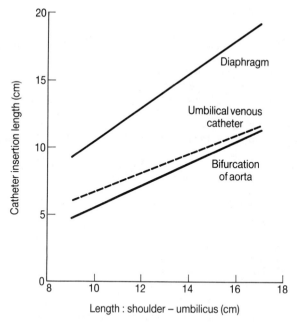

Fig. 26.2   Distances for insertion of umbilical arterial (solid lines) and venous (broken lines) catheters. (See text)

Insertion of arterial lines

Peripheral arterial lines

To be used for sampling or exchange transfusion, not to be used for giving drugs, parental nutrition, dextrose etc.

Site

Radial artery or posterior tibial artery. The temporal, brachial or femoral arteries should not be used, as they are end arteries.

Technique

The adequacy of the ulnar collateral flow to the hand should be assessed (see page 342).

Localize the artery by palpation or by transillumination with a fibre-optic light.

Cleanse the skin with antiseptic solution, and puncture the skin with a 21 G needle.

Hold the wrist or foot as for arterial blood sampling. Excessive flexion or extension will put traction on the artery and reduce flow.

Transfix the artery with a 22 G cannula with a luer-locking end by entering the skin through the puncture at an angle of $25°-30°$. Withdraw the stilette, and very slowly withdraw the cannula until the blood begins to flow freely up the cannula. Then gently advance the cannula up the artery, and quickly connect to a syringe of heparinized saline (1 unit/ml), or the prepared tubing. Gently flush the cannula.

Tape the wrist or foot so that the fingers and toes are clearly visible and any evidence of ischaemia may be observed.

Tape the cannula in position and firmly immobilize the extremity with an adequate sized splint.

NOTE: We only infuse heparinized saline (0.45% NaCl with heparin 1 unit/ml) and this must be taken into account in calculating the daily fluid and sodium requirements.

Umbilical arterial catheter

Technique

Use a full aseptic technique (gloves and gown). The cord and skin are cleansed with antiseptic solution and the abdomen is draped with sterile towels.

Tie a loose ligature around the base of the cord to prevent blood loss.

Cut the cord cleanly with a scalpel blade to a length of 1.0–1.5 cm and identify the vein and arteries. (1 vein – has large lumen and thin walls. 2 arteries – have small lumen and thick walls.)

Stabilize the cord between the second and third fingers of the non-preferred hand and fixate the edge of the cord with forceps. Tease the lumen of the artery open with a blunt dilator or a pair of fine forceps to a depth of 5 mm. Spread the tips of the forceps slightly for a minute or so to overcome arterial spasm.

Insert a heparinized, saline-filled 3.5 or 5.0 FG catheter into the artery, and then advance it slowly into the aorta. Success is indicated by blood flowing or being easily aspirated up the catheter.

The catheter tip should be located either between L3 and L4, i.e. just above the aortic bifurcation and below the origin of the inferior mesenteric artery, or between T8 and T10, i.e. well above the origin of the coeliac axis. The distance the catheter is inserted is estimated from the shoulder to umbilical length (see Fig. 26.2). The position of the catheter tip must be checked by X-ray.

The catheter is held in place by a pull-string suture and tape.

Keep the catheter patent with an infusion of 0.45% saline containing heparin 1 unit/ml at a rate of 0.5–1 ml/hour.

Problems

(1) Occasionally the catheter will not pass through into the aorta. This may be due to arterial spasm or else a false passage has been created.
(2) The catheter does pass into the aorta, but a 'white or blue leg' or 'blue toes' develop. This is due to vasospasm.

In either of these situations the catheter should be removed and the other artery catheterized.

Catheter removal

The infusion through the catheter is stopped approximately 1 hour prior to removal, and a ligature is tied around the umbilical stump.

The catheter is removed slowly over a period of approximately 5 min, to allow time for the umbilical artery to go into spasm and thus minimize bleeding.

The catheter tip should be sent for culture.

Lumbar puncture

Technique

The infant is placed on his or her side or in the sitting position, and held firmly at the buttocks and shoulders, so that the lower spine is curved. Care must be taken to keep the neck straight, so as not to cause airway obstruction during the procedure, and the spine horizontal.

Prepare a sterile field and drape the area with sterile towels.

Use a 22 G LP needle with trochar. Alternatively a 25 G butterfly needle can be used, but carries the risk of causing implantation dermoid cysts.

Using the iliac crests as a guide, insert the needle between the L3 and L4 spinous process and advance it in the direction of the umbilicus.

Usually a slight 'pop' is felt as the needle enters the subarachnoid space. The internal stilette should be withdrawn frequently and the needle gently rotated to check for CSF flow. It is easy to push the needle too far and enter the anterior vertebral venous plexus.

Once in the subarachnoid space, CSF should be collected into at least three containers.

After removal of the needle, swab the area with collodion and cover with a small adhesive dressing.

Ventricular tap

This should only be carried out by experienced staff.

Technique

Have an assistant firmly hold the baby supine with the nose upwards and the neck and face parallel to the mattress.

Mark the four corners of the anterior fontanelle with an ink marker and as accurately as possible estimate the midline of the fontanelle. Measure 6 mm to one side of the midline, in the line of the coronal suture: this is the point of entry.

Using a full sterile technique, pass a 22 G 4 or 5 cm LP needle through the marked point and advance it horizontally; and parallel to the midline axis, for a distance of 4 to 5 cm. Do not insert the needle beyond the level of the mid-point of the eye.

Always insert and withdraw the needle along the same track. Before reinserting the needle after a dry tap, always withdraw the needle fully.

Subdural tap

This should only be carried out by experienced staff.

Technique

The subdural space is entered with a 22 G LP needle at the lateral angle of the anterior fontanelle. Use a guard on the needle to limit insertion to 5 mm. As soon as the 'give' is felt (penetration of the dura) the stilette is withdrawn. If fluid is present it will flow out but may be viscid, so flow may be very slow.

NB   *DO NOT* attach a syringe and aspirate subdural fluid.

Suprapubic bladder tap
Technique

This should be performed at least 1 hour after the last wet nappy.

Use a 23 G needle attached to a 5 ml syringe.

Have an assistant hold the infant firmly, immobilizing the legs and pelvis.

Cleanse the area with an antiseptic solution and insert the needle in the midline, just superior to the pubic symphysis.

Advance the needle at right angles to the skin. The bladder is entered at a depth of 1 to 2 cm. Do not insert the needle more than 2 cm.

After withdrawing the needle cover the area with a small adhesive dressing.

A full bladder may be identified by ultrasound but runs the risk of stimulating micturation.

Intubation

Endotracheal intubation should be done as a controlled procedure in an infant who has been well oxygenated with a bag and mask.

Do not let the infant become hypoxic during the procedure. If this does occur, stop immediately and apply positive-pressure ventilation with a bag and mask.

Endotracheal tube (ETT) size

Baby's weight	ETT size (mm)
<1000 g	2.5
1000–2000 g	3.0
2000–3000 g	3.0 or 3.5
>3000 g	3.5

Technique

Ensure the head and neck are in line with the rest of the body and the neck is slightly extended.

Insert the laryngoscope blade over the tongue in the mid-line to the back of the pharynx.

Lift the epiglottis forward by exerting traction parallel to the handle of the laryngoscope (*NOT* by tilting the blade upward).

The vocal cords should then be visualized (Fig. 26.3). Brief suction may be needed to clear secretions. Gentle cricoid pressure with the 5th finger of the left hand (or by an assistant) may help.

Insert the ETT through the vocal cords, for a distance of about 2 cm. During nasotracheal intubation, Magill's forceps can be used to grasp the tube and guide it between the cords.

Auscultate the chest to check the tube position (equal air entry

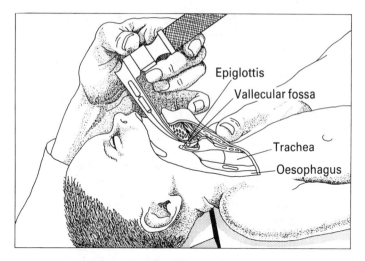

Fig. 26.3 The technique for endotracheal intubation.

on both sides) and then confirm with a chest X-ray. (Tip should be 1–2 cm above carina.)

If the infant does not respond to intermittent positive pressure ventilation (IPPV) within 30 sec, check that the tube is not blocked or dislodged.

Common errors

The condition of the infant is ignored during the procedure.

The vocal cords are not properly visualized before intubation is attempted.

The infant's upper gum may be lacerated by excessive pressure of the laryngoscope blade.

The ETT is inserted too far down and into the right main bronchus.

Thoracentesis
(a) Chest transillumination

In a low birthweight infant, a pneumothorax may be demonstrated by increased transillumination (using a fibre-optic light source in a darkened room or a dark cover over the incubator).

(b) Needling the chest

Used for the emergency drainage of a tension pneumothorax (or, less commonly, for draining a pleural effusion).

Technique

Attach a 21 G butterfly needle to a 10 ml syringe through a three-way tap. (For effusions use an i.v. 19 or 21 G i.v. cannula.)

Insert the needle in the third or fourth intercostal space in the mix-axillary line.

If free air is present it will aspirate easily. The three-way tap allows for repeated aspiration without disconnecting the syringe from the needle. If a pneumothorax is found, the tap should be connected to a sterile extension tube with its other end 2–3 cm under the surface in a bottle of sterile water (at least 20 cm below the level of the baby). The tap is then turned to allow drainage of the pneumothorax through this temporary system whilst a definitive drain is inserted.

(c) Chest drain insertion

Technique

See Fig. 26.4 for sites of insertion of chest drains.

(1) Anterior
   Second or third intercostal spaces in the mid-clavicular line. *The nipple and breast bud must be avoided.*
(2) Lateral
   Third to fifth intercostal spaces in the anterior axillary line.

The drains work best if the tip lies in the anterior pleural space. There is evidence that the anterior insertion site is more successful in achieving this and has a lower incidence of complications. (Allen **et al.**, 1981).

If time allows infuse a small amount of local anaesthetic.

Make a small incision through the skin with a scalpel blade, parallel to the rib.

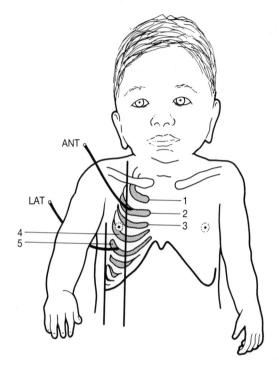

Fig. 26.4 Sites for insertion of chest drains to relieve pneumothorax.
Adapted from Allen R. W., Jung A. L., Lester P. D., *J. Pediatr*. 1981. **99**:
629–34.

With a pair of artery forceps blunt dissect through the intercostal
muscle down to and *including* the parietal pleura. A soft hiss of air
may be heard as the parietal pleura is breached.

Using a size 8, 10, or 12 FG chest drain, remove the trochar and grasp
the tip of the drain with a pair of curved artery forceps. Push the
forceps and drain through the chest wall.

Release the forceps and advance the chest drain, aiming anteriorly.

Connect the chest drain to an underwater seal drain; observe for air
bubbles and swinging respiration.

If necessary, connect the drain to a 10 cm water-negative suction
pressure (Fig. 26.5).

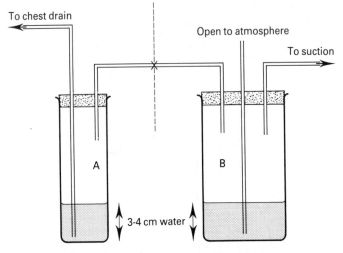

Fig. 26.5 Underwater seal drainage for pneumothorax. Bottle A must be at least 30 cm below the level of the baby. Tubing may be left open to atmosphere at point X or connected to a second bottle B if suction is required. The water level in bottle B must not exceed 10 cm.

Place suture adjacent to the incision and tie it around the chest drain. Finally, tape the tube in position.

Retransilluminate and X-ray the chest to check on tube position and effectiveness.

Removal of the chest drain

Once the chest drain has ceased to function, apply a clamp. If the clinical condition of the infant is unchanged, or X-ray shows no further reaccumulation of pneumothorax after 24 hours, the drain is removed.

Close the wound with steristrips. Do not use a purse-string suture because this will cause a permanent disfiguring scar.

Exchange transfusion

The most common indication for an exchange transfusion is severe hyperbilirubinaemia. Other indications include polycythaemia (Chapter 15, page 233) and septicaemia (Chapter 14, page 217). For hyperbilirubinaemia a 'two-volume exchange' is performed, i.e. the volume of blood exchanged equals twice the infant's blood volume, that is, 2×80 ml/kg = 160 ml/kg. This will replace approximately 80% of the infant's blood. 'Priming' the infant with albumin (1 g/kg given i.v. over 30–60 min as a 10% solution two hours before the exchange) may increase the removal of bilirubin.

Technique

Fresh blood (cytomegalovirus negative) should be used, less than 4 days old and cross-matched against mother's blood. It should be partially packed to a PCV of 60%. There are two ways of performing the procedure:

(a) In-out method

This used to be the commonest way of doing an exchange but is now used less often. Aliquots, 5 or 10 ml, of infant blood are withdrawn via an umbilical venous catheter and replaced by an equal volume of donor blood in a serial manner via a three-way tap. 10 ml out, 10 ml in, 10 ml out etc., until the calculated volume has been exchanged. This method has a higher incidence of complications.

(b) Continuous flow method

This is the preferred technique (See Fig. 26.6). Insert peripheral arterial and venous lines, if this is not possible umbilical artery and vein or a combination or peripheral and umbilical vessels can be used. Donor blood is infused at a constant rate through the vein via a blood warmer using a volumetric pump. Baby's blood is withdrawn at the same rate from the arterial line using a 50 ml syringe. It is essential to balance the rate of withdrawal with the infusion rate.

No matter which method is used, a two volume exchange (160 ml/kg) should take 1.5 hours to complete, i.e. a slower rate in a smaller baby. A deficit of 10 ml in the baby should be left at the end of the exchange.

Monitoring

One operator should record the volumes of the blood exchanged, and check vital signs, e.g. heart rate, respiratory rate and temperature, at regular intervals.

In sick, low birthweight infants, blood gas and blood sugar measurements should be checked once or twice during the exchange.

If there is evidence of hypocalcaemia (irritability, tachycardia,

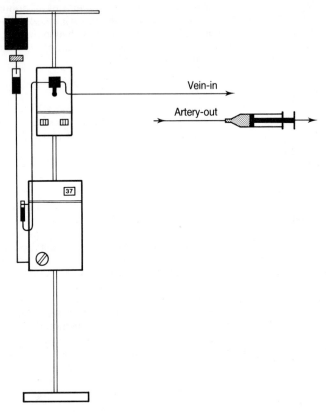

Fig. 26.6   Apparatus for exchange transfusion by the arterio-venous technique.

prolonged *Q–T* interval) the infant should be given 0.5 ml 10% calcium gluconate solution i.v. over 5–10 min. In the absence of such signs, the hazards of calcium administration (bradycardia or cardiac arrest) outweigh its usefulness.

Blood samples

The *first 10 ml* of blood removed should be sent for estimation of bilirubin, haematocrit and any other investigations needed (e.g. enzyme assays for glucose 6-phosphate dehydrogenase (G-6-PD) or galactosaemia, liver function tests etc.)

The *last 10 ml* of blood removed should be sent for blood sugar, electrolytes, bilirubin, calcium, blood gases and haematocrit.

Check capillary blood sugar 1, 2 and 4 hours after the exchange, as reactive hypoglycaemia may occur.

Feeding

Do not feed infants for 2–4 hours before exchange transfusion (to reduce risk of aspiration and for 2–4 hours afterwards (to reduce the risk of necrotizing enterocolitis). Give maintenance fluids i.v. during this period.

Complications

Vascular	Embolization (air or clots) and thrombosis
Cardiac	Arrhythmia; volume overload or depletion; arrest
Electrolyte	Hyperkalaemia, hypernatraemia, hypocalcaemia, acidosis or alkalosis
Infective	Bacteraemia, hepatitis B, CMV
Miscellaneous	Hypothermia, hypoglycaemia, necrotizing enterocolitis (metronidazole is sometimes given as a prophylaxis against necrotizing enterocolitis)

Pericardial aspiration

This is performed if cardiac tamponade due to pneumopericardium occurs.

Technique

(a) Use a 23 G needle connected via a three-way tap to a 10 ml syringe.
(b) Enter under the rib cage to the left of the xiphisternum and advance upwards and to the left at 45° to vertical and 45° to the mid-line while applying gentle suction.
(c) The pericardium is entered at a depth of about 1 cm and the air is withdrawn.

Intracardiac injection

The entry point is the same as for the pericardial aspiration. The needle is inserted until blood is easily aspirated. When the myocardium is reached, pulsation can be felt through the needle and syringe.

NB   In the treatment of cardiac arrest adrenaline may also be given down an endotracheal tube.

Cardiac massage
Technique

Hold the infant with one or both hands around the thorax, with the fingers supporting the spine.

The thumbs are placed at the junction of the middle and lower third of the sternum.

The sternum is depressed approximately two-thirds of the way to the vertebral column at a rate of 100 times per min. (Co-ordinate cardiac massage with IPPV: 4 cardiac compressions to each IPPV breath.)

Abdominal paracentesis

This can be performed via a mid-line or a lateral approach.

(a) **Mid-line approach**
   The bladder must be empty before proceeding. A 21 G needle is inserted vertically through the abdominal wall 1–2 cm below the umbilicus.
(b) **Lateral approach**
   The needle is inserted into either iliac fossa, keeping well lateral to the rectus muscle, as the inferior epigastric artery runs just underneath its lateral border. Take care to avoid enlarged liver or spleen.

Percutaneous 'long-line' insertion
Site

Antecubital fossa or long saphenous vein anterior to the medical malleolus.

Technique

Use a full aseptic technique (gloves and gown).

Perform a venepuncture with a 19 G needle.

Thread a long-line silastic cannula through the needle and into the vein, using a pair of sterile, fine, non-toothed dissecting forceps.

Position of the cannula

There are two possible positions:

(a) Insert the cannula 2–3 cm. In this position blood flow is fast enough to allow safe, long-term infusion of hypertonic fluids, but does not carry the risk associated with central venous lines.
(b) Insert the cannula so that the tip lies in the subclavian vein, superior vena cava, or inferior vena cava. The line will last for several weeks in this position if meticulous anti-infective measures are taken. If this 'central' position is used, the position of the cannula tip must be checked with an X-ray, if not radio-opaque; infuse 1 ml of a radio-opaque dye, e.g. sodium diatrizoate 45% w/v 'Hypaque 45', to check position on X-ray.

Once inserted to the required length, *gently* withdraw the needle and clamp the plastic protector over it. Connect the cannula to the i.v. infusion via a T-piece connector.

Tape the cannula in place and immobilize the limb or extremity.

Care of the long-line

Change the i.v. fluid containers, giving-set and tubing (excluding the T-piece) daily. (Use full aseptic technique.)

Spray the T-piece connector with iodine-containing antiseptic before connecting the new tubing.

Culture the i.v. fluid removed from the discarded tubing.

When the long-line cannula is removed, culture the tip.

Any infant with a percutaneous long-line should have a blood culture 2–3/week.

Bone marrow aspiration

This should be carried out by experienced staff only.

Site

There are three possible sites for this procedure:

(a) Tibia
(b) Anterior iliac crest
(c) Posterior iliac crest

Technique

Use a full aseptic technique.

Use a 19 G butterfly needle with syringe attached.

Tibia

(a) Hold the tibia firmly with the knee flexed.
(b) Enter the bone marrow at an angle perpendicular to the skin, just below and medial to the tibial tuberosity.

Anterior iliac crest

(a) Hold the infant firmly in the supine position.
(b) Locate the iliac crest by palpation, and enter at an angle perpendicular to the skin.

Posterior iliac crest

(a) Hold the infant in the lumbar puncture position.
(b) Enter the posterior iliac crest at right angles to the skin.

Bibliography

Allen, R. W., Jing, A. L. and Lester, P. D. (1981). Effectiveness of chest tube evacuation of pneumothorax in neonates. *J. Pediatr.*, **99**, 629–34.

Blumenfeld, T. A., Turi, G. B. and Blanc, W. A. (1979). Recommended site and depth of newborn heel skin punctures based on anatomical measurements and histopathology. *Lancet*, **i**, 230–3.

Cooke, R. W. I. (1982). *A Guide to Resuscitation of the Newborn Infant*. Basingstoke: Vickers Medical.

Dunn, P. M. (1966). Localisation of the umbilical catheter by post-mortem measurement. *Arch. Dis. Child.*, **41**, 69.

Philip, A. G. S. (1977). *Neonatology: A Practical Guide*, London: Henry Kimpton.

27

Follow-up after discharge

Infants requiring special follow-up
The follow-up appointment
Developmental assessment
Sensory testing
Immunization
Attendance at clinic
Follow-up checklist

Medical and neurodevelopmental follow-up of babies who have had perinatal problems is important:

To provide continuity of care and support for parents.

To detect and institute treatment for medical and neurodevelopmental problems.

To provide ongoing care for specific problems apparent at discharge (dislocated hips, anomalies etc.).

On occasions to give appropriate advice and counselling.

This care must compliment and not duplicate other community care which is provided by the primary care team. Nonetheless, having identified a group of children at particular risk it is important to ensure adequate follow-up within these contexts. Ideally follow-up should be organized at the community level but constraints of service provision rarely make it possible to hold clinics in local health centres.

Infants requiring special follow-up

Birthweight <2000 g
Gestation <34 weeks
Birthweight <3rd percentile for gestation
Head circumference <3rd percentile for gestation
Babies who have needed intensive care (see page 51)
Babies with recognized congenital anomalies
Babies with specific neonatally detected problems (e.g. congenital
  infection, heart murmur, dislocatable hips, urinary tract infection)

Within these groups special attention must be paid to the follow-up of children with recognized perinatal complications which have prognostic implications (e.g. cerebral ultrasound abnormality, bronchopulmonary dysplasia, retinopathy etc.).

Where appropriate, early referral to the relevant district paediatric speciality for assessment and therapy of specific disorders is essential.

The follow-up appointment

Parents

The consultation is an opportunity for parents to discuss their specific concerns and time should be allocated for this. Taking home a child who has received intensive care is a daunting prospect for many parents, who may find difficulty in the expression of their anxieties. It is important to be positive with respect to their child's progress and not deliberately overcautious.

Frequency

The frequency of follow-up visits is determined by the support needed by each family. Standard ages allow for familiarity with developmental patterns at each age. Visits should start within 4–6 weeks of discharge from hospital and subsequently, if all is well, children are seen at 4, 8, 12 and 24 months **post-term**, although earlier discharge is usual for those at low risk of long-term sequelae.

Correcting for prematurity

Calculation of age from expected date of delivery is essential for assessment of growth and development in infancy and early childhood.

Growth must be assessed at each visit and weight, length and use head circumferance plotted on percentile charts.

Physical examination should follow the developmental examination.

Developmental assessment

At each visit an assessment of the adequacy of developmental progress should be attempted. Formal estimation of developmental quotient is time consuming and unnecessary unless research data are being collected. A simple test such as the Denver II is a useful aide (Fig. 27.1) and should be combined with sensory assessment (see below) and interpreted in the context of everything one knows about the child.

Sensory testing

Vision

All babies <32 weeks' gestation should have an ophthalmic assessment before discharge as a screen for retinopathy (Chapter 23). Any child with a recognizable eye abnormality or a squint at follow-up should be referred for further assessment. Visual assessment is part of routine follow-up and an important component of the assessment of fine motor development (Fig. 27.1).

Visual acuity may be assessed from 6 to 7 months using graded white balls displayed against a black background. These may be presented rolling or on sticks. Alternatively, visual following or reaching for a 1 mm cake decoration ('hundreds and thousands') at 60 cm is a useful screening test.

Hearing

It is our practice to refer all children at high risk for hearing impairment to the district audiology services at discharge. Failure to respond to distraction testing is then followed by routine brain stem evoked potentials. Indications for referral (high risk) are: <32 weeks' gestation, moderate/severe birth asphyxia, recurrent seizures or exchange transfusion for hyperbilirubinaemia.

Hearing is assessed at each clinic visit using a Manchester (high frequency) rattle. Stilling to sound is observed at six weeks. Distraction tests become most reliable after six months. In a quiet room the infant is sat on mother's lap whilst the examiner attracts the child's

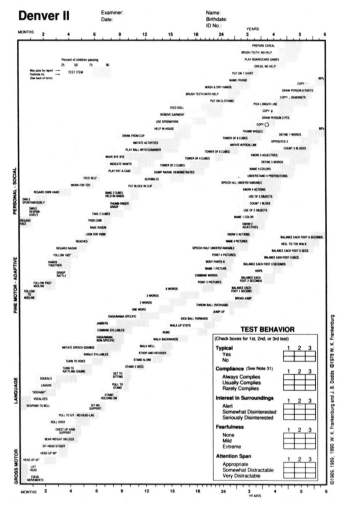

Fig. 27.1 Denver II developmental screening test (0–6 years). Reproduced by permission of Professor W K Frankenberg and Denver Developmental Materials Inc.

DIRECTIONS FOR ADMINISTRATION

1. Try to get child to smile by smiling, talking or waving. Do not touch him/her.
2. Child must stare at hand several seconds.
3. Parent may help guide toothbrush and put toothpaste on brush.
4. Child does not have to be able to tie shoes or button/zip in the back.
5. Move yarn slowly in an arc from one side to the other, about 8" above child's face.
6. Pass if child grasps rattle when it is touched to the backs or tips of fingers.
7. Pass if child tries to see where yarn went. Yarn should be dropped quickly from sight from tester's hand without arm movement.
8. Child must transfer cube from hand to hand without help of body, mouth, or table.
9. Pass if child picks up raisin with any part of thumb and finger.
10. Line can vary only 30 degrees or less from tester's line. |/
11. Make a fist with thumb pointing upward and wiggle only the thumb. Pass if child imitates and does not move any fingers other than the thumb.

12. Pass any enclosed form. Fail continuous round motions.

13. Which line is longer? (Not bigger.) Turn paper upside down and repeat. (pass 3 of 3 or 5 of 6)

14. Pass any lines crossing near midpoint.

15. Have child copy first. If failed, demonstrate.

When giving items 12, 14, and 15, do not name the forms. Do not demonstrate 12 and 14.

16. When scoring, each pair (2 arms, 2 legs, etc.) counts as one part.
17. Place one cube in cup and shake gently near child's ear, but out of sight. Repeat for other ear.
18. Point to picture and have child name it. (No credit is given for sounds only.)
    If less than 4 pictures are named correctly, have child point to picture as each is named by tester.

19. Using doll, tell child: Show me the nose, eyes, ears, mouth, hands, feet, tummy, hair. Pass 6 of 8.
20. Using pictures, ask child: Which one flies?... says meow?... talks?... barks?... gallops? Pass 2 of 5, 4 of 5.
21. Ask child: What do you do when you are cold?... tired?... hungry? Pass 2 of 3, 3 of 3.
22. Ask child: What do you do with a cup? What is a chair used for? What is a pencil used for?
    Action words must be included in answers.
23. Pass if child correctly places and says how many blocks are on paper. (1, 5).
24. Tell child: Put block on table; under table; in front of me, behind me. Pass 4 of 4.
    (Do not help child by pointing, moving head or eyes.)
25. Ask child: What is a ball?... lake?... desk?... house?... banana?... curtain?... fence?... ceiling? Pass if defined in terms of use, shape, what it is made of, or general category (such as banana is fruit, not just yellow). Pass 5 of 8, 7 of 8.
26. Ask child: If a horse is big, a mouse is __? If fire is hot, ice is __? If the sun shines during the day, the moon shines during the __? Pass 2 of 3.
27. Child may use wall or rail only, not person. May not crawl.
28. Child must throw ball overhand 3 feet to within arm's reach of tester.
29. Child must perform standing broad jump over width of test sheet (8 1/2 inches).
30. Tell child to walk forward, ⇐⇒⇐⇒⇐⇒→ heel within 1 inch of toe. Tester may demonstrate.
    Child must walk 4 consecutive steps.
31. In the second year, half of normal children are non-compliant.

OBSERVATIONS:

attention visually. The assistant then rolls the rattle gently on each side of the infant. At six months children turn to sounds presented level with each ear at a distance of 45 cm, and at nine months to sounds presented at 1 m.

Immunization

The current Department of Health recommendations are that all children should receive full immunization unless there are specific contraindications (DHSS, 1990). For preterm babies this should start at two months of age *UNCORRECTED for prematurity*. For some babies this will mean starting immunization before discharge from hospital. Premature babies form a special risk group who should be immunized as a matter of priority. Immunization with oral polio vaccine is delayed until the day of discharge from the SCBU.

A child with neurological abnormality during the neonatal period is considered to have a problem history (DHSS, 1990). It is our policy to offer pertussis immunization to all babies who have received intensive care, including those with intraventricular haemorrhage, periventricular leucomalacia and hydrocephalus. It is essential for babies who have bronchopulmonary dysplasia.

Attendance at clinic

Parents often find it difficult to attend clinic because of many reasons such as change of address, lack of transport or illness. Consideration should be given to special assistance if possible for those with particular problems. Clinic attendance may be less appealing if there is a poorly organized appointments system, a long wait, no play area for siblings or no literature is available.

Always arrange a further appointment (usually in 2–4 weeks). Further non-attendance should be followed up with a request for the GP or Health Visitor to visit the family. If families are persistent non-attenders with problems that deserve follow-up ensure that the GP is fully informed of the situation.

Follow-up checklist

Parental concerns
Growth (plotted on charts)
Diet and vitamin supplements
Medication
Recent illness/problems
Immunizations

Mother/infant interaction
Development
Vision
Hearing
Examination especially
   Neurology
   Murmurs
   Hips

Information given to parents
Next visit – necessary? when? who to see?

Bibliography

DHSS (1990). *Immunisation Against Infectious Disease*. Report of the Joint Committee on Vaccination and Immunisation. London: HMSO.

Egan, D. F., Illingworth, R. S. and Mac Keith, R. C. (1969). *Developmental Screening 0–5 Years*. Oxford: Heinemann Medical.

Illingworth, R. S. (1980). *The Development of the Infant and Young Child*, 7th Edn. Edinburgh: Churchill Livingstone.

28

Drugs and prescribing

Drugs in pregnancy
Drugs which can be given to breast-feeding mothers
Blood and blood products
Neonatal drug doses and administration
Antibiotic prescribing in the neonate
Antifungal agents

Drugs in pregnancy

Although only a few drugs have been shown to be definitely teratogenic, no drug should be regarded as completely safe particularly
during the first trimester. After the embryonic stage of development,
drugs may have toxic side-effects on the fetus, influencing growth and
development. Drugs given shortly before delivery may carry over
their effects into the newborn period. Remember that not all drugs
are prescribed; self-medication is common and drug abuse an increasing problem. Table 28.1 lists some of the drugs where adverse
effects are known or suspected. In some cases the benefits of maternal medication may outweigh the risk to the fetus, for example,
malarial prophylaxis or anticonvulsant therapy.

Drugs which can be given to
breast-feeding mothers

Most drugs are excreted in breast milk, but are usually present in tiny
amounts that are unlikely to harm the child (see references to Table
28.2). Studies have tended to use only a single dose which does not
reflect clinical use. The newborn metabolize and excrete drugs very
inefficiently. Preterm babies are at greater risk. Where practicable,
all drugs should be avoided during breast feeding and mothers should

Table 28.1 The effects on the fetus and neonate of maternal drugs during pregnancy. For a more detailed list see *British National Formulary*

Drug	Possible effect on fetus and neonate
Alcohol	Fetal alcohol syndrome (Chapter 1, page 7)
Aminoglycosides	Eighth nerve damage
Aminophylline	Neonatal irritability
Amiodarone	Goitre
Anticoagulants (oral)	Malformations; fetal and neonatal haemorrhage
Antimalarials:	Possibly teratogenic
Primaquine	Haemolysis; methaemoglobinaemia
Pyrimethamine	Possibly teratogenic
Quinine	Teratogenic in high doses
Aspirin	Fetal and neonatal haemorrhage; rash; kernicterus; metabolic acidosis. High doses could close ductus arteriosus in the fetus
β-Adrenoceptor blockers	Hypoglycaemia; bradycardia
Barbiturates	Neonatal withdrawal syndrome (Chapter 1, page 4)
Benzodiazepines	Respiratory depression; hypotonia; hypothermia
Carbimazole	Goitre; hypothyroidism
Chloramphenicol	Grey-baby syndrome
Clofibrate	Reduced fetal growth
Corticosteroids	High doses may cause adrenal suppression
Cytotoxic drugs	Teratogenic. Possible immune suppression
Diazoxide	Impaired glucose tolerance
Diuretics	Reduce placental perfusion
Ergotamine	Oxytocic effects, vomiting, convulsions
Flucytosine	Possibly teratogenic
Indomethacin	Closure of fetal ductus arteriosus and persistent pulmonary hypertension
Iodides	Goitre; hypothyroidism
Local anaesthetics	Large doses may cause respiratory depression, hypotonia and bradycardia
Lithium	Malformations; goitre; hypotonia and cyanosis
Narcotics	Respiratory depression; withdrawal syndrome
Naproxen	This and other non-steroidal anti-inflammatory drugs have the same effects as indomethacin
Phenobarbitone	Malformations; fetal and neonatal haemorrhage (Chapter 1, page 4 and Chapter 15, page 224); sedation
Phenothiazine derivatives	Occasional extrapyramidal effects
Phenytoin	Malformation; fetal and neonatal haemorrhage (Chapter 1, page 4 and Chapter 15, page 224)
Podophyllum	Possibly teratogenic; neonatal death
Propylthiouracil	Goitre; hypothyroidism
Radioiodine	Destruction of fetal thyroid
Reserpine	Bradycardia; nasal stuffiness

Drugs and prescribing

Table 28.1   *Continued*

Drug	Possible effect on fetus and neonate
Rifampicin	Neonatal haemorrhage
Sex hormones	Virilization of female fetus (Chapter 13, page
Sex hormones	198); possibly teratogenic
Stilboestrol	Vaginal carcinoma
Sulphasalazine	Haemolysis and jaundice
Sulphonamides	Haemolysis and methaemoglobinaemia; risk of kernicterus
Sulphonylureas	Hypoglycaemia
Tetracyclines	Retarded skeletal growth; enamel hypoplasia and stained teeth
Thiazides	Thrombocytopenia
Tricyclic antidepressants	Tachycardia; irritability; muscle spasms
Trimethoprim (and co-trimoxazole)	Possibly teratogenic; same effects as sulphonamides
Valproate sodium	Possibly teratogenic (Neural tube defects; see Chapter 1, page 4)

be warned about self-medication. Recommendations for a nursing
mother are probably over-cautious and mothers who need treatment
should not be prevented from breast feeding if the drug is likely to be
safe. Drugs that are known to have produced adverse effects include
cancer chemotherapy drugs, radiopharmaceuticals, carbimazole,
lithium, ergotamine and phenindione. Others are relatively contraindicated because they reach high concentrations in milk and/or have
effects which could harm the infant.

Table 28.2 gives information on drugs which nursing mothers *can*
use. It includes at least one drug for each condition likely to require
medication.

Table 28.3 gives information on drugs which can be given to
neonates.

Table 28.2 Drugs and breast feeding

Category (as in BNF)	Drugs which may be used	Comments *
(1) Gastrointestinal		
Antacids	Aluminium hydroxide; magnesium carbonate and trisilicate	Little absorbed by mother
Antispasmodics	Mebeverine; propantheline	
Ulcer-healing drugs	Cimetidine ⎫ Ranitidine ⎭	Significant amounts enter milk, but safety is not known
	Sucralfate	Not absorbed by mother
	De-Nol	Absorption of bismuth too low to do harm.
Antidiarrhoeals	Kaolin	Not absorbed.
	Codeine phosphate	Prolonged use of high doses could constipate and sedate infant, and cause dependence*
	Loperamide	Mother absorbs little
	Sulphasalazine	Risk of haemolysis in glucose 6-phosphate dehydrogenase (G6PD)-deficient infants, and of kernicterus in jaundiced infants*
Laxatives	Bran, methylcellulose	Not absorbed by mother
	Bisacodyl; senna	Large doses could cause diarrhoea in baby*
(2) Cardiovascular		
Cardiac glycosides	Digoxin	Minimal amounts in milk. Excretion of other glycosides unknown
β-Adrenoceptor	Atenolol; metoprolol; nadolol; oxprenolol; propranolol; sotalol ⎫⎬⎭	Look for signs of beta-blockade in infant (bradycardia, hypoglycaemia) if mother is on a large dose
Antihypertensives	Labetalol; methyldopa; hydralazine	
Diuretics	Bendrofluazide; chlorothiazide Frusemide (orally) ⎫⎬⎭	May decrease milk production Avoid parental use
Anticoagulants	Heparin	Not present in milk

Table 28.2 *Continued*

Category (as in BNF)	Drugs which may be used	Comments *
	Warfarin	No apparent effect on infant's haemostasis
Haemostatics	Tranexamic acid; ethamsylate	Present in milk

(3) Respiratory system and allergy

Category (as in BNF)	Drugs which may be used	Comments *
Bronchodilators	Salbutamol; isoprenaline	Use by inhalation if possible
	Theophylline; aminophylline	Can make infant irritable
Corticosteroids	Beclomethasone	Preferable to oral corticosteroids
Anti-asthmatics	Sodium cromoglycate	
Antihistamines (H_1)	Chlorphenir- amine; promethazine; clemastine	Infant may become drowsy
Nasal decongestants	Ephedrine; pseudoe- phedrine; xylometazoline	Irritability and disturbed sleep reported with *oral* ephedrine
Cough suppressants	Codeine; pholcodine	Small doses safe (see Section 1 above)

(4) Central nervous system

Category (as in BNF)	Drugs which may be used	Comments *
Hypnotics and sedatives	Benzodiazepines	Drowsiness and poor feeding occur with regular use or high doses
	Chloral hydrate; Dichloral- phenazone	May cause drowsiness
Antipsychotics	Chlorpromazine; fluphenazine; flupenthixol; haloperidol	Little in milk. Drowsiness and other CNS effects* may occur with high oral doses or parental preparations
Antidepressants	Amitriptyline; imipramine; mianserin	Very little in milk
Anti-emetics	Metoclopramide	Very little in milk
	Cyclizine; promethazine	Risk of drowsiness*
Anticonvulsants	Carbamazepine; phenytoin; phe- nobarbitone; primidone	May cause drowsiness. Control maternal blood levels closely
	Sodium valproate	Very little in milk
	Ethosuximide	Significant amounts in milk

Category (as in BNF)	Drugs which may be used	Comments *
Analgesics: Non-narcotic	Paracetamol ⎫ Aspirin ⎭	Safe for occasional use. Dosage exceeding 3 g/day risks metabolic acidosis. Regular use could affect platelet function and prolong the bleeding time*
Narcotic	Codeine Dihydrocodeine; pethidine; morphine	Avoid prolonged use of high doses; monitor infant for CNS depression
(5) Infections Antibacterials	Penicillins; cephalosporins	Induction of hypersensitivity* possible
	Aminoglycosides	Intestinal bacteria could develop resistance*
	Erythromycin; trimethoprim	Significant amounts in milk
	Sulphonamides	Avoid in G6PD-deficient infants
	Co-trimoxacole	Risk of kernicterus in jaundiced infants*
	Metronidazole	Makes milk taste bitter and child may stop suckling. Where single-dose therapy is suitable, a 24-hour break in breast feeding may avoid this
Urinary tract	Nitrofurantoin	Avoid in G-6-PD-deficient infants*
Antituberculous	Rifampicin	Present in milk but not known to harm
	Isoniazid	Significant amounts in milk. Risk of neurotoxicity.* Mother and baby should be given pyridoxine
	Ethambutol	Very little in milk. Risk of ocular toxicity*
Antifungals	Nystatin	Not absorbed from gut. Safety of systemic antifungals (amphotericin, flucytosine, miconazole etc.) unknown
Antimalarials	Chloroquine and proguanil	For prophylaxis
	Pyrimethamine	Avoid Maloprim and Fansidar in G6PD-dependent infants*
Anthelminitics	Mebendazole	Poorly absorbed from the gut

Table 28.2 *Continued*

Category (as in BNF)	Drugs which may be used	Comments *
(6) Endocrine system		
Antidiabetics	Insulins	
	Glibenclamide	Possible hypoglycaemia,* monitor infant's blood glucose
Thyroid hormones	Thyroxine	Might interfere with screening of infant for hypothyroidism*
Antithyroid drugs	Propylthiouracil	Probably too little in milk to affect infant, but use propanolol instead if possible
Corticosteroids	Prednisolone	Probably safe in doses not exceeding 10 mg/day. Larger doses might cause adrenal suppression*
Sex hormones		
Oestrogens	Ethinyloestradiol	Doses above 50 µg/day decrease milk production and may cause feminization in male infants
Oral contraceptives	Combined oestrogen/ progestogen	Established lactation is not affected by low-dose preparations (<50 µg ethinyloestradiol)
	Progestogen only	Do not suppress lactation. Too little in milk to affect baby
(7) Vitamins and minerals		
Vitamins	Vitamin A	High doses (>2500 units daily) risk hypervitaminosis
	Vitamin D	High doses (>500 units daily) risk hypervitaminosis
	Vitamin B group Ascorbic acid Folic acid	
Iron salts	Ferrous sulphate etc.	
(8) Musculoskeletal system		
Anti-inflammatory analgesics	Naproxen; ibuprofen Ketoprofen; mefenamic acid; fenbufen	Very little in milk

BNF, *British National Formulary*. Information about specific drugs (especially if marketed recently) can often be obtained from the manufacturer or the NHS Drug Information Centres. The BNF gives further information about drugs contraindicated during breast feeding. *Indicates a theoretical risk.

References
(1) Anderson, P. O. (1977). *Drugs Intell. Clin. Pharm.*, **11**, 208–23.
(2) Giacala, G. P. and Catz, C. S. (1979). *Clin. Perinatalol*, **6**, 181–6.
(3) Wilson, J. T., Brown, R. D., Cherek, D. R. **et al.** (1980). *Clin. Pharmoacokinet.*, **5**, 1–66.
(4) American Academy of Pediatrics (1982). *Pediatrics*, **69**, 241–4.
(5) Beeley, L. (1981). *Clin. Obstet. Gynaec.*, **8**, 291–5.
(6) Chaplin, S., Sanders, G. L. and Smith, J. M. (1982). *Adv. Drug React. Ac. Pois. Rev.*, **1**, 255–87.
(7) *Drug and Therapeutics Bulletin* (1982). **20**, 102–4.

Taken from *Drug and Therapeutics Bulletin*, Volume 21, Number 2, 1983, with permission of the Editor and the Consumers Association.

Bibliography
British National Formulary, Number 19, 1990, Prescribing in pregnancy, p. 28; Prescribing during breast feeding, p. 34.
American Academy of Pediatrics (1989). Transfer of drugs and other chemicals to human milk. *Pediatrics*, **84**, 924–36.

Blood and blood products

It is essential that all blood and blood products are tested and shown to be negative for cytomegalovirus, hepatitis B and HIV before administration.

Albumin

1.0 g/kg i.v. slowly
1.0 g albumin is contained in 4 ml of 25% salt-poor solution

Blood

6 ml of donor whole blood (3 ml of packed cells) per kg body weight will raise the haemoglobin of the baby by 1 g/100 ml

Volume of whole blood (packed cell volume, PCV = 40%) to be given = weight in kg × required rise haemoglobin (Hb) × 6

Volume of partially packed cells (PCV = 60%) = weight in kg × require rise in Hb × 4

Volume of packed cells (PCV = 80%) = weight in kg × required rise in Hb × 3

Drugs and prescribing

Platelets

One unit of platelets will raise the peripheral platelet count by approximately 50 000 (give no more than 20 ml/kg)

Plasma (fresh frozen)

For treating shock, 10–15 ml/kg, over a period of 1 hour
For replacing clotting factors etc., 10 ml/kg
For dilutional exchange, 20–30 ml/kg

Comment: Whole blood/packed cells/platelets should be given using a syringe pump or volumetric infusion pump but **NEVER** by peristaltic infusion pump.

Bibliography

Loeb, S., Hamilton, H. K. (1990). *Handbook of Pediatric Drug Therapy*. Pennsylvania: Springhouse.

Table 28.3 Suggested neonatal drug doses and administration

Drug	Single dose/kg	Frequency	Route	Comments
Acetazolamide	5 mg	Daily	oral; i.v.	As a diuretic
Acetylcysteine	10 ml	6 hourly	Gastric tube	5% solution used in treatment of meconium ileus
	20 ml	Daily	Enema	
Corticotrophin (ACTH) (aqueous)	1 mg	6 hourly	i.m.	
Adrenaline 1/10 000	0.5 microg	Per minute	i.v. infusion	For severe hypotension
	0.1 ml	Once	i.v. intracardiac Endotracheal	For cardiac arrest
Alfacalcidol (1-alpha-vitamin D)	0.05 microg	Daily	Oral	
Aminophylline	6 mg	Loading dose	Oral; i.v.	Alter dose according to blood levels Therapeutic range for neonatal apnoea 28–55 microg/L
	2 mg	12 hourly		
Atropine	0.01 mg	Once	i.v.; i.m.	
Calcium gluconate (10%)	1–2 ml (0.2–0.4 mmol)	Once	Slow i.v. infusion	Use ECG monitoring (see page 197)
		8 hourly	Oral	

Drugs and prescribing

Table 28.3 *Continued*

Drug	Single dose/kg	Frequency	Route	Comments
Captopril	0.3 mg	8–12 hourly	Oral	See manufacturer's literature
Chloral hydrate	10–30 mg	8 hourly PRN	Oral	
Chlorothiazide	12.5 mg	12 hourly	Oral	
Cimetidine	10 mg	8 hourly	i.v.	H$_2$ antagonist
Chlorpromazine	1 mg	8 hourly	Oral	For drug withdrawal symptoms
Clonazepam	0.1 mg 25 microg	Once 12 hourly	Slow i.v. i.v., oral	For status epilepticus Dosage may be gradually increased to 250 microg/kg/day
Cortisone	0.5 mg	12 hourly	Oral	
Dexamethasone	0.2 mg	8 hourly	i.v., oral	7 day course for bronchopulmonary dyplasia (BPD). A further tapering 9 day course may be needed
Diazoxide	5 mg	8 hourly	Oral	Na$^+$ retention. Oedema. Hyperglycaemia
Digoxin	**Term baby** 5 microg **Preterm baby** 4 microg	12 hourly 12 hourly	Oral Oral	Check blood levels, toxicity uncommon below 3.5 ng/ml
Dobutamine	2–10 microg	per minute	Continuous i.v. infusion	Start with lowest dose

	Dose	Frequency	Route	Notes
Dopamine	**Low dose** 1–2 microg	Per minute	Continuous i.v. infusion	Vasodilation of mesenteric, renal, coronary and cerebral blood vessels. No cardiac effect
	Medium dose 2–10 microg	Per minute	Continuous i.v. infusion	Increases cardiac output Recommended dose 5 microg/kg/min
	High dose Over 10 microg	Per minute	Continuous i.v. infusion	Vasoconstriction Increase in blood pressure High dose may cause gangrene
Doxapram	0.5–1.5 mg	Per hour	i.v. infusion	See *Pediatrics*, 1987, **80**, 22
Edrophonium	0.5 mg	Once	i.m./slow i.v.	Test of myaesthenia If causes bradycardia, antidote is atropine
Ethamsylate	12.5 mg	6 hourly for 16 doses	i.m.; i.v.	To reduce risk of cerebral haemorrhage in preterm baby
Frusemide	1 mg	12 to 24 hourly	Oral, i.m., slow i.v.	Potentiates toxic effects of aminoglycocides Calciuric
9-α Fludrocortisone	100 micrograms total dose	Daily	Oral	See page 200
Glucagon	0.1 mg	4 hourly	i.v.	May cause rebound hypoglycaemia

Drugs and prescribing

Table 28.3 *Continued*

Drug	Single dose/kg	Frequency	Route	Comments
Heparin	100 units	12 hourly	i.m.	Modify dose according to clotting studies
Hydrocortisone	2.5 mg 25 mg	6 hourly Once	i.v., i.m. i.v.	For shock
Hydralazine	0.5 mg	8 hourly	Oral, i.m., i.v.	Modify dose according to response. Beware of hypotension
Indomethacin	0.1 mg	24 hourly to a maximum of 6 doses	i.v., oral	For closure of patent ductus arteriosus (PDA) Renal toxicity See page 127
Insulin	0.1 unit	According to blood glucose levels	s.c., i.m., i.v. infusion	Beware hypoglycaemia
Isoprenaline	0.1–0.5 microg	Per minute	Continuous i.v. infusion	For bradycardia and hypotension
Lignocaine	1 mg 20 microg	Once Per minute	i.v. slowly Continuous i.v. infusion	For cardiac arrythmia
Magnesium sulphate (50%)	0.2 ml	12 hourly Maximum of 3 doses	i.m.	0.2 ml (= 0.6 mEq of magnesium)

Mannitol (20%)	2 ml	Once	i.v. infusion over 30 min	For management of cerebral oedema see Chapter 10
Methyldopa	2.5 mg	8 hourly	Oral, i.v.	Increase up to 5 mg/kg according to response
Morphine	0.1 mg 5–20 microg	6 hourly Per hour	i.v., i.m. Continuous i.v. infusion	For sedation of babies on ventilation
Naloxone (neonatal)	10 microg	Once, but may be repeated at 2–3 min intervals	s.c., i.m., i.v.	Narcan Neonatal contains 20 microg/ml
Neostigmine	0.04 mg 1 mg	Once 6 hourly	i.m. Oral	Myasthenia test Maintenance
Nitroprusside (sodium)	0.5 microg	Per minute	Continuous i.v. infusion	Beware of severe hypotension and thiocyanate toxicity. (Benitz et al. J. Pediat. 1985, **106**, 102–10)
Pancuronium	0.05 mg	As required	i.v.	
Paraldehyde	0.1 ml 1 ml of 5% solution made up in 5% glucose	Once Per hour	Deep i.m. Continuous i.v. infusion Change syringe every 12 hours	Use glass syringe Up to 3 ml/kg/hour may be needed to control status epilepticus. Protect from light
Pethidine	1 mg	12 hourly	i.m.	Beware respiratory depression

Drugs and prescribing

Table 28.3 *Continued*

Drug	Single dose/kg	Frequency	Route	Comments
Phenobarbitone	10 mg	2 doses 30 min apart	i.v. over 5–10 min	See Chapter 10 for control of convulsions
	2 mg	12 hourly	i.m., oral	Maintenance
Phenytoin	20 mg	Once	i.v. over 15 min	Monitor ECG, may cause arrhythmia. See Chapter 10 for control of convulsions
	2.5 mg	12 hourly	Oral	Maintenance
Prednisolone	0.5 mg	6 hourly	Oral, i.m., i.v.	
Propanolol	0.05 mg	Once	i.v.	
	0.2–0.5 mg	8 hourly	Oral	Maintenance
Prostaglandin E_2	10 ng	Per minute	Continuous i.v. infusion	May be increased up to 50 ng/kg/min see page 122
Prostacyclin (Epoprostenol)	5–10 ng	Per minute	Continuous i.v. infusion	Beware of hypotension. Change infusion every 12 hours
Protamine	1 mg/100 units of last dose of heparin	Once	i.v.	
Pyridoxine	50 mg total dose	Once	i.v.	

Spironolactone	1.5 mg	12 hourly	Oral	
Theophylline	5 mg 1–2 mg	Once 8 hourly	Oral, i.v. Oral, i.v.	Loading dose Adjust dose according to blood levels
Thyroxine	*Preterm* 8–10 microg *Term* 5–8 microg	Daily	Oral	See Chapter 13
Tolazoline	1 mg 0.1 mg	Once Per hour	i.v. Continuous i.v. infusion	Beware of hypotension, GI bleeding. May increase infusion rate to 1.0 mg/kg/hour according to response
ANTIBIOTICS				
Amikacin	10 mg 7.5 mg	Once 12 hourly	i.v. i.v.	Loading dose
Ampicillin	30 mg	<7 days old 12 hourly >7 days old 8 hourly	Oral, i.m.	50 mg/kg/6 hourly for meningitis
Azlocillin	*Preterm* 50 mg *Term* 100 mg	12 hourly { <7 days old 12 hourly >7 days old 8 hourly }	i.v. i.v.	Must not be mixed in same syringe or infusion as aminoglycosides

Drugs and prescribing

Table 28.3 *Continued*

Drug	Single dose/kg	Frequency	Route	Comments
Cloxacillin } Flucloxacillin	25 mg	<7 days old 12 hourly >7 days old 8 hourly	Oral, i.m., i.v.	
Cefotaxime	25 mg	12 hourly	i.m., i.v.	In severe infections 150–200 mg/kg/day may be given
Ceftazidime	30 mg	12 hourly	i.m., i.v.	Half life is 3–4 times that in adults
Cefuroxime	15 mg	12 hourly	i.m., i.v.	100 mg/kg/day should be given for meningitis
Chloramphenicol	25 mg	All infants <14 days old 24 hourly Infants >14 days old 12 hourly	oral, i.v.	Always monitor blood level Therapeutic range 15–25 mg/l Toxic level 50 mg/l Total daily dose should not exceed 25 mg/kg for infants <2.0 kg regardless of age
Erythromycin	12 mg	6–8 hourly depending on severity of infection	Oral, i.v.	Excreted by liver so use with caution in presence of jaundice or immaturity
Fucidic acid	5 mg	6 hourly	Oral, i.v.	For i.v. use dissolve powder in buffer provided and infuse dose over 6 hours

Drug	Dose	Interval	Route	Comments
Gentamicin	2.5 mg	*Preterm and term* <7 days old 12 hourly *Term* >7 days old 8 hourly	i.m., i.v.	Monitor blood levels Peak 4–8 microg/ml Trough <2 microg/ml
Isoniazid	5 mg	12 hourly	Oral	Pyridoxine supplement should be given
Metronidazole	7.5 mg	8 hourly	Oral, i.v.	
Netilmicin	3 mg	*Preterm and term* <7 days old 12 hourly *Term* >7 days old 8 hourly	i.m., i.v.	Monitor blood levels Peak 6–12 microg/ml Trough <2.5 microg/ml
Penicillin G (benzylpenicillin)	15 mg	12 hourly for infants <7 days old 8 hourly for infants >7 days old	i.m., i.v.	Give 30 mg/kg/dose for streptococcal infection
Piperacillin	50 mg	12 hourly	i.m., i.v.	
Rifampicin	5 mg	12 hourly	Oral	Use with caution in jaundiced infants
Trimethoprim	4 mg 3 mg 2 mg	12 hourly 12 hourly Daily for prophylaxis	Oral i.v. Oral	Not recommended in first 14 days

Drugs and prescribing

Table 28.3 Continued

Drug	Single dose/kg	Frequency	Route	Comments
Tobramycin	2 mg	12 hourly for infants <7 days old 8 hourly for infants >7 days old	i.m., i.v.	Monitor blood levels as for gentamicin
Vancomycin	15 mg	12 hourly	i.v. infusion over 1 hour	Monitor blood levels Peak 25–40 microg/ml Trough 5–10 microg/ml
ANTI-FUNGAL AGENTS				
Amphotericin B	0.1 mg increasing over 7 days to 1.0 mg	Daily	i.v. infusion over 6 hours	Reduced renal function is a common side-effect 4–6 weeks treatment may be needed for systemic fungal infections
5-Flucytosine	50 mg	6 hourly	Oral	Usually given in combination with amphotericin
Miconazole	10 mg	12 hourly	i.v. infusion over 1 hour	Also available as 2% gel for oral or topical use
Nystatin	100 000 units (1 ml)	6 hourly	Oral (not absorbed) from GI tract	Also available as cream for topical use

Units for drug doses: 1 gram (g) = 1000 milligrams (mg); 1 milligram = 1000 micrograms (microg); 1 microgram = 1000 nanograms (ng). When prescribing doses in micrograms or nanograms, these should be written out in full and not abbreviated.

29

Medical audit

Neonatal documentation
Standardization of data collection
Perinatal definitions
Perinatal statistics
Perinatal audit
Perinatal mortality statistics
Audit of neonatal workload
Medical audit

Neonatal documentation

The neonatal period is the first and often the most critical chapter in the life of a new individual and client of the National Health Service. It is essential that it should be well documented for medical and also for legal reasons. Therefore, as the Korner Committee recommended in 1987, *every baby should be identified administratively and documented* as a patient at birth with an independent medical record, unit number and, eventually, a neonatal discharge record.

The neonatal record should be initiated following the first clinical examination on the first day of life, updated as necessary, and completed when the infant is examined within 24 hours before leaving hospital, or at around the 8–10th day.

As several members of the medical team may be involved in the care of each infant, it is essential that notes are written promptly and clearly, and that the doctor writing them signs his name legible.

The neonatal discharge record should be completed by the doctor undertaking the discharge examination. Copies should be made available to the GP and other members of the primary health care team (midwife/health visitor), the obstetrician and the District Health Authority or other body responsible for keeping perinatal data and statistics. A copy should also be retained in the infant's record.

Standardization of data collection

In order to collect clinical data and prepare statistics that are comparable within and between all health districts, it is important that a standard methodology (including definitions) should be used. Standard national forms are available for the notification of birth (within 36 hours), birth registration (within 6 weeks), neonatal death certifications, and the neonatal discharge record (see Dunn, 1980). The minimum data set for mother and baby recommended by the Körner Committee (1982) may be found in Table 29.1.

Perinatal definitions (see Fig. 29.1)

Livebirth

Signs of life observed after complete expulsion from the mother, irrespective of duration of pregnancy. Signs of life include breathing, heart beat, cord pulsation or voluntary movement.

Stillbirth (or late fetal death)

A fetal death prior to complete delivery of a baby born after the 28th week of pregnancy (196 days after the first day of the last menstrual period, LMP).

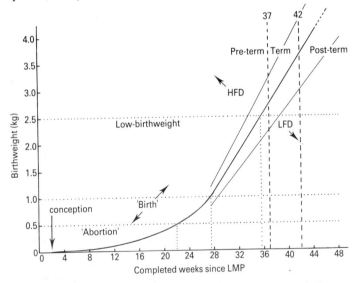

Fig. 29.1   Definitions relating to birthweight and gestational age (JFD = heavy-for-dates; LFD = light-for-dates)

Abortion

A conceptus born without signs of life before the end of the 28th week of pregnancy (<196 days from the LMP).

Birthweight

The first weight of the fetus or newborn infant obtained after birth (preferably measured within the first hour).

Low birthweight

A birthweight of less than 2500 g.

Gestational age

The duration of gestation measured from the first day of the last normal menstrual period and expressed in complete days or weeks.

Preterm

Less than 37 completed weeks (less than 259 days).

Term

From 37 to less than 42 completed weeks (259–293 days).

Post-term

Forty-two completed weeks or more (294 days or more).

The neonatal period

The first 28 days after delivery.

Lethal congenital malformation

Death due primarily to congenital malformation (see Chapter XIV of the WHO *International Classification of Diseases*).

Heavy- or light-for-dates infants

Usually classified as infants above the 90th percentile or below the 10th percentile of birthweight distribution at any given gestational age. The standard birthweight-for-gestation reference chart shown in Fig. 29.2 may be used in the perinatal period. More extended standard birthweight-for-gestation reference charts, including head circumference and length may be found in Chapter 19.

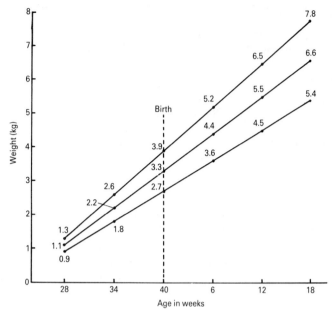

Fig. 29.2 Bristol perinatal growth chart with lines representing the 10th, 50th and 90th percentiles of weight-for-age of an average caucasian population from 28 weeks gestation to 18 weeks after term. Weights are shown at 6-week intervals. (Dunn, 1979, *Perinatal Medicine*, Stuttgart: Georg Thieme Verlag.)

Perinatal statistics

The stillbirth rate

The number of stillbirths per 1000 infants delivered.

The neonatal mortality rate

The number of infants dying in the neonatal period per 1000 live-births.

The perinatal mortality rate

The number of stillbirths and first-week deaths per 1000 total deliveries.

Perinatal audit

In order to compute mortality rates and evaluate other relevant

Table 29.1   Maternity data items and methods of collection

(a) Data items in the minimum data set collected by methods used for all patients

Mother	Each baby
Number/identifier	Number/identifier
—	Sex
Address code	Address code
Date of birth	Date of birth
Marital status	—
Category of patient	—
GP code	GP code
Method of admission	Method of admission
Source of admission	Source of admission
Date of 1st antenatal assessment	—
Intended management	—
Wards occupied	Wards occupied
Operative procedures	Operative procedures
Method of discharge	Method of discharge
Destination on discharge	Destination on discharge
Consultant/GP codes	Consultant/GP codes
ICD diagnoses	BPA diagnoses (ICD compatible)

(b) Data items collected by notification of each birth

Mother	Baby	Delivery	Identifiers
Parity	Birth order	Place of delivery	Mother's number/identifier
	Live/stillbirth	Original intention	Mother's date of birth
	Birthweight	Reason for change	Baby's number/identifier
	Resuscitation	Number of babies	Baby's date of birth
		Length of gestation	Baby's time of delivery
		Method of labour onset	
		Method of delivery	

(c) Data items obtained from the registration of each birth

Parental occupation   Baby's NHS number

(d) Data items in the clinical options

Mother	Delivery	Each baby
Height	Length of 1st stage	Head circumference at birth
Blood group	Length of 2nd stage	Birth length
Previous pregnancies	Pain relief given	Apgar score
	Presentation of fetus	Hips examination
		Jaundice presence
		Type of feeding established
		PKU + BCG performed
		Gestation (paediatric assessment)
		Additional diagnoses
		Follow-up arrangements

Körner Committee Recommendations (1982).
ICD, International Classification of disease.
BPA, British Paediatric Association
PKU, phenylketonuria.

information it is necessary to obtain corresponding information on all births (see Table 29.2) so that population statistics may be produced. The importance of obtaining post-mortem confirmation of the cause of death, including histology, cannot be over-emphasized.

Perinatal Mortality and Morbidity Committees are desirable at local, as well as at regional and national levels, with representation from the following disciplines: obstetrics, paediatrics, pathology, midwifery/nursing/health visiting, epidemiology and administration. The mother's GP should also be invited to attend or express his opinion. In some areas a midwife or health visitor seeks the mother's view of the events leading up to the death of her child; this often provides a valuable new insight into health-care management. Most hospitals or Districts arrange monthly meetings to discuss perinatal deaths which occurred in the previous month while memories are fresh. The consolidated findings of each year may then be prepared as an annual report, after removing all identification that might lead to a break in confidentiality.

Perinatal mortality statistics

The World Health Organization has recommended that *national* perinatal statistics should include all fetuses and infants delivered weighing at least 500 g or, when birthweight is unavailable, the corresponding gestational age (22 weeks) or body length 25 cm crown–heel), whether alive or dead.

Table 29.2 Livebirth, stillbirth and neonatal death certification

	Record linkage
	Methodology
Birth certificate	**Perinatal death certificate**
Name/address of mother	Name/address of mother
Date/hour of birth	Date/hour of birth
Place of birth	Place of birth
Single/multiple birth	Single/multiple birth
Sex of infant	Sex of infant
Birthweight	Birthweight
Live/still born	
	If stillborn:
	Died before labour/during labour/not known
	If neonatal death:
	Date/hour of death
	Necropsy: Yes/No
	Lethal malformation observed: Yes/no

It is recommended that national statistics should include fetuses and infants weighing between 500 g and 1000 g, both for their inherent value and because their inclusion improves the completeness of reporting at 1000 g and over. Inclusion of this group of very immature births, however, disrupts international comparisons because of differences in national practices concerning their registration. Another factor affecting international comparisons is that all liveborn infants, irrespective of birthweight, are included in the calculation of rates, whereas some lower limit of maturity is applied to infants born dead.

Table 29.3 FIGO recommendations. Perinatal statistics for a specific population

---

Information required

Number of: Total births ≥ 500 g
Stillbirths ≥ 500 g
Early (first week) neonatal deaths
Late (2–4th weeks) neonatal deaths

Number of: Births < 1 kg
Stillbirths < 1 kg
Early neonatal deaths < 1 kg
Late neonatal deaths < 1 kg

Number of: Infants with lethal malformations
Stillbirths with lethal malformations
Early neonatal deaths with lethal malformations
Late neonatal deaths with lethal malformations

Number of: Infants < 1 kg with lethal malformations
Stillbirths < 1 kg with lethal malformations
Early neonatal deaths < 1 kg with lethal malformations
Late neonatal deaths < 1 kg with lethal malformations

Perinatal statistics
Lethal malformation rate per 1000 total births
Stillbirth rate per 1000 total births
Neonatal mortality rate per 1000 livebirths
Perinatal mortality rate per 1000 total births

Excluding lethal malformations (includes < 1 kg)
Stillbirth rate per 1000 total births
Neonatal mortality rate per 1000 livebirths
Perinatal mortality rate per 1000 total births

Excluding births < 1 kg (includes malformation)
Stillbirth rate per 1000 total births
Neonatal mortality rate per 1000 livebirths
Perinatal mortality rate per 1000 total births

Excluding lethal malformations and births < 1 kg
Stillbirth rate per 1000 total births
Neonatal mortality rate per 1000 livebirths
Perinatal mortality rate per 1000 total births

In order to eliminate these factors, it is recommended that countries should present, solely for *international* comparisons, 'standard perinatal statistics' in which both the numerator and denominator of all rates are restricted to fetuses and infants weighing 1000 g or more or, where birthweight is unavailable, the corresponding gestational age (28 weeks) or body length (35 cm crown–heel). Table 29.3 shows a standard form of presentation for such statistics, as recommended by FIGO.

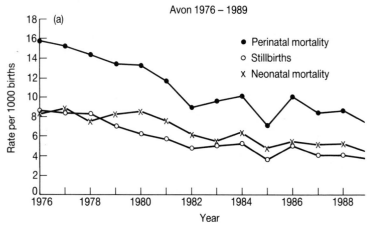

Fig. 29.3a   Perinatal and neonatal mortality rates.

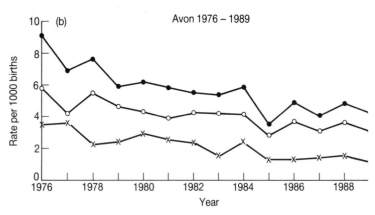

Fig. 29.3b   Perinatal and neonatal mortality rates (excluding malformations and less than 1o00 g)

Perinatal mortality statistics
for Avon County and the UK

The perinatal mortality in the UK in 1989 was approximately 8 per 1000 births, half being stillborn and half being first-week deaths. About a quarter of these perinatal deaths were due to lethal malformations and another quarter involved infants weighing less than 1 kg at birth. Figures 29.3a,b shows the perinatal neonatal mortality rates for babies born to Avon County residents over the period 1976–1989 (total number of births = 138 962).

The post-neonatal infant mortality rate (1 month to 1 year) is similar to the neonatal mortality rate, but has fallen very little in the period 1984–1989.

The breakdown of the major groups of conditions contributing to infant mortality (birth to 1 year) in Avon County over the six-year period 1984–1989, inclusive, is shown in Fig. 29.4 (mean infant mortality rate 9.7/1000 live births).

Figure 29.5 shows survival by gestation in 1989 in the two Bristol maternity hospitals.

Audit of neonatal workload

In order to establish the staffing and facilities required for neonatal care in a unit, infants may be grouped into one of three categories:

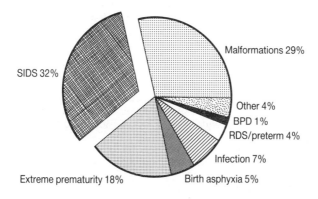

$n = 600$

Fig. 29.4 Avon infant mortality study 1984–1989. Summary of 'causes' of infant deaths.

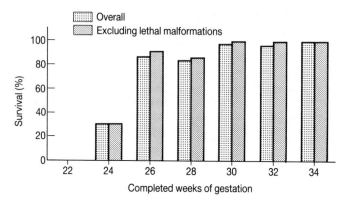

Fig. 29.5   Survival rates by gestation for infants born in the two University of Bristol teaching hospitals in 1989. For infants without lethal malformations born at or beyond 30 weeks gestation survival was >99%.

intensive, special and routine care. Examples are given below. Audit may be undertaken during each nursing shift, or one a day on the basis of the previous 24 hours' experience. All babies using the facilities or staff of the unit should be counted, including those being transferred or undergoing surgery. The count should include babies in the postnatal wards. Babies who require a level of care which cannot be provided because of lack of staff or facilities should be included in the category reflecting the level of care required (British Paediatrics Association/British Association for Perinatal Paediatris, 1984).

Intensive care

'Care given in a special or intensive-care nursery which provides continuous skilled supervision by nursing and medical staff.'

The following groups should be considered to be receiving intensive care:

Babies receiving assisted ventilation: intermittent positive-pressure ventilation (IPPV), intermittent mandatory ventilation (IMV), constant positive airway pressure (CPAP), and in the first 24 hours following its withdrawal.

Babies receiving total parental nutrition.

Babies with cardiorespiratory disease which is unstable, including recurrent apnoea requiring constant attention.

Babies who have had major surgery, particularly in the first 24 postoperative hours.

Babies of less than 30 weeks' gestation, during the first 48 hours after birth.

Babies who are having convulsions.

Babies transported by the staff of the unit concerned. This would usually be between hospitals, or for special investigations or treatment.

Babies undergoing major medical procedures such as arterial catheterization, peritoneal dialysis, or exchange transfusions.

Special care

'Care given in a special care nursery or on a postnatal ward which provides observation and treatment falling short of intensive care but exceeding normal routine care.'

The following groups of babies should be considered to be receiving special care:

Babies who require continuous monitoring of respiration, heart rate, or by transcutaneous transducers.

Those receiving additional oxygen.

Babies receiving intravenous glucose and electrolyte solutions.

Babies who are being tube fed.

Those who have had minor surgery in the previous 24 hours.

Babies with a tracheostomy.

Dying babies.

Babies who are being barrier nursed.

Babies receiving phototherapy.

Babies who receive special monitoring (for example, frequent glucose or bilirubin estimations).

Babies receiving antibiotics.

Those with conditions requiring radiological examination or other methods of imaging other than routine screening.

Normal care

'Care given, usually, by the mother in a postnatal ward with supervision by a midwife and doctor but remaining minimal medical or nursing advice.'

All babies not included in the above special or intensive care groups may be regarded as receiving 'normal care'.

Medical audit

This provides a mechanism for assessing and improving the quality of patient care; enhancing medical education by promoting discussion between colleagues about practice; and identifying ways of improving the efficiency of clinical care.

Three main categories of clinical care should be measured.

Structure: the quantity and type of resources available.

Process: what is done to the patient.

Outcome: the result of clinical intervention.

To improve clinical practice it is necessary to:

Observe practice: what actually happens.

Set a standard of practice: what should happen.

Compare observed practice with standard practice

Implement changes

Observe practice after changes implemented

Feedback information: to health care team.

All systems of medical audit should be educational and relevant to patient care; should be controlled by clinical peers with voluntary participation; should be set up locally by participating clinicians; should be non-threatening, interesting, objective and respectable; should be cheap, simple and cause minimal disturbance; should involve adequate and easily retrievable clinical records.

Medical audit and its outcome may be summarized by the following words:

Ascertainment, objectives, standards, organization, education, prevention, therapy, evaluation and *information feedback* to which should be added the catalysts of *goodwill, friendship, co-operation* and *service.*

Bibliography

British Paediatric Association/British Association for Perinatal Paediatrics (1984). *Categories of Babies receiving Neonatal Care.* London.

Dunn, P. M. (1979). Perinatal terminology, definitions and statistics. In: *Perinatal Medicine*, pp. 1–19 (6th European Congress, Vienna 1978). Ed. O. Thalhammer, K. Baumgarten and A. Pollak, Stuttgart: Georg Thieme Verlag.

Dunn, P. M. (1980). A standard neonatal discharge record. In: *Perinatal Audit and Surveillance*, pp. 93–105. Eds I. Chalmers and G. McIlwaine. London: Royal College of Obstetricians and Gynaecologists.

International Federation of Gynecologists and Obstetricians (1983). *Report of the FIGO Committee on Perinatal Mortality and Morbidity* (Workshop on Monitoring and Reporting Perinatal Mortality and Morbidity, Heidelberg, March, 1982). Geneva: FIGO.

Mutch, L. M. M., Brown, N. J., Speidel, B. D. and Dunn, P. M. (1981). Perinatal mortality and neonatal survival in Avon, 1976–79. *Br. Med. J.*, **282**, 119.

NHS/DHSS Steering Group on Health Services Information (1982). *First Report*, pp. 24, 29, 45–49. Chairman Mrs E. Korner. London: HMSO.

Report of the Royal College of Physicians (1989). *Medical Audit. A First Report. What, Why and How.* London: Royal College of Physicians of London.

World Health Organization (1979). Perinatal mortality. Definitions and recommendations. *International Classification of Diseases*, 9th edn, Volume 1, pp. 731–7, 763–8. Geneva: WHO.

30

Medical ethics and the severely malformed or handicapped infant

---

General principles
Guidelines on decisions to withhold or withdraw support

General principles

A doctor has two main duties: to act in the interest of the patient and to preserve life and health. When these two duties are in conflict, they give rise to ethical dilemmas of great complexity and difficulty, especially in relation to infants with severe malformation, those with brain death, and those of extreme prematurity. Modern medicine provides the means to prevent death in circumstances in which prolonged life may not be considered to be in the interests of the patient. While adults in sound mind may exercise their right to refuse life-saving treatment, such a right does not exist in law for children and newborn infants. In practice in the UK (and in many other countries) doctors and parents have always used their discretion and the law has been content to permit this, provided no direct action is taken to end life. In recent years, though, concerned pressure groups have sought to deny this discretion and hence deprive infants of the 'right-to-die' from natural causes. However, attempts to invoke the strictest interpretation of the law to prosecute doctors for murder in such circumstances have been unsuccessful, and society has indicated its wish to leave these difficult decisions in the hands of the parents and their medical advisers as long as they act responsibly and within the consensus view of what is currently considered acceptable (Fig. 30.1). The view of society in this respect is not immutable but evolves in response to changing attitudes and conditions, such as advances in medical care.

It has been suggested that the law should be modified to protect doctors involved in the withholding or withdrawing of medical care from the severely malformed or handicapped infant. The problem is

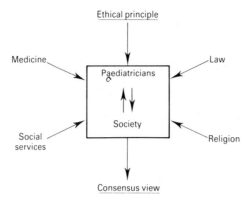

Fig. 30.1 Parties involved in a consensus view.

that there are so many variables between and within each individual case, that such a law would be most difficult to frame and interpret. Probably it is preferable for doctors to continue to strive to serve their patients' interests in these ethical dilemmas, knowing at the same time that they may be called upon to defend and justify their actions before the law.

Another suggestion that has been made is that decisions in individual cases should be decided by ethical committees. However, experience has shown that such committees tend to be ponderous and insensitive and also tend to err on the side of continued life-support. The wider discussion and even publicity that may result is also capable of causing great distress to the already grief-stricken family. While parents and doctors may wish to seek advice from a variety of sources (Fig. 30.2), their final and usually agonizing decision is best reached after private discussions.

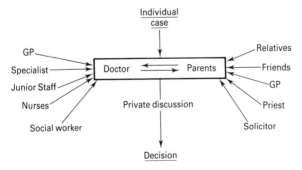

Fig. 30.2 Parties involved in private decision making.

Guidelines on decisions to withhold or withdraw support

Advice and decisions on the withholding (or withdrawal) of medical/ surgical measures required to preserve life should be made by the most senior doctor available, usually the consultant.

In an emergency, as at resuscitation in the delivery room, a junior doctor must exercise his/her clinical judgement. If in any doubt, resuscitation care should be provided until further investigations can be made and the opinion of a senior doctor sought.

Advice and decisions on the withholding of medical care should be based on careful clinical examination, supplemented by appropriate special investigations. The findings should always be carefully documented. Photographs are an important part of the record.

Whenever possible, a second opinion should be sought from another senior doctor. This is particularly desirable when the patient's medical problem would normally necessitate assistance from another discipline (e.g. spina bifida and neurosurgery; see Chapter 10, page 148).

The doctor responsible for the patient would also be wise always to discuss his thoughts on the management options with his own medical and nursing teams, and in turn listen to their views. They, too, are involved in the outcome of any ethical decision, even though it is the leader of the team who takes final responsibility for the decision.

Whenever possible the parents should be fully informed of their baby's condition and prognosis and also of the management options. They should be encouraged to seek advice, if they so wish, from others such as their GP (see Fig. 30.2) and should always have the opportunity to talk together alone before reaching a decision. In many instances the doctor will not be seeking a decision but will rather be trying as sensitively as possible to gain insight as to the parents' wishes should some life-threatening event arise. A skilful and sensitive doctor prepared to spend time with the parents can acquire this knowledge while sparing them much avoidable distress and feelings of guilt (see Chapter 20).

In reaching a decision to withhold medical care, both doctor and parents should have only one aim in mind – *to act in the interests of the baby*. While the interests of the family cannot be completely discounted, those of society should be. In obtaining the considered views of the parents, the doctor should convince himself that their decision is a loving one in their child's interest, as well as being medically justifiable.

The withholding of medical or surgical care, which may be partial or complete according to the circumstances, does not of course imply withdrawal of love or of the routine non-medical care to which all human beings are entitled. Parents should be encouraged to maintain close contact with their child. They will of course need continuing support.

The pain and distress of a severely malformed or handicapped infant may be such that parents may ask their doctor to take active steps to end life. Such appeals should be sympathetically but firmly resisted. Neither medical ethics nor the law permits doctors to undertake actions which have the intention of shortening the life or killing the patient, however much it may appear to be in his or her interest. On the other hand, no patient should be allowed to suffer unnecessarily and in the circumstances under discussion it would be wrong to withhold drugs capable of relieving pain or distress (even though they may also on occasion shorten life).

The reasons for the decision to withhold care and the outcome of discussions with the parents should be carefully documented. The clinical progress should be regularly annotated, as should the reasons for giving drugs such as analgesics or sedatives.

In the event of the baby's death, permission should be sought from the parents for a post-mortem examination. The results of the latter are required not only to confirm that the decision to withhold treatment was correct but also to enable optimal advice to be given to the parents concerning the likely outcome of future pregnancies.

Most maternity hospitals with Special Care Baby Units hold regular perinatal mortality conferences attended by all members of the health-care team, at which the individual circumstances of all infants dying in the perinatal period are presented and discussed in confidence. It is particularly important that cases involving ethical dilemmas and decisions should be fully and frankly discussed at such meetings.

Bibliography

Berseth, C. L. (1983). A neonatologist looks at the baby Doe rule: ethical decisions by edict. *Pediatrics*, **72**, 428.

British Medical Association (1983). *Handbook of Medical Ethics*. As modified: *Brit. Med. J.*, **2**, 1593. (Medical Ethics: Severely Malformed Infants).

Campbell, A. G. M. (1982). Which infants should not receive intensive care? *Arch. Dis. Child.*, **75**, 569.

Campbell, A. G. M. (1983). The right to be allowed to die. *J. Med. Ethics*, **9**, 136–40.

Duff, R. S. and Campbell, A. G. M. (1973). Moral and ethical dilemmas in the special care nursery. *New Engl. J. Med.*, **289**, 890.

Dunn, P. M. (1985). Fetal viability: a perinatal viewpoint. In:

Preterm Labour and its Consequences, pp. 295–301. Ed. R. W. Beard, and F. Sharp. London: Royal College of Obstetricians and Gynaecologists.

Illingworth, R. S. (1974). Some ethical problems in paediatrics. In: *Modern Trends in Paediatrics*, pp. 329–57. Ed. J. Apley. Guildford: Butterworth Scientific.

Lorber, J. and Salfield, S. A. W. (1981). Results of selective treatment of spina bifida cystica. *Arch. Dis. Child.*, **56**, 822.

Report of a Working Party (1975). Ethics of selective treatment of spina bifida. *Lancet*, **i**, 85.

31

Normal laboratory and physiological data

Normal values for laboratory investigations in the newborn
Drugs – therapeutic range
Normal physiological values in the newborn

Normal values for laboratory investigations in the newborn

Clinical chemistry

Test and reference range	Comment
Alanine aminotransferase 9–44 IU/l	Not always available as a routine test since it adds no further information than aspartate aminotransferase (*qv*).
Albumin 24–36 g/l at birth 34–46 g/l 0–3 months	
Alkaline phosphatase 70–260 IU/l	Reference range depends on the method used and will vary in different hospitals. Serum is the preferred specimen. Anticonvulsants cause raised values, and transient hyperphosphatasaemia is well recognized in infancy. Although a widely measured

Test and reference range　　*Comment*

estimation, it is of little value on its own.

Alpha-l-antitrypsin
　1.3–4.0 g/l all infants
　2.0–4.5 g/l full term

May be low in respiratory distress syndrome (RDS) and low birthweight infants. The genotype should be assessed if the level is below 2 in infants with prolonged jaundice.

Alpha-fetoprotein
　13–86 mg/l at birth

Levels decline rapidly after birth: plasma half-life = 3.5 days. May remain increased in neonatal hepatitis, biliary atresia and tyrosinosis. May become elevated with certain tumours (e.g. hepatoblastoma in Beckwith Syndrome).

Amino acids
Approximate upper limit of
　normality (μmol/l)
0–21 days

Quantification is usually done to confirm an inborn error in which levels of individual acids may be up to ten times higher. Minor increases are of doubtful significance and should not be a cause for concern except in infants undergoing treatment for a specific amino acid disorder. Interpretation is difficult (impossible) in infants receiving hyperalimentation.

　　30 Aspartic acid
　　　Citrulline
　　　Methionine

　　100 Arginine
　　　Glutamic acid
　　　Histidine
　　　Isoleucine
　　　Phenylalanine
　　　Taurine

　　150 Cystine
　　　Leucine
　　　Ornithine
　　　Serine
　　　Threonine
　　　Tyrosine

Test and reference range   *Comment*

  200 Lysine
      Valine

  300 Glycine
      Proline

  400 Alanine

  500 Glutamine

Ammonia
  10–40 µmol/l
  (venous samples)

May rise to 150 µmol/l
  capillary samples even when
  analysed within 30 min of
  collection. (Arterial samples
  may be easier to interpret.)

EDTA sample is usually
  required. Ammonia
  continues to rise after sample
  collection and rapid
  separation and analysis is
  essential. Thus, this test must
  be arranged with the
  laboratory. Results are
  usually above 200 µmol/l, in
  Reye's syndrome. It is often
  slightly raised in all sick
  infants, and often raised in a
  number of organic acidaemias
  in addition to urea-cycle
  disorders. This is an
  important, often
  under-requested,
  investigation in sick infants.

Anion gap
  6–14 mmol/l

Calculated as the sum of sodium
  and potassium, less the sum
  of chloride and bicarbonate.
  A raised level is highly
  suggestive of the presence of
  an unmeasured organic acid
  anion, e.g. lactate,
  methylmalonate etc.

Aspartate aminotransferase
  3–60 IU/l

Haemolysis causes elevated
  results. Turbidity and severe
  icterus interfere with
  laboratory methods.

Normal laboratory and physiological data

Test and reference range

Comment

Laboratory method used will affect reference range.

Bicarbonate
  18–22 mmol/l

Usually measured as total CO_2 liberated from plasma when included with other electrolytes, otherwise see notes on acid–base studies.

Bilirubin
  1–12 hour 15–115 μmol/l
  12–24 hour 20–170 μmol/l
  24–48 hour 10–180 μmol/l
  76–96 hour 20–170 μmol/l
  1–4 weeks 0–100 μmol/l
  (see Fig. 31.1)

Increased values are caused by dextrans (technical) and lower values by phenobarbitone (pharmacological). Bilirubinometer results may correlate poorly with chemical methods in infants receiving phototherapy.

β-Hydroxybutyrate
  0.03–0.78 mmol/l

Usually measured with lactate (*qv*). Requires special container and prior arrangement with the laboratory staff.

Calcium
Breast fed
  1 day 1.77–2.29 mmol/l
  8 days 1.72–2.64 mmol/l
Artificial feeds
  1 day 1.88–2.28 mmol/l
  8 days 2.14–2.46 mmol/l
  1–6 weeks 2.25–2.80 mmol/l

Increased by thiazides and vitamin D and decreased by phenobarbitone, phenytoin and insulin. There is often a marked fall immediately after birth lasting for 2–3 days especially in RDS, acidosis and associated with maternal diabetes. Approximately half of the total calcium is ionized but prediction of the true ionized fraction is not possible from the total concentration even if pH, protein and albumin concentrations are known.

Test and reference range   *Comment*

Chloride
92–109 mmol/l

Cholesterol
1.0–5.6 mmol/l

Copper
12–27 µmol/l

Cortisol
0–700 nmol/l

There is a steady rise to the adult range of 280–700 nmol/l by the end of the first week of life. The reference range is markedly method-dependent.

Creatine kinase
40–470 IU/l

Apparent activity is increased by haemolysis due to adenylate kinase. There is a rapid rise and fall in plasma activity in the first three days of life. Birth asphyxia causes a marked increase in all CK isoenzymes. The reference range is dependent on the method used and temperature of incubation.

Creatinine
28–60 µmol/l

Results in the newborn period are often unreliable for methodological reasons (see Chapter 16).

Ferritin
Birth 65–395 µmol/l
2 weeks 90–630 µmol/l
4 weeks 140–400 µmol/l

Increased by haemolysis. Rapid changes occur in the neonatal period.

Folic acid
4–24 nmol/l

Gamma glutamyl transferase
0–260 IU/l

The reference range is dependent on the temperature at which the assay is done. It is high at

Test and reference range	*Comment*
	birth, with a steady predictable fall with age. This is a more interpretable enzyme than alkaline phosphatase in liver disease, except that it may be induced by some drugs such as anticonvulsants.

Glucose
   2.8–4.5 mmol/l
   1.7–3/6 mmol/l

Although lower concentrations may be found in premature or low birthweight infants, their interpretation as 'normal' is debatable. A glucose less than 2 mmol/l is cause for concern.

17-Hydroxyprogesterone
   0–36 hours <50 nmol/l
   Subsequently <18 nmol/l

The sample must be separated promptly. It is usually best to arrange this test with laboratory staff.

Immunoglobulins
IgA
   0–1 week 0–0.05 g/l
   1–4 weeks 0–0.22 g/l
IgG
   0–1 week 7.0–19.0 g/l
   1–4 weeks 4.0–11.2 g/l
IgM
   0–1 week 0.2–0.4 g/l
   1–4 weeks 0.2–0.6 g/l

Iron
   14–22 μmol/l

May be much higher at birth, up to 60 μmol/l, with a rapid fall in the first few hours, followed by a modest steady rise over the next few weeks. Ferritin is a more reliable index.

Test and reference range   *Comment*

Lactate
  1.4–2.8 mmol/l

May be higher shortly after birth falling into the reference range by the end of the first week. Requires prior arrangement with laboratory staff as plasma needs to be separated rapidly.

Lactate dehydrogenase
  0–1500 IU/l

Very variable activity of this enzyme makes it less useful in newborn infants than it is in adults.

Magnesium
  0.7–1.0 mmol/l

May be lower at birth and in infants with RDS or macrosomia due to maternal diabetes. Haemolysis elevates values. Neuromuscular symptoms do not usually occur unless less than 0.5 mmol/l.

Osmolality
  Plasma 270–285 mosmol/kg

Sodium salts are the principal contributors to osmolality. There are more than 20 formulae in the literature for calculation of osmolality from other parameters, but a figure representing twice the sodium concentration approximates to the true osmolality sufficiently well for practical purposes, provided that urea or glucose are not grossly raised, except in very premature infants where the usual relationships of sodium, water and renal tubular function may not hold.

Normal laboratory and physiological data

Test and reference range   *Comment*

Phosphate
  1.2–2.78 mmol/l   Affected by dietary intake and
                                             the type of milk feeds.
                                             Increased by haemolysis.

Potassium
  3.6–4.6 mmol/l   Usually higher in capillary
                                             samples; up to 6.6 mmol/l in
                                             newborn infants. Affected by
                                             haemolysis and elevated in
                                             acidosis.

Protein (total)
  54–74 g/l

Pyruvate
  Up to 120 μmol/l   May be measured with lactate
                                             (qv) but very unreliable and
                                             of doubtful value.

Sodium
  133–143 mmol/l   30% of very low birthweight
                                             infants may have a sodium
                                             level less than 130 mmol/l.
                                             Concentration depends on
                                             intake. Term infants receiving
                                             3 mmol/kg/24 hour at 2–6
                                             weeks should have a sodium
                                             level above 130 mmol/l (see
                                             Chapter 17, page 251).

Thyroxine (T_4)
  0–1 week   145–325 nmol/l
  1–16 weeks 110–220 nmol/l

Thyroid-stimulating hormone
  (TSH)   This test is included with the
  0–10 U/l   phenylketonuria (PKU)
                                             screening test (see Chapter
                                             13, page 203).

Triglycerides
  0.35–1.15 mmol/l

Urea
  1.4–5.4 mmol/l   Upper limit of reference range
                                             may be increased to 7.5 for
                                             infants on cows' milk

Test and reference range

Comment

formulae and may be lower than 1.4 in the first few days of life in low birthweight infants.

Uric acid
60–240 µmol/l

There is a transient increase in the first few days of life.

Vitamin A
0.4–2.1 µmol/l

Arrange with laboratory. Specimen must not be exposed to daylight and must be sent to the laboratory immediately.

Vitamins B_1, B_2, B_{12}, and E

Adequate information in newborn infants is not available.

Zinc
9.2–29.1 µmol/l

Clotted samples give higher values.

Drugs – therapeutic range

Digoxin
1–2.5 nmol/l

Therapeutic dose may be higher than that used in adults. Blood levels also tend to be higher relative to dose but are better tolerated. Blood levels must be assessed when blood and tissue concentrations are in equilibrium – usually 4–6 hours after intramuscular dose.

Phenobarbitone
45–110 µmol/l

Although 50% is protein bound in older children this is not the case in jaundiced neonates where up to 70% of

Normal laboratory and physiological data

Test and reference range	*Comment*
	the drug may be free. Cerebrospinal fluid concentrations approximate to the free plasma concentration. Toxicity levels are poorly defined.
Phenytoin 40–80 μmol/l	Only 10% or less of the drug is free in plasma. Newborn infants have diminished capacity to eliminate phenytoin, especially if premature.
Theophylline 25–80 μmol/l	The distribution of this drug is equal between red cells and plasma so that haemolysed samples can be assayed unless haemolysis directly interferes with the assay – ask the laboratory staff.
Valproic acid (sodium valproate) 350–700 μmol/l	There is no recognizable relationship between blood levels and therapeutic effect, although there is for toxic effects.

Haematological values in the newborn

NB   See Chapter 15 for investigation of bleeding/clotting disorders. Table 31.1 shows mean haematological values in term infants and Table 31.2 shows differential counts in term and preterm infants.

Cerebrospinal fluid values in infants without meningitis

Table 31.3 shows CSF values in infants without meningitis.

Table 31.1 Mean haematological values during the first two weeks of life in term infants (95% ranges given in brackets)

Value	Cord blood	Day1	Day 3	Day 7	Day 14
Haemoglobin* (g/dl)	16.8	18.4	17.8	17.0	16.8
	(13.7–20.1)	(14–22)	(13.8–21.8)	(14–20)	(13.8–19.8)
Venous haematocrit % (= PCV) (capillary values 2–3% higher)	53	58	55	54	52
Red cells (10^3 mm³)	5.25	5.8	5.6	5.2	5.1
MCV (fl)	107	108	99	98	96
	(96–118)				
MCH (pg)	34	35	33	32.5	31.5
	(33–41)				
MCHC (%)	31.7	32.5	33	33	33
	(30–35)				
Reticulocytes (%)	3–7	3–7	1–3	0–1	0–1
Nucleated RBC/mm³	500	200	0–5	0	0
Platelets (10^3/mm³)	290	192	213	248	252
	(150–400)				

MCV, Mean corpuscular volume.
MCH, Mean corpuscular haemoglobin.
MCHC, Mean corpuscular haemoglobin concentration.
†Nucleated RBC counts may rise very rapidly with stress (e.g. fetal distress, birth asphyxia, infection, RDS) as well as after haemorrhage. Counts may rise to 10,000/mm³ within six hours (R. R. Slade, 1990).
*Haemoglobin values in preterm AGA infants are lower (mean cord Hb 15 g/dl at 32 weeks' gestation) and values in SGA infants are commonly higher (see Chapter 15, page 228).
From Oski and Naiman (1982) *Haematologic Problems in the Newborn*, 3rd edn, London: W. B. Saunders.

Table 31.2 Differential white cell counts in term and preterm infants (10^3 cells/mm³)

Age (hours)	Total WBC	Neutro-philis	Bands Metas	Lympho-cytes	Mono-cytes	Eosino-philis
Term infants						
0	10.0–26.0	5–13	0.4–1.8	3.5–8.5	0.7–1.5	0.2–2.0
12	13.5–31.0	9.0–18.0	0.4–2.0	3.0–7.0	1.0–2.0	0.2–2.0
72	5.0–14.5	2.0–7.0	0.2–0.4	2.0–5.0	0.5–1.0	0.2–1.0
144	6.0–14.5	2.0–6.0	0.2–0.5	3.0–6.0	0.7–1.2	0.1–0.8
Preterm infants						
0	5.0–19.0	2.0–9.0	0.2–2.4	2.5–6.0	0.3–1.0	0.1–0.7
12	5.0–21.0	3.0–11.0	0.2–2.4	1.5–5.0	0.3–1.3	0.1–1.1
72	5.0–14.0	3.0–7.0	0.2–0.6	1.5–4.0	0.3–1.2	0.2–1.1
144	5.5–17.5	2.0–7.0	0.2–0.5	2.5–7.5	0.5–1.5	0.3–1.2

From Xanthou (1970) Leucocyte blood picture in healthy full-term and premature babies during the neonatal period. *Arch. Dis. Childh.* **45**, 242.

Normal laboratory and physiological data

Table 31.3   Cerebrospinal fluid values in infants without meningitis

	Term infants	Preterm infants
Total white blood cell count (cells/mm³)		
Mean	8.2	9.0
Median	5	6
Range	0–32	0–29
± 2 SD	0–22.4	0–25.4
mean % polymorphonuclear cells	61.3%	57.2%
Protein (g/l)		
Mean	0.9	1.15
Range	0.2–1.7	0.65–1.5
Glucose (mmol/l)		
Mean	2.9	2.8
Range	1.9–6.6	1.3–3.4
CSF/blood glucose (%)		
Mean	81	74
Range	44–248	55–105

From Sarff, Platt and McCracken (1976) *J. Pediatr.*, **88**, 473.

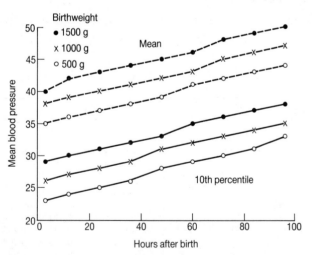

Fig. 31.1   Mean and 10th percentile values for mean blood pressure in infants of different birthweights. From Weindling A. M. (1989), Blood pressure monitoring in the newborn. *Arch. Dis. Childh*; **64**, 444–7.

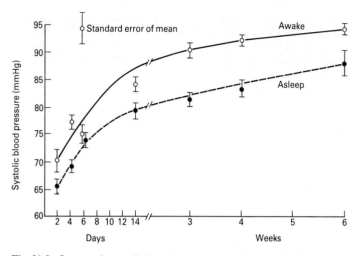

Fig. 31.2 Increase in systolic blood pressure in healthy, term infants awake and asleep between the ages of two days and six weeks. From: Earley, Fayer, Ng, Shinebourne and de Swiet. *Arch. Dis. Childh*, **55**, 755–757, 1980. With permission of the authors and publishers.

Normal physiological values in the newborn

Blood pressure

See Figs 31.1 and 31.2 for blood pressure values.

Blood gases

Normal values in healthy term infants

Age (hours)	1–4	12–24	24–48	48–168
PaO_2 (mm Hg)	50–75	60–80	65–85	70–85
(kPa)	6.5–9.8	7.8–10.4	8.5–11	9.1–.fifi
$PaCO_2$ (mm Hg)	30–45	30–40	30–40	30–38
(kPa)	3.9–5.9	3.9–5.2	3.9–5.2	3.9–4.9
Arterial pH	7.30–7.34	7.30–7.35	7.35–7.40	7.35–7.40

NB   Values obtained for $PaCO_2$ and pH on arterialized capillary blood are close to those given. For PO_2 arterialized capillary values are usually 5–10 mm Hg (0.65–1.3 kPa) lower than arterial values for PaO_2 <60 mm Hg (7.8 kPa). Above this value capillary PO_2 does not reflect arterial PO_2. Capillary blood gases are unreliable in conditions of hypotension, poor peripheral perfusion, and cold stress.

Index

Abdomen,
   birth trauma 44
   masses 240
   paracentesis 358
   wall defects 178, 181
Aberdeen splint 77, 78
ABO incompatibility 269
Abortion 389
Achondroplasia 72
Acidaemias, organic 194
Acidosis 243
Acrodermatitis enteropathica 301
Acropustulosis 302
Adrenal hyperplasia 198
Adrenaline 30
Adrenal insufficiency 256
Adrenocortical crisis 200
AIDS 5
Air leaks 88
Airway,
   care of at birth 27
Alanine aminotransferase 405
Albinism 315
Albumin 375
   normal value 405
   priming in exchange
      transfusion 266
Alcohol
   pregnancy and 7
Alkaline phosphatase 405
Alpha-fetoprotein 11
   in neural tube defects 12
   normal value 406
   screening limitations 13
Alpha-1-antitrypsin 406
Alport's syndrome 238

Alveolar rupture 88
Amblyopia 310
Amelia 71
Amino acidaemias 194
Amino acids
   normal values 406
Aminoglycosides
   dose and administration 382
   effect on kidney 237
Aminophylline 106
   dose and administration 377
   effect on kidney 237
Ammonia 407
Amniocentesis 11
Amphetamine abuse 8
Anaemia 33, 34, 231–2
   definition 231
   during ventilation 101
   early 231
   late 232
   management 231
   in renal disease 242
Anencephaly 150
Anion gap 407
Aniridia 315
Aniscoria 315
Anocutaneous fistula 186
Anomalous origin of left
      pulmonary artery 126
Ano-rectal anomalies 108, 186
Antecubital fossa
   long line insertion in 358
Anterior chamber cleavage
      syndrome 314
Antibiotics
   breast feeding and 373

Antibiotics – *cont.*
  dosage and administration 382
Anticoagulants
  in pregnancy 4
Anticonvulsant drugs 136
  affecting fetus 4
Antidiuretic hormone 237, 254
Antifungal drugs
  breast feeding and 373
  dosage and administration
    386
Anti-inflammatory agents
  breast feeding and 374
Aorta, coarctation of 112, 124
Aortic arch
  anomalies of 123
Aortic valve stenosis 124, 128
Apert syndrome 68, 72
Apgar score 25–6
Aplasia cutis 67
Apnoea
  at birth 27
  recurrent 94, 105, 106
Apnoea monitors 55
Arnold-Chiari malformation 142
Apts test 225
Arrhythmias 129–30
Arterial lines
  insertion of 346
  sampling blood from 342
Arthrogryposis multiplex
    congenita 72
Artificial feeding 158–67
  comparison of milks 158, 159
  composition of milks 162, 163
  low birth weight 159–60
  milks 158
  special formulae 159, 162–5
  techniques 166
Aspartate aminotransferase 407
Asphyxia 26, 28, 29
  assessment of 143
  cerebral intensive care and 143
  fetal 24
  management of 144
  in small-for-gestational age
    babies 59
Association for all Speech Impaired
    Children 285
Association for Children with
    Artificial Arms 289

Association for Spina Bifida and
    Hydrocephalus 285
Association for the Improvement of
    the Maternity Services 285
Atelectasis
  primary 89
  resorption 99
Atrioventricular canal 112
Atrioventricular septal defect 125
Autoimmune
    thrombocytopenia 230

Baths and bathing 50
BCG vaccination 3
Beckwith-Widemann syndrome 68,
    182, 193
Bicarbonate
  values 408
Biliary atresia 267
Biliary obstruction 261, 267
Bilirubin
  levels 408
  toxicity 261
Bilirubin encephalopathy 262
Biotin deficiency 306
Birth
  airway obstruction at 27
  assessment of clinical status 25
  cardiac massage at 30
  care of airway 27
  division of cord 26
  management of 25–32
  resuscitation at 28
  thermal care at 25
Birth defect
  definition of 63
Birth trauma 39–45
  See also specific injuries etc
  of large infants 60
  obstetric events predisposing
    to 39
  presentation and 40
Birthweight
  definition of 389
Bladder
  abnormalities 241
  enlarged 240
  exstrophy 241
  suprapubic tap 349
Bladder Exstrophy Association
    286

Bleeding disorders 225
   diagnosis of 225, 226
   hereditary 228
Blepharophimosis 313
Blistering 300
Bloch-Sulzberger syndrome
   316
Blood
   arterial sampling 342
   capillary samples 341
   normal values 224, 415
   transfusion 375
   sampling 341
   venous samples 341
Blood clotting disorders 225
   screening tests 226
Blood diseases 224–34
   diagnosis of 229
Blood gases
   measurement of 93
   monitoring 55
   normal values 417
Blood glucose 56, 145
Blood plasma
   transfusion 376
Blood platelets 224–5
   transfusion 375
Blood pressure
   before transport 83
   measurement 93
   monitoring 56
   normal values 416–17
Blood products 375
Blood sugar
   checks before transport 83
   monitoring 64
Blood tests
   for high risk infants 56
Blood transfusion 375
   exchange 265, 354
Blue asphyxia 26, 28, 29
Bockdalek, foramen of 178
Bone marrow aspiration 359–60
Bottle feeding 158
Bowel obstruction 49, 187–8
Brachial artery
   blood sampling from 343
Brachial plexus injury 42
Bradycardia
   at birth 30
   fetal 16

Brain
   haemorrhagic lesions 138, 139,
      140
   ischaemic lesions 141
   oedema 145
   periventricular haemorrhage 138
   persistent ventricular
      enlargement 141
   subcortical leucomalacia 141
   tumours 142
   ultrasonic scanning 137–8
Branchial sinus 67
Breast feeding 47, 152–8
   antenatal preparation 153
   AIDS and 5
   clinical problems 155
   comparison of milks 160–1
   diuretics affecting 2
   drug abuse and 9
   engorgement of breast in 157
   hypotensive drugs and 2
   lactation problems 156
   mastitis and blocked ducts in 157
   maternal drugs and 368–75
   maternal problems 157
   physiology of 153
   postnatal considerations 153
   preterm infants 154
   routine management 154
   special considerations 154
   in tuberculosis 3
   viral infections and 158
Breast milk,
   compared with other
      milks 160–1
   composition of 160–1
   contaminants 157
   impaired release 156
   initiation of 153
   insufficiency 156
   production of 153
   pumps 154
British Heart Foundation 286
Bronchopulmonary dysplasia 89,
   103, 181
Bruising at birth 45
Bubble test 187
Bullous dermatosis of
   childhood 307
Bullous impetigo 300, 306
Burns 301

Caesarean section for preterm
    infants 35
Calcium levels 195, 408
Calcium requirements 165
Candidiasis 222, 303, 304, 306
Caput succedaneum 40
Carbohydrate in intravenous
    feeding 168
Cardiac arrhythmias 129–30
    see also Heart disease
Cardiac massage 358
    in birth resuscitation 30
Cardiac tamponade 357
Cardiomyopathy 61
Cardiorespiratory monitors 55
Cardiotochograph 16
Cardiovascular drugs
    breast feeding and 371
Cardiovascular problems in
    preterm infants 59
Care
    medical audit and 389–99
    special *See Special care*
Carpenter's syndrome 68
Cataract 316
Catecholamine drive 244
Catheterisation
    umbilical artery 346
    umbilical vein 344
Cavernous haemangioma 66
Central nervous system
    drugs and breast feeding 372–3
Cephalhaematoma 41
Cerebral oedema 145
Cerebrospinal fluid values 414,
    416
Cervical spine
    birth fracture 43
Chest
    drain insertion 352
    needling 352
Chignon 40
Chlamydial infections 220
    of eye 310
Chloride values 409
Choanal atresia 68
Cholesterol 409
Chorion villous biopsy 11
Choroid
    disorders of 317
Christmas disease 228

Chromosomal abnormalities 59,
    324
    detection of 12
Chromosomal analysis 326
Chromosomal inheritance 322
Chromosomal syndromes 72–4
Cigarette smoking in pregnancy 9
Citrullinaemia 306
Clavicle
    fracture of 42, 43
Claw hand 43
Cleft lip and palate 69
    complicating breast feeding 155
    with hypopituitarism 203
Cleft Lip and Palate
    Association 286
Clinic,
    attendance at 366
Club foot 78
Coarctation of aorta 112, 123
Cocaine 8
Cold stress 54
    *See also Heat loss, Thermal care
    etc.*
    adverse effects of 53
    at birth 25
    during transport 80
    prevention of 29, 46, 48, 52
Collodion baby 305
Coloboma 313, 315, 316
Compassionate Friends 286
Congenital abnormalities 63–79
    antenatal diagnosis 178
    care of parents 281
    definitions 63
    examination of 64
    incidence of 64
    inheritance patterns 322–5
Congenital deformations 65, 74,
    320–8
    characteristics 66
    definition 63
    diagnosis 320
Congenital dislocation of hip 75–8
Congenital heart block 130
Congenital heart disease
    *see also Heart disease and specific
    lesions*
    asymptomatic murmurs 128
    cyanotic 117–22
    heart failure in 122

incidence of 108
management of 121
maternal factors in 109
Congenital malformations 64, 66, 74
See also Congenital abnormalities, Congenital deformations etc.
anticipation of 24
characteristics of 66
definition 63, 389
ethics and 400
genetics of 320
guidelines for decision making 402
in infants of diabetic mothers 61
infections associated with 213
recurrence risks 327
Congenital postural scoliosis 75
Congenital sternomastoid torticollis 74
Congenital talipes 78
Conjunctivitis 310
Continuous positive airway pressure 94–6
management of baby 96
methods 95
Contraceptives, oral
breast feeding and 374
Convulsions 84, 133
categories of 133
causes of 134
drug therapy 136
investigation of 135
management of 136
prognosis 136
Copper 409
Corectopia 315
Cornea
dermoid tumours 314
opacities 314
ulcers 311
Cornelia de Lange dwarf 72
Coronary artery
anomalous 126
Coroners 331, 336
Cor pulmonale 181
Corpus callosum
agenesis of 150
Cortisol 409
Cor triatriatum 125

Craniostenosis 67
Creatine kinase 409
Creatinine 409
excretion 235, 236
Cretinism 201
Crouzon syndrome 68
Cryptophthalmos 313
Cryptorchidism 241
Cutis aplasia 41
Cyanosis 117–22
common causes 117
traumatic 42
Cystic adenomatoid malformation 89
Cystic fibrosis 49, 188
bowel obstruction in 188
Cystic Fibrosis Research Trust 286
Cystic hygroma 67
Cystic periventricular leucomalacia 140
Cytomegalovirus infection 211, 212, 304

Dandy Walker malformation 142
Data,
collection of 388
maternal 391
Death of baby
care of parents 282
cause of 329
reporting to coroner 331
Definitions 388
Delivery 20–38
anticipation of common conditions 23
complications of 15
high risk 14
management of placenta 37
obstetric history and 21
preparation before 21
presentation and birth trauma 40
resuscitation equipment 22
Delivery room 20–38
aftercare in 36
care of parents in 280
management of diaphragmatic hernia in 178
management of exomphalos in 181
neonatal medical team in 20
organization 20

Delivery room – *cont.*
  precautions against AIDS and
    hepatitis 5
  record keeping 37
  respiratory care in 91
  resuscitation in 20, 24, 30, 36
  routine care 46
Denver Developmental Screen
  364–5
Dermal sinuses 67
Dermatitis 306
Developmental assessment 363–7
Dexamethasone 104
Diabetes insipidus 238
Diabetes mellitus
  in small-for-dates babies 192
Diabetic mother,
  infant of 60, 61
Dialysis 250–1
Diaphragmatic hernia 34, 84,
    178–81
  diagnosis 179
  follow-up 181
  management of 179
  postoperative care 180
  respiratory symptoms 89
Diarrhoea
  congenital 176
  differential diagnosis 175
Digoxin 127
Discharge
  examination 50
  record 387
Disseminated intravascular
    coagulation 225
Diuretics
  affecting breast feeding 2
  chronic lung disease 103
  heart failure 126
DNA analysis 328
Documentation 389
Dopamine 122
Dorsalis pedis
  blood sampling from 343
Down's syndrome 68, 72, 316
  congenital heart disease with 108
  duodenal atresia with 187
  maternal age and 12
Down's Syndrome Association 286
Drugs 368–86
  affecting kidney 237

breast feeding and 371–4
causing convulsions 134
dosage and
  administration 377–86
in pregnancy 369–70
therapeutic range 413–14
Drug abuse in pregnancy 8–9
Drug eruptions 306
Duodenal atresia 187
Dwarfism 72

Ears,
  anomalies of 68
Ebstein's malformation 111, 120,
  129
Echocardiography 115
ECHO virus infection 221
Edward's syndrome 73, 316
  heart disease in 109
Electrocardiography 115
Electrolytes
  in asphyxia 145
Electrolyte therapy
  See Fluid and electrolyte therapy
Emphysema 88
  acquired lobar 90
  congenital lobar 90
  interstitial 103
Encephalitis 212
Encephalocele 150
Encephalopathy
  causing convulsions 134
  from asphyxia 144
Endocrine problems 198, 203
Endocrine system
  drugs and breast feeding 371–4
Endotracheal intubation 350
  suctioning 297
  tubes 350
Epidermal naevus 67
Epidermolysis bullosa 300
Epidermolytic hyperkeratosis 301
Epilepsy
  maternal 4
Epispadias 241
Erb's palsy 43, 79
Erythema neonatorum 300
Erythrodermas 304
Erythropoiesis
  increased intrauterine 233
Ethics 400–3

Exchange transfusion 265, 354
Exomphalos 108, 181
Eyes 309–19
  birth trauma to 314, 317
  capillary haemangioma 314
  congenital anomalies of 68
  dermoid cyst 314
  examination of 309
  external disorders 313
  globe size 318
  internal disorders 315
  tumours of 314
Eyelids
  disorders of 313

Face
  birth injury to 42
  congenital anomalies of 67
Facial palsy 79
  from birth injury 42
Fallot's tetralogy 119
Family
  care of 280–91
  of dying baby 283
Family Fund 287
Fat requirements 168
Feeding 47
  See also Breast feeding, Artificial feeding
  additives 160
  exchange transfusion and 357
  gastric 166
  high risk infant 54
  intravenous *See Intravenous feeding*
  of infant of diabetic mother 61
  transpyloric 166
Feet
  deformities 78
  plantar creases 275, 277
Femoral vein
  blood sampling from 342
Ferritin 409
Fetal abnormalities
  detection of 11–13
  from anticonvulsants 4
Fetal alcohol syndrome 7
Fetus
  anaemia 33
  asphyxia 24

  assessment of growth and well-being 10, 14
  biophysical assessment 11
  blood loss 33
  blood pH 117
  concussion 23
  foot length 337
  heart rate in labour 14
  high risk delivery 14
  postural deformities 9
  sedation of 23
Fingers,
  malformations of 72
Floppy infant 146–8
Fluid and electrolyte
  therapy 253–59
Fluoride supplements 165
Folic acid 409
  requirements 166
Follow-up 361–8
  appointment 362
  assessment at 363–6
  attendance at clinic 366
  check list 367
  reasons for 361
  special 362
Foundation for Study of Infant Deaths 287
Fractures at birth 43, 44
Frusemide 237, 379
Fungal infections 221–3

Galactosaemia 194
Gamma glutamyl transferase 409
Gastric content
  aspiration of during transport 83
Gastric feeding 166
Gastroenteritis 175, 219
Gastrointestinal drugs
  breast feeding and 371
Gastrointestinal problems 172–6
  in premature infants 58
Gastro-oesophageal reflux 172, 185
Gastroschisis 183
  transport of patient 84
Genetics 321–8
  autosomal dominant conditions 322, 323
  autosomal recessive patterns 322, 324
  inheritance patterns 322–5

Genetics – *cont.*
  mitochondrial inheritance 323,
    325
  microdeletion syndromes 326
  multifactorial inheritance 322,
    324
  prediction in neonate 326
  skin biopsy in 328
  tests 326
  X-linked dominant
    inheritance 324
  X-linked recessive patterns
    in 323, 324
Genetic counselling 327
Genitalia
  anomalies 70, 241
  ambiguous 198–9
  birth trauma 44
Gestational age
  assessment 272
  definition 389
  neurological assessment 276,
    278, 279
  organ weights and 335
Gingerbread 287
Glaucoma 314, 318
Glomerular filtration rate 235, 236,
  246
Gluconeogenic disorders 192
Glucose
  see also *Hyperglycaemia,*
    Hypoglycaemia
  rate calculator 196
  values 410
Glycogen storage disease 193
Glycosuria 254
Goldenhaar's syndrome 313
Gonococcal ophthalmia 310, 311
Gonococcal ulceration of
    cornea 314
Graves' disease 202
Group B streptococcal disease 217
Growth charts 273–4

Haemangiomata 66
Haematemesis 225
Haematocrit 224
Haematological problems 224–34
  diagnosis 225
Haematological values 415
Haematuria 242

Haemofiltration 251
Haemoglobin
  normal values 224
Haemoglobinopathies,
  maternal 6
Haemolysis 231, 232
  acute intravascular 261
Haemolytic anaemia
  Vitamin E deficient 165, 232
Haemolytic disease 264
  iso-immune 264
  rhesus 269
Haemophilia 228
Haemophilia Society 287
Haemophilus influenzae 214
Haemorrhage
  in preterm infants 58
Haemorrhagic disease of
    newborn 227
  Vitamin K and 40, 46, 227
Handicapped infant
  ethics and 400
Harlequin fetus 304
Head,
  charts 273–4
  circumference of 131
Hearing
  testing 363
Heart
  injection into 357
  massage 30, 358
Heart block
  congenital 130
Heart disease 108–30
  See also Heart failure and specific
    lesions
  assessment of infant 109
  congenital *See Congenital heart*
    disease
  ECG in 113
  echocardiography 115
  examination in 109
  incidence of 108
  investigation of 113
  presentation 115
  radiology 113
Heart failure 122–8
  at birth 34
  causes of 122
  signs of 122
  treatment of 126

Heart murmurs 128
Heat loss
  prevention of 54
  thermal core 52
  thermal neutral ranges 55
Heavy-for-dates babies 388
Heel prick sampling 341
Hemimelia 71
Hepatitis (neonatal) 267
Hepatitis B 213
  maternal 6
Hernia
  diaphragmatic *See Diaphragmatic
    hernia*
  inguinal 191
Heroin 8
Herpes infection 211, 212, 301, 304
Herpes simplex 307
High-risk infant
  care of 51–62
  feeding 54
  minimal handling 57
  monitoring 55, 292
  thermal care 52
Hip,
  congenital dislocation of 75–8
Hirschsprung's disease 49, 189
Histiocytosis X 307
Holoprosencephaly 150
Horner's syndrome 42, 313, 315
Hydranencephaly 90, 151
Hydrocele 71
Hydrocephalus 142–3
  causes of 142
  ex vacuo 143
  management of 143
  post-haemorrhagic 140
  postinfection 142
Hydrops fetalis 33, 71
Hydrometrocolpos
  congenital 71
β-Hydroxybutyrate 408
17-Hydroxyprogesterone 410
Hymen,
  imperforate 71
Hyperaldosteronism 258
Hyperammonaemia 208
Hyperbilirubinaemia 363
  conjugated 260, 266
  exchange transfusion for 354
  unconjugated 266

Hyperglycinaemia
  non-ketolic 195
Hyperkalaemia 258
  in asphyxia 145
Hypernatraemia 257
Hyperoxia 94
  test 115
Hypertelorism 150
Hypertension 242–5
  drug therapy affecting infant 2
  in pregnancy 1
Hyperthyroidism
  maternal 2
  neonatal 202
Hypocalcaemia 195, 196
Hypoglycaemia 182, 192
  artificial feeding and 158
  asymptomatic 193
  at birth 34
  causes of 192
  definition 192
  in infant of diabetic mothers 60
  investigation 204
  late 195
  in small-for-gestational age
    infant 59
  symptomatic 193
Hypokalaemia 258
  in asphyxia 145
Hypomagnesaemia 197, 198
Hyponatraemia 256
  in asphyxia 145
  late 257
Hypoparathyroidism 201
Hypopituitarism 208
Hypoplasia of left heart 111
Hypoplastic left heart
  syndrome 123
Hypospadias 241
Hypotension during ventilation 101
Hypotensive drugs
  affecting infant 2
Hypothyroidism 208
  screening for 208
Hypotonia 147
Hypovalaemia 24, 33
Hypoxia 94
  refractory 102

I:E ratio 98
Ichthyoses 305

Immunization 366
Immunoglobulins 410
Impetigo 303
Inadvertant positive end-expiratory
    pressure 98
Inborn errors of metabolism 192–8
Incontinentia pigmentia 301, 316
Incubator 54, 295
Indomethacin
    in patent ductus arteriosus 127
    renal effects of 237
Infections 211–23
    antibiotics for 218, 382
    causing convulsions 134
    congenital 23, 211
    during ventilation 101
    early onset 213
    fungal 221–3
    general management 217
    in high risk infants 57
    intrapartum 213
    investigation of 214
    isolation of infant 295
    late onset 214
    maternal 213
    neonatal 213
    organisms causing 218
    in preterm infants 59
    prevention of 48, 294
    risk factors 214
    signs suggestive of 215
    skin 303
    superficial 215
    systemic 215
    treatment 217, 218
    viral 221
Inguinal hernia 191
Inherited disease
    chromosomal anomalies 321
    collection of samples 327
    genetic patterns of 322, 323
    genetic tests for 326
    inborn errors of
        metabolism 192–8, 206–9
    prediction of 326
Insect bites 301
Intensive care
    babies receiving 396
    *See also Neonatal intensive care
        unit*
Intertrigo 306

Intestine
    atresia and stenosis 187
    malrotation and volvulus 189
Intracardiac injection 357
Intracranial pressure
    raised 145, 244
Intralipid 168, 169
Intramuscular injections 343
Intrauterine growth retardation 59
Intrauterine pressure
    neurapraxia 42
Intravenous feeding
    administration 170
    cautions 170
    indications 167
    monitoring 171
    regimen 168
Intravenous lines
    insertion of 344
Intraventricular haemorrhage 101,
    137–41
Intubation 295–8, 350–1
    at birth 29
Iris
    disorders of 315
Iron,
    requirements 166
    values 410
Iso-immune thrombocytopenia
    228
Iso-valeric acidaemia 195

Jaundice 41, 260–71
    conjugated 266
    from ABO incompatibility 269
    from rhesus haemolytic
        disease 268
    management of 264
    pathological 261
    pathophysiology of 261
    phototherapy in 265
    physiological 260
    in preterm infants 58
    prolonged 266
Jugular vein
    blood sampling from 342

Kasai procedure 267
Kearns Sayre syndrome 323
Keratoglobus 318
Kernicterus 262

Kidney
   See also Renal
   abnormalities 239
   disease *See Renal disease*
   drug dosage and 237
   multicystic 240
   normal physiological values 236
   physiology of 235
Klumpke's paralysis 43

LSD 9
Laboratory data 405–18
Labour,
   cardiotocographs during 16
   complications of 15
   fetal well-being during 14
   inhibition of 18
   preterm 17–18
Lactate
   normal value 411
Lactate dehydrogenase 411
Lactation 152
   See also Breast feeding
   failure of 156
   insufficient 156
Lactose intolerance 176
Ladd's bands 189
la Leche league 287
Large-for-gestational age babies,
   care of 60–2
Laryngomalacia 155
Leiner's disease 305
Lens
   disorders of 316
Leucocoria 315
Leukocyturia 243
Light-for-dates babies 388
Limbs,
   fractures at birth 44
   malformations of 71–2
   tone of 133
Listeriosis 220
Livebirth 392
   definition 388
Liver
   impaired cellular function 261
Liver disease 206
Long line
   insertion 358
Low birthweight babies
   care of 51–60

   in delivery room 20–37
   hyperglycaemia in 194
   meconium passage in 49
Lumbar puncture 348
Lung 86–107
   chronic disease of 103–4
   congenital hypoplasia 103
   cystic adenomatoid
     malformation 89
   haemorrhage 88
   hypoplasia 90

Macroglossia 68
Magnesium 197, 198, 411
Malrotation and volvulus of
   intestine 189
Mannitol 146, 378
Maple syrup urine disease 192, 208
Marijuana 9
Marriage Guidance 288
Mastitis 157
Mastocytosis 301
Maternal conditions
   affecting infant 1–19
   drugs 369–75
   see also pregnancy etc
Mean airway pressure 97
Meconium,
   passage of 59
Meconium aspiration 32, 87
Meconium ileus 188
Meconium plug 49
Medical audit 387–99
Medical ethics 400–4
   general principles 400
   guidelines 402
Megalencephaly 150
Megalocornea 318
Melaena 227
Membranes
   premature rupture of 18
Meningitis 218, 219
   in listeriosis 219
   viral 221
Meningomyelocele 149–51
   assessment 149
   definition 148
Metabolic acidosis 26, 30
   in congenital heart disease 22
Metabolic causes of
   convulsions 134

Metabolic problems 192–8
  in preterm infants 58
  screening for 205
Metabolism, inborn errors of 192,
    206–9
  clinical features 192, 205
  investigations 204
  neurological deterioration in 205
  postmortems in 335
Metatarsus varus 78
Methadone abuse 8, 9
Microcephaly 151
Microcolon 188
Microdeletion syndrome 326
Microphthalmos 319
Milia 300
Miliaria 300
  pustular 302
  rubra 305
Milks
  comparisons 160–1
Milroy's oedema 71
Minerals
  requirements 169
Monitoring 292
  high risk infants 55
Morphine abuse 8
Mortality statistics 392, 393, 395
Mouth
  thrush 156, 221
Movement
  examination of 132
Mucus gland retention cysts 69
Mumps 213
Muscle biopsy
  in floppy infant 148
Musculoskeletal system,
  congenital malformations of 71
Myasthenia gravis 4
Myelocele 149
Myeloschisis 149
Myocarditis 221
Myopathies
  floppy infant in 146
Myotonic dystophy 146–8

Naevi 66
Naevus flammeus 66
Naloxone 29, 379
Napkin dermatitis 306
Nasolacrimal duct obstruction 311

National Association for Deaf
    Blind and Rubella
    Handicapped 290
National Association for the
    Welfare of Children in
    Hospital 288
National Childbirth Trust 288
National Council for One Parent
    Families 288
National Deaf Children's
    Society 288
Neck and truncal tone 133
Necrotizing enterocolitis 159,
    173–5, 357
  aetiology 173
  complications and prognosis 175
  management 174
Neonatal death certification 387
Neonatal intensive care unit,
  admission of infant 53, 296
  definition 50
  nursing care in 295
  transfer to 37
Neonatal medical team 20
Neonatal mortality rate 394
Neonatal period
  definition of 386
Neonatal workload
  audit of 395
Nephrotic syndrome 238, 241
Nervous system
  assessment 131
  developmental defects 148–51
  examination of 132
Neural tube defects 12
Neurapraxias 42, 43, 79
Neurological disorders 131–51
  in preterm infants 58
  skin signs 133
Norrie's disease 323
Nose
  obstruction 156
Nursing care 292–8
  intensive care unit 295
  intubated baby 296
  minimal handling 91, 294
  routine 47
  special care baby unit 295
Nutrition 152–77
  *See also Breast feeding, Artificial
    feeding etc*

Observation and monitoring 55, 292
Oedema 243
Oesophageal atresia 84, 108, 183
Oesophageal reflux 171, 185
Oesophagitis 172
Oligohydramnos
effects of 9, 70, 72, 238
Oliguria 241
Omphalocele 84, 181
Ophthalmia neonatorum 310
Ophthalmic disorders 309–19
Ophthalmoscopy 309
Opiate antagonists 29
Orbit
lesions of 314
Organ weights
by body weight 338
by gestational age 339
Organic acidaemias 195
Osmolality 411
Osteomyelitis 219
Oxygen 92–3, 99
inspired concentration 56
low flow 104
Oxygen saturation 56, 94

Palatal defects 69
breast feeding and 155
Pallister-Killian syndrome 321
Paraldehyde 136
Parents
care of in pregnancy 280
explanations to 38
in special care unit and intensive care unit 282
Patau's syndrome 73, 108, 316
Patent ductus arteriosus 125, 127, 158, 181
Pathology 329–39
Peak inspiratory pressure 97
Penis
see Genitalia
Perianal dermatitis 306
Pericardial aspiration 357
Perinatal audit 383
Perinatal mortality committees 392
Perinatal mortality statistics 390, 392, 395
Perinatal statistics 390
for specific population 393–4

Peripheral veins
intravenous lines in 344
Peritoneal dialysis 244, 250
Periventricular haemorrhage 140
Persistent fetal circulation 91, 121
Persistent pulmonary hypertension 91, 121
pH measurements in respiratory care 93
Phenobarbitone 136, 413
Phenylketonuria 205
Phenytoin 136, 414
Phocomelia 71
Phosphate
dietary supplement 165
values 412
Phosphorus requirements 165
Phototherapy 265
Phrenic nerve
birth injury 42
Physiological values 405–13
Pierre Robin syndrome 69
breast feeding in 155
Pigmented naevi 66
Pilonidal sinus 67
Pityriasis rubra pilaris 305
Placenta
management of 37
Plasma
fresh frozen 376
Platelets 375
Pleural effusion 89
Pneumomediastinum 88
Pneumonia 217, 218
congenital 88, 217
in listeriosis 220
treatment of 219
Pneumopericardium 357
Pneumothorax 32, 88
CPAP and 96
thoracentesis in 351
Polycoria 315
Polycythaemia 233
exchange transfusion for 354
in small-for-gestational age infants 60
Polydactyly 72
Polyhydramnios 10, 83
diaphragmatic hernia and 34
Polyuria 241
Porencephalic cysts 151

Porencephaly 141, 151
Port wine stain 66
Positive end expiratory pressure 98
Positive pressure ventilation at
    birth 29
    see Resuscitation
Posterior tibial artery
    blood sampling from 343
Postmortem examination
    consent to 330, 335
    purpose of 329
    reports 336
    request form 332
    requirements for 334
    special 335
Postnatal ward
    care of parents in 281
    routine care in 46
Postural deformities 65
Posture 132
Potassium 145, 258
    intake 255, 258
    normal values 412
Potters' syndrome 9, 70, 238
Practical procedures 340–60
Prader-Willi syndrome 147
Pre-auricular sinus 67
Pre-eclampsia 1
Pregnancy
    alcohol consumption in 7
    anticoagulants in 4
    care of family during 280
    cigarette smoking during 9
    drug abuse in 8–9
    drugs in 368–70
    epilepsy in 4
    haemoglobinopathies in 6
    high risk 1
    hypertension in 1
    infections during 211–13
    myasthenia gravis in 4
    systemic lupus erythematosus
        in 4
    thyroid disease in 2
    tuberculosis in 3
Prescribing 368–86
Preterm infant 23
    blepharophimosis 313
    breast feeding of 154
    caesarean section 35
    care of parents 281

chronic pulmonary insufficiency
    in 103
definition of 389
delivery of 17
feeding 54, 158
immunization 366
infections in 213
inguinal hernia in 191
jaundice in 264
patent ductus arteriosus in 127
problems of 57
skin of 299
special food additive
    requirements 165
Proptosis 314
Prostaglandin E therapy 122, 380
Protein
    normal values 412
    requirements 169
Proteinuria 240
Prune belly syndrome 90
Psoriasis 305, 306
Ptosis 313
Pulmonary atresia 118
    with intact septum 110, 118
    with VSD 110, 118
Pulmonary dysmaturity 89, 103
Pulmonary haemorrhage 88
Pulmonary hypoplasia 9, 90
Pulmonary oedema 113
    haemorrhagic 88
Pulmonary stenosis 128
    critical 118
    with VSD 111
Pulmonary trunk
    anomalous origin of left coronary
        artery from 125
Pulmonary venous connection
    anomalous 119
Pupils
    disorders of 315, 316
Pustular disorders 302
Pustular melanosis 302
Pyloric stenosis 190–1
Pyruvate 412

Queckenstedt's test 143

Radial artery
    blood sampling from 342
Radial hypoplasia 71

Radial nerve injury 43, 79
Ranula 69
Recto-urethral fistula 186
Rectovaginal fistula 186
Rectum
  lesions of 186
Recurrent apnoea 94, 105, 106
Red blood cells
  decreased production 231
  defects 231
  normal values 415
  transfusion 233
Reflexes
  examination of 133
Renal disease 235–52
  See also Renal failure
Renal enlargement
  causes of 240
Renal failure,
  acute 246
  causes of 246
  dialysis in 250
  hypocalcaemia in 195
  hyponatraemia in 256
  intrinsic 247, 248
  investigations 247
  management of 248
  polyuria in 241
  postrenal 246, 247
  in preterm infants 58
  symptoms and signs 245
Renal tubular acidosis 244
Renal tubular disorders 256
Renal tubular function 237
Renal vein thrombosis 242
  in infants of diabetic mothers 61
Respiration
  monitoring in asphyxia 145
Respiratory care in transport 83
Respiratory distress
  anticipation of 23
  causes of 86, 87
Respiratory distress syndrome 86,
    214, 244
  care of baby with 91
  CPAP in 94
  in infant of diabetic mothers 60
  steroids and 18
  ventilation and 96
  water balance and 253
Respiratory monitors 55, 293

Respiratory problems 86–107
Respiratory system (maternal)
  drugs and breast feeding 372
Restricted Growth Association 289
Resuscitation 20
  aftercare 36
  at birth 28
  difficulty 30
  failed 31
  medical ethics 400
  special problems 32
Retina
  disorders of 317
  haemorrhage 317
Retinoblastoma 317
Retinopathy of prematurity 312
Rhesus haemolytic disease 268
  management of 269
Routine care 46–50
  in delivery room 46
  first-day assessment 47, 48
  postnatal ward 46
Royal National Institute for the
    Blind 289
Royal National Institute for the
    Deaf 289
Royal Society for Mentally
    Handicapped Children and
    Adults 289
Rubella (congenital) 211, 212
Russel Silver dwarf 72

Salt and water retention 244
Saphenous vein
  long line insertion in 358
Scabies 303
Scalded skin syndrome 300, 305
Scalp
  birth injuries to 40
  fetal blood sampling 41
  lesions from electrode clips 41
Scalp veins
  intravenous lines in 344
Scalpel incisions
  accidental 42
Scleroderma 301
Scoliosis
  congenital 75
Scrotum
  birth trauma 44
  in gestational age assessment 277

Sebaceous gland hyperplasia 300
Sebaceous naevi 67
Seborrhoeic dermatitis 305, 306
Seckel's bird head dwarf 72
Self help organizations 285–91
Sensory testing 363–6
Septicaemia 217, 218, 219
Sex
   ambiguous 198, 199
'Short gut' syndrome 183
Sickle-cell disease and trait 7
Skin
   disorders of 299–308
   marbling 299
   signs of neurological problems
      in 133
   viral infections 304
Skin biopsy in genetics 328
Skull
   birth trauma 41
   depressed fracture of 41
Small-for-gestational age infants
      23
   care of 59–60
   diabetes in 195
Small left colon syndrome 61
Sodium
   in asphyxia 145
   balance 255
   deficit 256
   excess 257
   intake 255, 256
   values 412
Sodium bicarbonate in
      resuscitation 30
Spastics Society 290
Special care
   babies receiving 397
   definition 51
Special care baby unit
   care of parents in 282
   definitions 51
   indications for admission 52,
      296, 397
   nursing care in 292
   respiratory care in 91
   transfer to 37
Spina bifida 148–50
   assessment of 149
   definition 147
   occulta 148

Spine
   birth fracture 43
Squint 310
Statistics
   perinatal 390, 392, 395
STEPS 290
Steroids
   in chronic lung disease 104
   effect on lung maturation 18
   respiratory distress syndrome
      and 18
Stillbirth 392
   definition 388
Stillbirth and Neonatal Death
      Association 291
Stillbirth rate 390
Stork mark 66
Strawberry nevus 66
Streptococcal (Group B)
      disease 217
Subaponeurotic haemorrhage 41
Subarachnoid haemorrhage 139
Subdural haemorrhage 138
Subdural tap 349
Sucking and swallowing reflex
   immaturity of 61
Suprapubic bladder tap 349
Supraventricular tachycardia 129
Surfactant
   deficiency of 60, 86, 87
   replacement of 99
Surgical problems 178–91
Survival rates 396
Syndactyly 72
Syphilis 213, 303, 307
Systemic lupus erythematosus 4
   Congenital heart block and 130

Tachycardia 129
   fetal 16
Tachypnoea of newborn 87
Talipes 78
Teeth,
   congenital 69
Temperature monitoring 52, 56
Temporal artery
   blood sampling from 343
Testis
   birth trauma 44
   congenital torsion 44
Tetralogy of Fallot 118

Thalassaemia 7
Theophylline 414
Thermal care 48, 52, 294
  See also Heat loss, Cold stress etc.
  at birth 25, 29
  during transport 82, 83
  in delivery room 46
  of high-risk infant 52
  of small-for-gestational age
    infants 59
Thoracentesis 351
Thrombocytopenia 226, 228, 242
  maternal 230
Thrush 221, 222
Thymus
  enlarged 112
Thyroid disorders 201-2
Thyroid stimulating hormone 412
Thyrotoxicosis 2, 202
Thyroxine 412
Tolazaline
  effect on kidney 237
  in persistent pulmonary
    hypotension 121
  in refractory hypoxia 102
Tongue tie 68
  breast feeding and 155
TORCH infections 208
  associated conditions 211
Torticollis 74
Total anomalous pulmonary venous
    connection 119
Towne's syndrome 238
Toxic epidermal necrolysis 300
Toxoplasma infection 212, 316
Tracheo-oesophageal fistula 84,
    183-5
  complications 185
  diagnosis and management 184
  H type 185
Transient tachypnoea of
    newborn 87
Transport of sick infant 80-5
  monitoring 83
  necessary equipment 81
  organization of service 80
  stabilization of patient 82
  team 82
  with special problems 84
Transposition of great arteries 117
  with intact septum 111

Transpyloric feeding 166
Tricuspid atresia 110, 119
  with high pulmonary flow 110
Triglycerides 412
Trisomy 13-15 *See Patau's
    syndrome*
Trisomy 18 *See Edward's syndrome*
Trisomy 21 *See Down's syndrome*
Truncus arteriosus 112, 126
Tuberculosis 3
Tuberous sclerosis 133
Turner's syndrome 73, 316
  heart disease and 108
Twins 40
Twins and Multiple Births
    Association 291
Tyrosinaemia 193

Ultrasound
  cerebral scanning 137
  detecting fetal abnormalities 11
  echocardiography 115-16
Umbilical arterial catheter 346
Umbilical cord
  blood pH 26
  division of 26
Umbilical hernia 181
Umbilical veins
  intravenous lines in 344
Umbilicus
  infections of 215
Urea 412
Urea cycle disorders 195
Uric acid 413
Urinary tract infection 245
  treatment 219
  with anorectal anomalies 186
  obstruction 240, 243
Urine
  obstruction to flow 49
  osmolality 236
  passage of 49
  testing 57
Urological tract anomalies 70
Urticara pigmentosa 301

Vacuum extraction 40, 41
Valproic acid 414
Varicella zoster 213, 304
Venous lines
  insertion of 344

Ventilation
    Resuscitation at birth 29 *See also
        Continuous positive airway
        pressure*
Ventilation, mechanical 96–103
    fighting against 101
    principles of 96
    settings 99
    weaning off 102
Ventricular hypertrophy 114, 115
Ventricular septal defect 110, 111,
        125, 128
Ventricular tap 348
Vesico-ureteric reflux 238
Virus infections 221, 304
    breast feeding and 158
Visceral trauma at birth 44
Vision
    testing 363
Vitamins 159, 169
    breast feeding and 374
    values 413
Vitamin D 165
Vitamin E requirements 165
    prophylaxis for intracranial
        haemmorhage 140
Vitamin K 46
    haemorrhagic disease and 227
Vitreous
    disorders of 316
Voluntary Council for
        Handicapped Children 291

Volvulus 189
Vulva
    haematoma at birth 45
von Rosen splint 77, 78
von Willebrand's disease 228

Water
    balance 253–4
    intake 254, 255
    loss of 254, 257
    overload 256
    therapy 254
Weighing 48
    breast feeding and 155
    high risk infants 57
Werding-Hoffman disease 147
White asphyxia 26, 29, 33, 37
White cell count 224, 416
Wilms' tumour 315
Wilson-Mikity syndrome 89, 103
Wolff-Parkinson-White
        syndrome 129, 130

Xray
    chest 86–91
    heart 110–13
XO syndrome *See Turner's
        syndrome*

Zinc 413
    deficiency 307
Zoster immune globulin 213